ACUPUNCTURE & MOXIBUSTION

ACUPUNCTURE & MOXIBUSTION

David Tai MD (Peking)
Acupuncture Services Pty Ltd
142 Clarence Street
Sydney, New South Wales 2000
Australia

Foreword by:
Jim Cairns MD
Canberra

Gower Medical Publishing   LONDON · NEW YORK

Distributed in Australia and New Zealand by
Harper & Row (Australasia) Pty Ltd
Corner Frederick Street and Reserve Road
P.O. Box 226
Artarmon, NSW 2064

Distributed in all countries except
Australia and New Zealand by
Harper & Row International
10 East 53rd Street
New York, NY 10022, USA

© Copyright 1987 by David Tai.
All rights reserved. No part of this publication may be
reproduced, stored in a retrieval system or transmitted in
any form or by any means electronic, mechanical,
photocopying, recording or otherwise, without the prior
written permission of the publisher.

ISBN: 0-397-44564-4

Project Editor: Sharyn Wong

Designers: Ian Spick
            Mehmet Hussein

Illustration: Lynda Payne

Printed in Hong Kong by Imago Publishing Ltd.
Typeset in Plantin by TNR Productions, London N7.

FOREWORD

In the lifetime of Albert Einstein, Matter began to disappear as it was replaced by Energy as the central or vital factor in human (Western) thinking and behaviour. Prior to that time, Matter and its philosophy, Materialism, dominated the West and the rest of the world set out rapidly to follow. The result was alienation, acquisitiveness and violence unprecedented in human history and prehistory till, finally, it became a recognised threat to survival of the species and of life on this planet.

The revolution in human thinking, however, and the one implied in human behaviour, has not gone as far. Scientists still, almost completely, live in a pre-Einstein world. Theology finds it no easier to make the shift because human energy is disturbingly organic and sexual while philosophy wrestles with what Gregory Bateson called 'Cartesian dualism'. It could be expected that medical doctors would be amongst the first to begin the shift from matter to energy, with all its biological implications, but they are not.

Acupuncture raises the question of Energy in the human body and the necessity for it to be able to function within – as activity rising to a high point, then subsiding or relaxing, then rising again. The oscillation of Energy is the pulse of life. This principle of Yin and Yang, it appears, is the essence of the philosophy of Chinese Medicine – both ancient and modern – and of Chinese philosophy as a whole.

Energy within the body cannot be compartmentalized, or considered or treated as being in the mind only or in the body only. It cannot be comprehended by a science or philosophy which is reductionist or positivist. The fact that Energy exists means that the human body, although constantly changing and fluctuating, is one living unit. It is not separable, either, from what is not within it, that is to say, from its environment, especially the human parts of that environment.

Health and, we may say, personal and human growth depend upon an energetic flow of experience between the individual and others (close body contact or intimacy, and the need for this may be the strongest of all animal instincts) and with the natural environment. In Western culture, it may be that artificial ('intellectual' and repressive) separations are now more damaging than ever before in human history.

In his book, Dr. David Tai explains, better than has been done previously, the significance of the theory of human energy and its use in diagnosis and clinical practice, which embodies 'anatomy, physiology, pathology, biochemistry, clinical syndromes' and other medical concepts. He adds to it as well the significance of Emotions.

It may be that acupuncture, more than any other branch of medical practice, will show the importance of Energy and the holistic philosophy and practice. No other single aspect may be as important for the field of medicine and no other may help as much in opening up ways of creating personal and social health in our society. David Tai is well equipped to assist in this development and this book is an example of what needs to be done, because it is first of all a book of education for the healers and for those who need to be healed.

Jim Cairns, MD
Canberra, 1987

PREFACE

Acupuncture and moxibustion are ancient Chinese arts of healing which have proved successful in the prevention and treatment of disease. Over many centuries, knowledge and experience of acupuncture and moxibustion have been extended, but the principles and fundamental theories have not changed; these two ancient healing arts have retained their efficacy in treating the illnesses of the modern world. Understanding of these treatments, however, is at the same time very simple and very complex, and no one yet has been able to expound the mystery surrounding them.

This book was conceived with the intention of assembling all aspects of acupuncture and moxibustion into one volume, of correcting errors that have been perpetuated as new books have appeared and, more importantly, of introducing new information that has not been published before.

Philosophy is an integral part of Chinese Medicine, and the philosophy of Yin and Yang is one of its most important aspects. This philosophy (as regards acupuncture treatment) should be applied in a practical sense as a way of life, for with it comes an understanding of the relationship between the human body and nature which, in turn, engenders the serenity of mind that is so essential for a healthy body and for the control of one's own life.

According to the Chinese philosophers, the theory of Zang and Fu was one which viewed the whole body with the combined considerations of anatomy, physiology, pathology, biochemistry, clinical syndromes and philosophy. Nowadays, one issue which seems to be overlooked – or at best given only superficial attention – is that of Emotion. In ancient China, medical thought recognized man as a whole entity, and the physical and emotional elements were inseparable. As emotional disturbances can be a cause of disease, more emphasis should be placed on the importance of philosophy as a means of relieving the tensions and pressures of life. Instead of a dependence on drugs, exercise, food or even on treatment, it is a case of exercising the mind to cultivate the emotions. What safer and more effective means of restoring health?

On the always interesting subject of pulse diagnosis, the pulse-reading methods of Dr. Pin Hoo Lee (1518–1593) have been used in China for four centuries and are still in use today. This book gives a complete record of pulse reading methods as well as a carefully compiled description in detail of the twenty-eight individual pulses.

Medically, the Chinese concept of the Meridians and body energy flow provides a vehicle for acupuncture treatment and is itself a fascinating subject for investigation. The illustrations and the comprehensive data on the Fourteen Meridians follow the 'HUANG-DI NEI-JING' (*The Yellow Emperor's Classic of Internal Medicine*, 500–300 BC) and show how the energy flow connects one Meridian to the other Meridians, to the organs and to the acupuncture points.

A thorough knowledge of the acupuncture points is essential for acupuncture practice. There is no simple way to discover the exact functions and symptoms of each point nor is this information easily collated from the many different books written on the subject. However, through personal long-term practical experience, acupuncture points can be individually proved to be reliable and effective when subjected to comparative results in the clinic. Dependable information from Dr. Yang's book, *Compendium of Acupuncture and Moxibustion* (AD 1600), has also been included where appropriate.

Complete details of the location and anatomical structure of each acupuncture point are listed, giving clear emphasis to the points forbidden for needle insertion and moxibustion treatment and to the precautions necessary in clinical practice.

Needle techniques must always stem from personal experience. In this work, the detailed descriptions of acupuncture and moxibustion techniques from the simple to the complex, and the accompanying illustrations, have rarely appeared in Western publications. (Of course, the complex techniques are used only by highly skilled and experienced practitioners.)

After studying many books on the subject and having seen the results of treatment in my patients, I have put my research and observations into writing. I hope this book will provide not only an insight into oriental culture and the acupuncture knowledge of ancient China, but will also serve to separate the factual from the fictitious. If, in addition, it can be of benefit to students of acupuncture or other practitioners in their treatment of patients, it will have been worthwhile.

I would like to thank Audrey Deakin, without whose help it would have been impossible to write this book, and all of my patients who have been so helpful to me.

Although care has been taken to make this book as accurate as possible, misconceptions and errors may have been included because of the still limited knowledge of acupuncture and moxibustion which is available. I would, therefore, be glad to receive from readers any suggestions or criticisms which will help in improving this book.

David Tai
Sydney, 1987

CONTENTS

Foreword	v
Preface	vi
1 Yin and Yang	**1**
Balance on a regular level	3
Balance on a lower level	3
Balance on a higher level	3
2 Zang and Fu	**6**
1. Heart and Small Intestine	6
2. Liver and Gall Bladder	12
3. Spleen and Stomach	16
4. Lungs and Large Intestine	20
5. Kidneys and Bladder	25
6. Pericardium and Three Heater	31
7. The Extra Fu	33
3 Pulse Diagnosis	**35**
General knowledge	35
Pulse diagnosis procedures	38
Pulses of the body	40
Pulse diagnosis of children	42
Female pulses	42
Pulses and environment	43
Pulses and emotion	45
Individual pulses	46
1. Floating pulse	46
2. Sunken or Deep pulse	47
3. Slow pulse	47
4. Rapid pulse	48
5. Slippery pulse	48
6. Choppy pulse	49
7. Empty pulse	49
8. Full pulse	50
9. Long pulse	50
10. Short pulse	50
11. Overflowing pulse	50
12. Minute pulse	51
13. Tight pulse	51
14. Unhurried pulse	52
15. Hollow pulse	52
16. Bowstring pulse	52
17. Leather pulse	53
18. Firm pulse	53
19. Weak/Floating pulse	54
20. Weak pulse	54
21. Scattered pulse	55
22. Fine pulse	55
23. Hidden pulse	55
24. Moving pulse	56
25. Hasty pulse	56
26. Knotted pulse	56
27. Intermittent pulse	57
28. Hurried pulse	57
4 Fourteen Meridians and Acupuncture Points	**59**
The Meridian Complex	59
Acupuncture points	62
1. *Ah-Shi* Points	62
2. New Acupuncture Points	62
3. Extraordinary Points	62
Naming of points	63
Point location	63
1. Following body structure	63
2. Proportional measurement	63
3. Finger-length measurement	66
Point anatomy and physiology	66
Functions and symptoms	67
Specific points	67
1. *Shu* (Five Element Acupuncture) Points	67
2. *Yuan* (Source) Points	69
3. *Luo* Points	70
4. *Xi* (Cleft) Points	70
5. Eight Confluent Points of the Eight Extra Meridians	71
6. Eight Influential Points	71
7. Back-*Shu* Points	72
8. Front-*Mu* Points	72
9. Meeting (or Crossing) Points	73
10. *He*-Sea Points	73
Points of the Fourteen Meridians	
1. Lung Meridian of Hand-*Tai* Yin	73
2. Large Intestine Meridian of Hand Yang-*Ming*	80
3. Stomach Meridian of Foot Yang-*Ming*	92

4. Spleen Meridian of Foot *Tai*-Yin	112
5. Heart Meridian of Hand *Shao*-Yin	123
6. Small Intestine Meridian of Hand *Tai*-Yang	129
7. Bladder Meridian of Foot *Tai*-Yang	139
8. Kidney Meridian of Foot *Shao*-Yin	168
9. Pericardium Meridian of Hand *Jue*-Yin	181
10. Three Heater Meridian of Hand *Shao*-Yang	187
11. Gall Bladder Meridian of Foot *Shao*-Yang	199
12. Liver Meridian of Foot *Jue*-Yin	219
13. Governor Vessel Meridian (*Du Mai*)	228
14. Conception Vessel Meridian *Ren Mai*	240

5 Acupuncture and moxibustion techniques — 253

Moxibustion	253
Needle technique	254
Filiform needle	255
Sterilization	255
Patient posture	255
Needle insertion techniques	256
Needle direction and depth	256
Acupuncture sensation and causes of pain	258
Manipulation techniques	259
Needling the *Luo* Meridian (bleeding technique)	263
Principal methods of reinforcement and reduction	266
Simple needle techniques	266
Complex needle techniques	267
1. 'Fire Burning the Mountain'; Pure reinforcement technique	267
2. 'Penetration of Celestial Freshness'; Pure reduction technique	268
3. 'Shadow of Yin between the Yang'; Combination of reinforcement and reduction techniques	268
4. 'Shadow of Yang between the Yin'; Combination of reduction and reinforcement techniques	269
5. 'Battle of the Dragon and Tiger'; Combination of reduction and reinforcement techniques through needle rotation	270
6. 'Descent and Ascent of the Dragon and Tiger'; Combination of reinforcement and reduction techniques through needle rotation and lift and thrust	270
7. 'Pounding the Meridian in Mortar'; Combination of reinforcement and reduction techniques through needle rotation and simultaneous lift and thrust	271
8. 'Wagging the Tail of the Dragon'; Reinforcement through manipulation of the tail of the needle	271
9. 'White Tiger Shakes His Head'; Reduction through manipulation of the tail of the needle	272
10. 'Tortoise Detects the Point'; Multidirectional placement of needle for reinforcement	272
11. 'Peacock's Fantail'; Reinforcement technique	273
Needle numbers	273
Single needle	273
Double needles	273
Triple needles	275
Plum-blossom needles	275
Multiple needles	275
Accident management	275
Needle sticks in tissue	275
Needle bends in tissue	275
Needle breaks in tissue	276
Fainting	276
Needle punctures vital organ	276
Clinical needle techniques	277
Needling criteria	
When acupuncture and moxibustion are forbidden	277
Depth of needle insertion	278
Point selection	279
Formula	282

Index — 284

1 YIN AND YANG

We can see beauty in beauty
Only because there is ugliness.
   Tao Te Ching

One of ancient China's most important philosophies encompasses the unique principle of Yin and Yang. This philosophy holds that all sciences, arts and technologies on all levels are manifested in the theory of Yin and Yang. Although embracing physiology, pathology and clinical therapeutics, Chinese medicine is largely philosophical; acupuncture particularly appears to be quite incomprehensible.

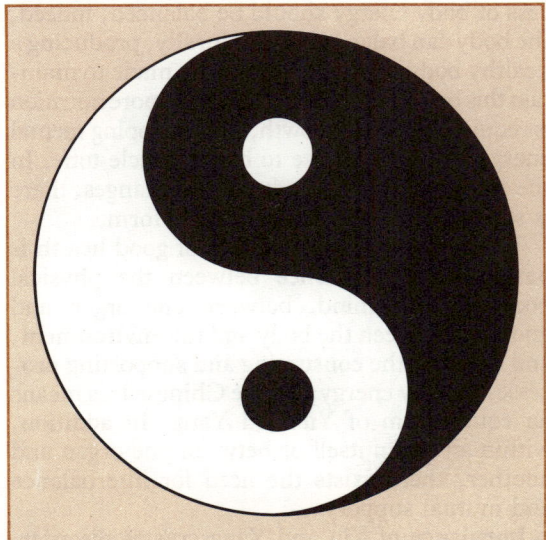

Fig. 1.1. *T'ai Chi t'u'*, the traditional Chinese symbol of the concept of energy (Life Force), shows Yin and Yang in perpetual balance.

It is from the relationship between the 'Negative Terminus' and the 'Grand Terminus' that the creation of all things in the universe and the principle of Yin and Yang (Darkness and Light) are understood (Fig. 1.1). When the Grand Terminus acts, it forms Yang. When activity reaches its extreme point it becomes inactive, and inactivity forms Yin; likewise, extreme inactivity eventually changes and becomes activity, which forms Yang. Thus, activity is the cause of inactivity and *vice versa*.

The principle of Yin and Yang also embodies the belief that everything in the universe is divisible *ad infinitum*, and that each entity has two opposite aspects: one is Yin and one is Yang.

YIN	Earth	Female	Cold
YANG	Heaven	Male	Heat
YIN	Internal	Downward	Negative
YANG	External	Upward	Positive
YIN	Front	Zang	Blood
YANG	Back	Fu	Energy
YIN	Inhibition	Deep	Slow
YANG	Stimulation	Floating	Rapid

Yin and Yang natures exist only by comparison; they are relative and not absolute:

- When comparing the neck with the head, the neck is Yin and the head is Yang; but when comparing the neck with the chest, the neck is Yang and the chest is Yin.

- The Liver is Yin when compared with its partner, the Gall Bladder, which is Yang; but within the Liver itself, Liver energy is part of Liver Yang and Liver blood is part of Liver Yin.

YIN AND YANG

- What is the chest? Relative to the back, the chest is Yin but if compared with the abdomen, the chest is Yang. Hence, the chest (and all other things) may be Yin or Yang depending on its position relative to that with which it is being compared.

In Chinese diagnosis, the method for analyzing disease syndromes is based on the philosophy of Yin and Yang and involves eight separate groups of syndromes: exterior; interior; heat; cold; excess; deficiency; Yang; Yin.

Exterior + Heat + Excess	YANG
Interior + Cold + Deficiency	YIN

For example, when external causes of disease (such as wind, cold or damp) attack the body, the body's protective system (*Wei-Qi*) prevents the disease from directly invading deep into the internal organs. Symptoms present superficially (on the exterior of the body), thus revealing the struggle by the body's defence system.

The treatment prescribed for Yang disorders should include the use of Yin-type herbs (Yin balances Yang). In acupuncture treatment of Yang disorders, the disease factors should be removed as soon as possible. Needle technique should be shallow, avoiding deep penetration.

The concept of Yin and Yang provides the key to directing methods of treatment.

- Points on the front of the body are used for treating disorders of the back;

- Points on the surface of the body, such as Front-*Mu* Point CV 22 or Back-*Shu* Point Bl 18, are used for balancing the functions of the internal organs (for example, gastric disorders);

- Points on top of the head, such as GV 20, are used for treating disorders in the perineum (such as prolapse of the rectum);

- Points on the right elbow are used for complaints of the left elbow;

- Point Bl 23 (Bladder Yang) can be used to treat Kidney (Yin) disorders.

In general, body energy is supported by prenatal energy inherited from the parents and by postnatal energy derived from air, water, food, sunshine and the harmonious functioning of healthy organs. Body energy is consumed by mental and physical work, living/working conditions (personal environment), association/relationships with people, climatic changes (heat and cold) and the normal functioning of body tissues and organs (metabolism).

This fundamental consuming/supporting process of body energy should be balanced; indeed, the body can balance itself naturally, producing a healthy body, and efforts must be made to maintain this balance. During childhood, more nutrition is required for body growth, for developing mental energy and for exercise to build muscle tone. In the elderly, although body energy changes, there is still the need to keep it in good form.

The essence of maintenance of good health is harmonious coexistence between the physical body and the mind, between one organ and another, between the body and the environment, and between the consuming and supporting processes of body energy. To the Chinese this means an equilibrium of Yin and Yang. In addition, within an organ itself or between one organ and another, there exists the need for interbalance and mutual support.

Imbalance of Yin and Yang creates disorder. Unbalanced organs, however, are capable of balancing themselves without medical treatment. In these circumstances, Yin and Yang can be

YIN AND YANG

balanced at any of three levels: regular; lower; and higher. When the functions of the organs have readjusted there is always a point (over the maximum or under the minimum) where the balance is again broken. The body then has great difficulty in balancing itself once more as the disorder will have become more serious.

BALANCE ON A REGULAR LEVEL

Nutrients are absorbed by the Spleen and are transformed by Spleen energy (through a biochemical function) into blood. The entire blood circulation is regulated by Heart and Liver energies (Heart Yang and Liver Yang), and is protected by Spleen Yang which controls its flow to the blood vessels.

Blood nourishes the organs and the organs produce energy. Only when there is an abundant blood supply are the organs themselves able to produce energy. Both mental and physical work consume blood and energy while their loss is made up for by nourishment and rest. In this consuming/supporting process, Yin and Yang are relatively well balanced (on a regular level), although absolute equilibrium does not exist.

BALANCE ON A LOWER LEVEL

After a major operation, the whole body is in trauma because of blood and energy loss. In these cases it is absolutely essential that the patient remains quietly in bed, peaceful in mind, in order to conserve energy and help the body regain the balanced functioning of its internal organs. Once energy has been replenished, exercise should be introduced gradually and nourishment increased to enable all physical functions to be rejuvenated. Mental energy too can help to speed recovery of the physical body. Balance on the lower level of Yin and Yang eventually returns to the regular level; the body is then completely recovered.

BALANCE ON A HIGHER LEVEL

Mental and emotional stress can cause severe diseases and always disturb the functions of the Heart and Liver, particularly by increasing their activities:

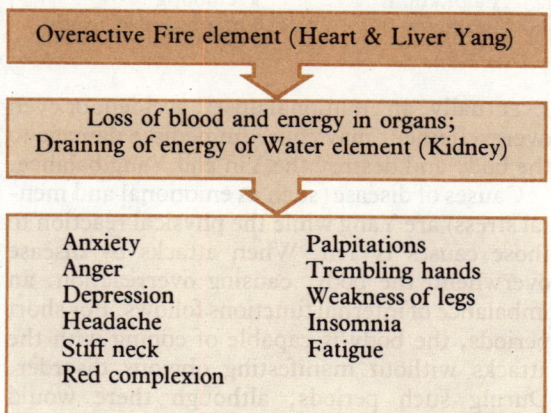

Overactive Fire element (Heart & Liver Yang)

↓

Loss of blood and energy in organs;
Draining of energy of Water element (Kidney)

↓

Anxiety	Palpitations
Anger	Trembling hands
Depression	Weakness of legs
Headache	Insomnia
Stiff neck	Fatigue
Red complexion	

Any of these symptoms can cause physical illness, but what of the mind? Society has created the need to consume (amongst other things) coffee, tobacco and alcohol, and encourages overeating; the result is an acceleration of Spleen functions and increased stimulation of blood and energy flows. In order to cope with this overload (needed by the Fire element), the Kidney must supply extra energy at the cost of increased demands upon itself. Forced to use its prenatal energy for support, the Kidneys thus run the risk of becoming enlarged.

When the causes of disease continue to affect the body (for example, enlargement of the Heart, Liver and Kidney), the consequent increased Spleen function eventually leads to further structural changes throughout the body. Prolonged organ changes (and age) make it impossible for the body to withstand mental and physical stress indefinitely. Symptoms become more pronounced:

YIN AND YANG

Severe headache	Chest pain
Irritability	Shortness of breath
Restlessness	Obesity
Stiff neck & back	Body heaviness
Bloodshot eyes	Fatigue
Palpitations	Trembling or
Insomnia	numbness of hands

Eventually, an emotional upset, accident or even overexcitement may cause immediate damage to the body and destroy the Yin and Yang balance.

Causes of disease (such as emotional and mental stress) are Yang while the physical reaction to those causes is Yin. When attacks by disease overwhelm the body, causing overreaction, an imbalance of internal functions follows. For short periods, the body is capable of coping with the attacks without manifesting obvious disorder. During such periods, although there would appear to be a balance between the causes of disease (Yang) and the physical body (Yin), it is, in fact, a false balance. If the causes of disease are not relieved, the imbalance of Yin and Yang will progress to physical deterioration. The disease will eventually so damage the body as to break the Yin and Yang balance.

Thus, a very important aspect of treatment is observing and understanding the balance of the body when under attack by disease. All treatment should concentrate on removing the causes as well as relieving the symptoms.

We are all aware of the impossibility of existence without our society and environment, the earth, sun and universe. As the universe is Yang and the human body is Yin, mankind should endeavour to live harmoniously within it. Food, air, sunshine, water, people, all have an influence on man and his life; hence, we should always seek to be in harmony with our world.

In the celebrated '*HUANG-DI NEI-JING*' ('The Yellow Emperor's Classic of Internal Medicine, 500–300 BC), the lesson entitled 'Treatise on the Natural Truth in Ancient Times' states:

'In ancient times those who understood *Tao* modelled themselves upon the balanced principles of Yin and Yang. In their ordered and well regulated daily lives they harmoniously cultivated their bodies and minds, were moderate in eating and drinking habits, practised no excesses and wasted none of their physical energy ... The sages of ancient times taught their followers that weakness, noxious influences and injurious winds should be avoided at specific times. They themselves [the sages] were tranquilly content in nothingness, and the true vital force accompanied them always. As their vital (original) Spirit was preserved within, how could illness overtake them?'

Philosophy is a key to open the Heart, the Mind and the Spirit.

Knowing others is wisdom,
Knowing oneself is enlightenment.

Mastering others requires force,
Mastering oneself needs strength.

See simplicity in the complicated,
Achieve greatness in little things.

TAO TE CHING

2 ZANG AND FU

The theory underlying traditional Chinese medicine, including diagnosis and clinical practice, is based on one precept: that the human body, although constantly changing and fluctuating, is one living unit. This theory, called Zang and Fu, embodies anatomy, physiology, pathology, biochemistry, clinical syndromes and other medical concepts in the idiom characteristic of the ancient Chinese philosophers.

When speaking of the unity of the human body, these early philosophers believed that 'although all organs are hidden in the body, their condition can be observed externally'. Their reasoning was based on countless observations of interactions between the internal and external body and the emotions. No organ is an island; each continually modifies, and is being modified by, the internal body and its external environment. Within the body these interactions are mainly effected through energy channels which the Chinese called *Jing-Luo* or Meridians. This is the medium through which the body stores, transforms, transports and expels energy. The Meridians connect exterior to interior and upper to lower; they are the foundation of physical acupuncture treatment.

The Zang and Fu are organs only in the Chinese sense of the word; they are the passive and active principles of physiological energy. The Zang are solid organs, viscera, which produce and store energy to nourish the whole body. They are relatively more passive than the Fu and are considered Yin. The Fu are hollow organs, bowels, whose activities regulate and transform energy throughout the entire body. As the Fu are engaged in keeping the energy moving, they are considered Yang.

Each Zang organ has its Fu counterpart. Their complementary characteristics, passivity and activity, work in pairs:

ZANG		FU
Lungs	&	Large Intestine
Spleen	&	Stomach
Heart	&	Small Intestine
Kidneys	&	Bladder
Pericardium	&	Three Heater
Liver	&	Gall Bladder

Zang and Fu partnerships are evident in the energy pathway of the Twelve Main Meridians:

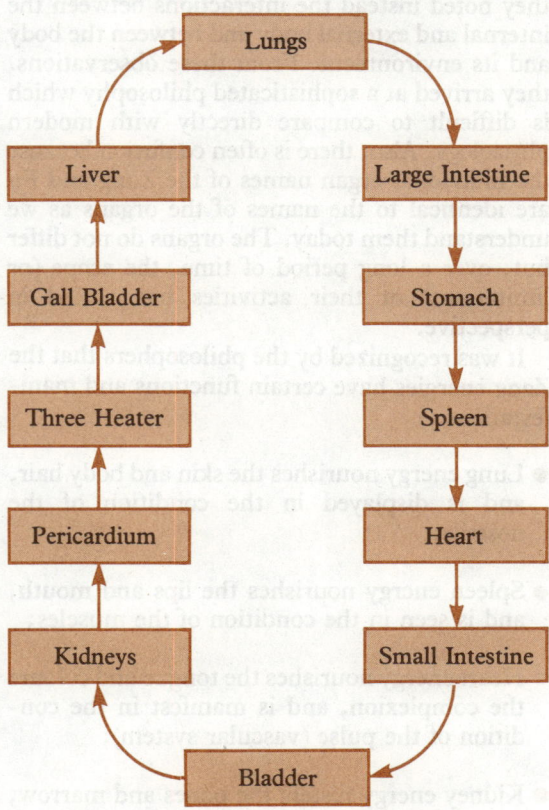

ZANG AND FU

The relationship between the Zang and Fu is also reflected in the Five Elements:

ELEMENT	ZANG	FU
Fire	Heart	Small Intestine
Fire	Pericardium	Three Heater
Metal	Lungs	Large Intestine
Earth	Spleen	Stomach
Water	Kidneys	Bladder
Wood	Liver	Gall Bladder

As Chinese philosophers were unable to study the body scientifically (autopsies were forbidden), they noted instead the interactions between the internal and external body and between the body and its environment. From these observations, they arrived at a sophisticated philosophy which is difficult to compare directly with modern physiology. Also, there is often confusion because the individual organ names of the Zang and Fu are identical to the names of the organs as we understand them today. The organs do not differ but, over a long period of time, the scope (or limitations) of their activities has varied in perspective.

It was recognized by the philosophers that the Zang energies have certain functions and manifestations:

- Lung energy nourishes the skin and body hair, and is displayed in the condition of the nostrils;

- Spleen energy nourishes the lips and mouth, and is seen in the condition of the muscles;

- Heart energy nourishes the tongue and colours the complexion, and is manifest in the condition of the pulse (vascular system);

- Kidney energy fosters the bones and marrow, and is apparent in the condition of the hair, ears, anus and urethra;

- Liver energy nourishes the tendons and nails, and its condition is mirrored in the eyes.

Each Zang generates its own special emotion:

- Joy is from the Heart;

- Fear is from the Kidneys;

- Reminiscence is from the Spleen;

- Gloom is from the Lungs;

- Anger is from the Liver.

Normally the emotions respond to natural daily and seasonal variations; but habitual emphasis on any one emotion interferes with the activities of the related Zang and, over a period of time, eventually leads to pathological disorder.

The emotions, the five senses and some body activities are interdependent on the condition of the Zang, but have no direct relationship to the Fu. Indeed, like most body activities, the Fu is dependent for nourishment and support on the condition of the Zang. Thus, Zang is truly the foundation of physiological activity and, accordingly, is given the most emphasis in the following account.

1. HEART AND SMALL INTESTINE
Heart
The Heart is Zang, a Yin organ, one of the five viscera and belongs to the Fire element. Its Main Meridian is the Heart Meridian of Hand *Shao* (Lesser)-Yin and its Fu partner is the Small Intestine.

Heart energy controls the blood and blood vessels, affects the complexion, nourishes the tongue and is a focus for the Spirit (*Shen*). It is through the Spirit that the Heart guides the activities of the Zang and Fu (in a manner analogous to the conductor of an orchestra).

The Chinese perception of the Heart relates primarily to the activities of the central nervous system (CNS), but is also connected to the autonomic nervous system (ANS) and vascular system (circulation).

Blood and blood vessels
The Spleen and Heart (Zang) energies respectively form and circulate the blood, one of the principal carriers of nutrients through the body. Because the activities of these two organs are closely bound together by the blood, a disorder in one very quickly causes disorder in the other. For example, a state of overconsumption of Heart energy, as in a disorder of the Spirit (mental illness), will also cause the Spleen to overwork to replenish Heart blood; eventually both organs are weakened, and purpura and haemorrhage may develop. Other symptoms common to these disorders include dizziness, palpitations, amnesia, insomnia, a pallid complexion and loss of appetite.

In Chinese philosophy, the relationship of blood and energy equates with Yin and Yang:

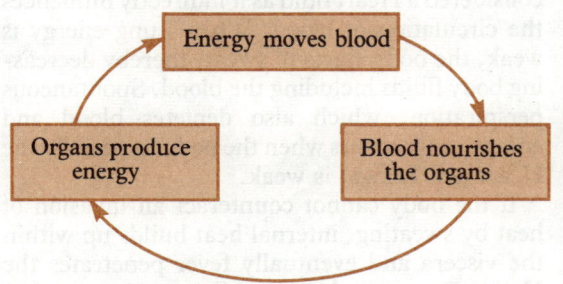

Active energy flow creates a regular blood circulation whereas obstruction in the energy flow correspondingly causes stasis in the circulation.

- The pushing force of the Heart (Heart energy) regulates the blood circulation;

- The volume of blood in the Heart and blood vessels (Heart blood) nourishes the Heart itself as well as all other organs and tissues.

A healthy Heart has an abundance of blood and energy from which evolve a smooth, strong and regular pulse beat and a lustrous complexion. Indications that these two vital forces are lacking or obstructed are a violet complexion, irregular pulse beat, cold extremities or a propensity to palpitations. If such a condition remains unchecked, vertigo, mental fatigue, shortness of breath and sweating will follow.

Emotion
Exponents of Western medicine define the emotions as a product of the central nervous system; the Chinese consider them to be the physical animation of the condition of the Zang, especially of the Heart and Liver.

As already stated, each Zang generates its own emotion in response to natural daily and seasonal stimuli. Very often, however, there is an overemphasis of one particular emotion which may then trigger off severe emotional stress or even physical imbalance.

Joy is the special emotion which inspirits and enlivens the Heart, strengthens its blood and energy flows, nurtures its physical structure, helps circulate its 'essences' and, most important of all, intensifies the awareness of life. When joy becomes excessive, Heart energy may become sluggish and, on occasions, the Spirit will defect. Loss of consciousness, hysteria, palpitations and insomnia are common symptoms of this state.

Spirit (Shen)
It is clear that, in Chinese philosophy and clinical practice, the Spirit (*Shen*) has its roots in the

ZANG AND FU

Heart. It is through the *Shen* that all thoughts and emotions relate back to the Heart. (The Heart influences the emotions and intellect through the Spirit and through its direction of the activities of the Zang and Fu.)

Strengthening the functioning of the Heart is essential for the preservation of health. A quiet and peaceful environment gives strength to the *Shen* and the mind. Indeed, mental exercises may be more important than merely physical ones.

When all the Zang and Fu organs function in accord, the *Shen* is strengthened; conversely, a strong and healthy *Shen* results in the whole body, physically and mentally, working harmoniously. In addition, clear vision, good concentration, creativity and confidence are largely dependent upon a strong *Shen*.

Emotional stress and physical tension not only increase Heart Fire and drain Heart energy but, because the Kidney supports Heart function, Kidney energy, the Will Power and *Shen* are also weakened.

The *Shen* and Zang and Fu are nurtured when Heart blood and energy are abundant, ensuring a strong intellect, discernment and good memory. Initially with Heart blood and energy deficiency, there is a decrease in the intellect and memory, eventually leading to syncope, constant drowsiness, continuous laughter, amnesia and coma as the condition becomes worse.

Relationship to Pericardium
The Pericardium envelopes the Heart and protects it from physical and emotional stress. Many mental illnesses and cardiovascular disorders, although basically considered Heart malfunctions, are often caused by a breakdown of Pericardium function. Regardless of whether the problem is initially of the Pericardium or of the Heart, treatment often entails strengthening the Pericardium to balance both functions.

Complexion and tongue
With a detailed knowledge of tongue diagnosis, the internal condition of the body is easily understood; but, as a whole, the tongue represents the condition of the Heart. Good health is indicated when the colour of the tongue is fresh and red and its movement is unrestricted. The state of Heart energy can be reliably tested by the ability of the tongue to distinguish the five tastes: pungent, salty, sweet, sour, and bitter. (The bitter taste especially correlates to the Heart.)

A scarlet tongue with ulcers on the tip is generally caused by insufficient Yin or excess Heart Fire. A pale or violet tongue indicates a Yang deficiency. A scarlet tongue with dark spots on the tip may be due to stasis of Heart blood. The presence of a speech impediment and a stiff tongue suggests an inflamed Heart through excessive body heat.

The condition of the Heart function is also manifested in the complexion. Good health is apparent when the complexion is fresh and glowing. With deficient Heart energy, the complexion can be pale or violet and dark; a deep red colour in the cheeks always indicates a Heart disorder.

Perspiration
Although controlled by the Lungs, perspiration is considered a Heart fluid as it indirectly influences the circulation of blood. When Lung energy is weak, the body starts to sweat, thereby decreasing body fluids including the blood. Spontaneous perspiration, which also depletes blood and energy, only occurs when the body (especially the Heart and Lungs) is weak.

If the body cannot counteract an invasion of heat by sweating, internal heat builds up within the viscera and eventually fever penetrates the Heart. Drugs, herbs or needles are then used to induce sweating. However, because the body is weak or deficient in Heart energy, induced sweating may lead to a severe loss of body fluids (including blood) and may result in shock or coma. In clinical practice, therefore, it is very important to determine the most appropriate method to induce sweating and to carefully monitor the reactions of the patient.

Heart Yin and Heart Yang
Heart Yang primarily regulates the rhythm of the Heart, strengthens the Heart beat, facilitates the circulation of blood and energy, and supports the emotional excitement factor. Heart Yang, therefore, correlates with and includes Heart energy and has a special function of self-defence against disease.

Heart Yin supports the emotional inhibition factor and has a significant association with Heart blood. Heart Yin as Yin fluid is an important part of the *Jing* blood system and also relates to Lung and Kidney Yin. Internal heat symptoms are always created when the body has a (Heart, Lung or Kidney) Yin deficiency caused by insufficient Yin fluid.

Heart Yin and Yang together equilibrate the Heart beat and are complementary and necessary components of the entire Heart function. Supported by Heart blood and energy, their solidarity secures strong Heart activity.

When Heart Yang is deficient, blood and energy (heat) decrease, resulting in the body becoming prone to cold disorders. Conversely, when Heart Yin is deficient, blood and energy increase, giving a predisposition to heat disorders.

Disorders
In Chinese medicine the differential diagnosis of Zang and Fu is an important method of disease identification. The following is a basic description of Heart disorders and disturbances.

ZANG AND FU

CHINESE DIAGNOSIS

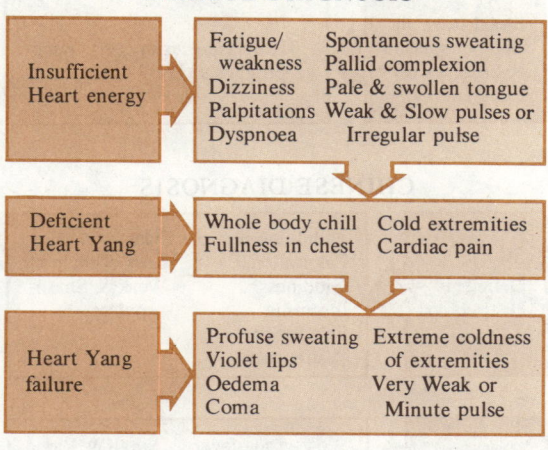

WESTERN DIAGNOSIS

Neurasthenia   Angina pectoris
General weakness   Heart failure
Arrhythmia cordis   Peripheral circulation failure

GENERAL CONSIDERATIONS

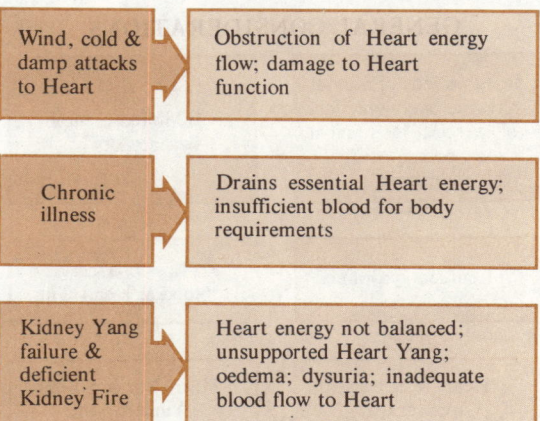

9

ZANG AND FU

Blood stasis in Lung or sputum obstruction of Lung energy → Heart Yang exhausted; poor prognosis

CHINESE DIAGNOSIS

Deficient Heart blood →
- Pallid complexion
- Palpitations
- Giddiness
- Insomnia
- Pale tongue
- Restlessness
- Fear
- Loss of memory
- Weak & Small pulses

Deficient Heart Yin →
- Low-grade fever
- Red-tipped tongue
- Night sweats
- Small & Rapid pulses

WESTERN DIAGNOSIS

- Malnutrition
- Tachycardia
- Hyperthyroidism
- Arrhythmia cordis
- Anaemia

GENERAL CONSIDERATIONS

Long periods of mental/physical overwork; lack of exercise; insufficient rest; poor nutrition; distress → Inhibited mental activity → Loss of Heart blood & Heart Yin → Spleen energy drained → Heart & Spleen overworked → Heart Yin & Spleen Yin deficient

CHINESE DIAGNOSIS

Hyperactive/overactive Heart Fire →
- Anxiety
- Overt anger
- Actual fear
- Restlessness
- Insomnia
- Headache
- Stiff neck
- Red complexion
- Red-tipped tongue
- Dry mouth
- Tongue ulcers
- Rapid & Floating pulses

WESTERN DIAGNOSIS

Psychiatric disturbances such as:
- Situation disorder
- Depression
- Neurosis
- Schizophrenia

GENERAL CONSIDERATIONS

- Poor nutrition
- Fatigue/exhaustion
- Physical trauma
- Domestic emotional stress
- Frustration
- Guilt
- Fright
- Lack of recreational outlet
- Anxiety

→ Drains Heart blood & energy; saps Kidney *Ching*; disturbs *Shen*

According to Chinese philosophy, the *Shen* is conceived by prenatal energy, nourished and developed by postnatal energy, and supported and maintained in these functions by Heart blood and energy. Deficiency of Kidney *Ching* with loss of Heart blood and energy disturbs Heart function and unbalances the *Shen*, especially in emotional struggles. The threat comes from unrecognized conflicts within. Stress manifested externally indicates an inability to adjust without showing evidence of instability.

ZANG AND FU

When hyperactivity is acute, the need for extra Heart blood is supplied by the Liver (which stores blood), thereby leading to an overactive Liver Yang. Heart Fire and Liver Fire result, thus making the condition worse.

Small Intestine

The Small Intestine is Fu, a Yang organ, one of the six bowels and belongs to the Fire element. Its Main Meridian is the Small Intestine Meridian of Hand *Tai* (Greater)-Yang and its Zang partner is the Heart.

The main function of the Small Intestine is to complete digestion; ingested nutrients and water are absorbed through its walls into the blood. Residual food matter is also transported by the Small Intestine to the Large Intestine. (Spleen energy absorbs and transports essential nutrients and water to all organs and tissues.) Small Intestine energy will transfuse (some) water to the Bladder.

The Small Intestine fulfils its objectives only when it works in collaboration with its Zang partner and overseer, the Heart. If the Small Intestine is too hot it will inflame the Heart, causing mouth ulcers and a red-tipped tongue. Conversely, an overheated Heart will inflame the Small Intestine, causing haematuria.

The main disorders of the Small Intestine are related to indigestion and malabsorption with symptoms such as abdominal pain and distention, diarrhoea, decreased urination and enuresis.

Common disorders of the Heart and Small Intestine

The most common disorders of Heart energy involve the blood vessels and *Shen*. Through clinical practice it has been confirmed that a disorder of the blood vessels is traceable to either a deficiency of Heart Yin or Yang or to a stasis in blood circulation.

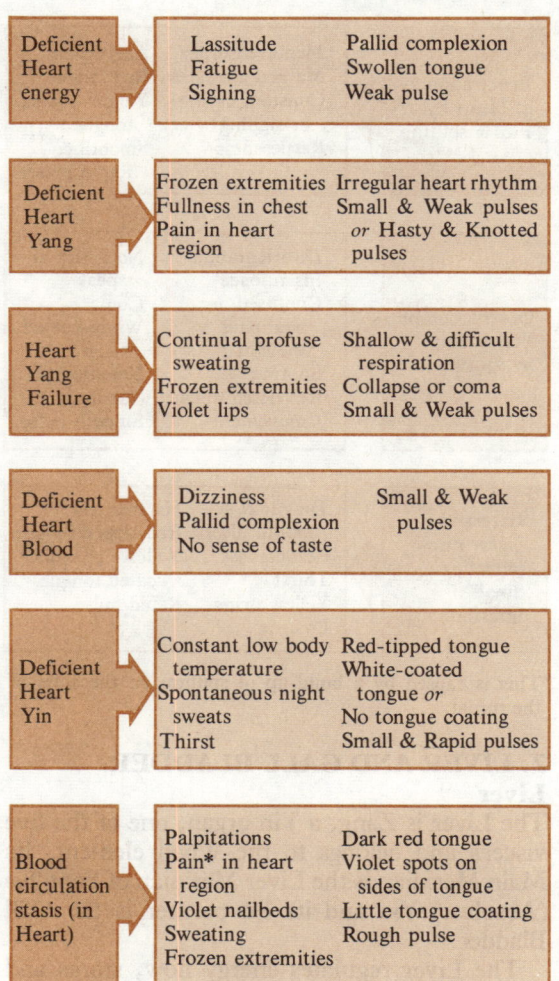

Deficient Heart energy	Lassitude Fatigue Sighing	Pallid complexion Swollen tongue Weak pulse
Deficient Heart Yang	Frozen extremities Fullness in chest Pain in heart region	Irregular heart rhythm Small & Weak pulses *or* Hasty & Knotted pulses
Heart Yang Failure	Continual profuse sweating Frozen extremities Violet lips	Shallow & difficult respiration Collapse or coma Small & Weak pulses
Deficient Heart Blood	Dizziness Pallid complexion No sense of taste	Small & Weak pulses
Deficient Heart Yin	Constant low body temperature Spontaneous night sweats Thirst	Red-tipped tongue White-coated tongue *or* No tongue coating Small & Rapid pulses
Blood circulation stasis (in Heart)	Palpitations Pain* in heart region Violet nailbeds Sweating Frozen extremities	Dark red tongue Violet spots on sides of tongue Little tongue coating Rough pulse

*The degree of pain indicates the severity of the disease.

A disorder of *Shen* is often caused by penetration of Fire or sputum into the Heart. By obstructing the Pericardium, sputum can indirectly affect the Heart. Emotional stress causes a direct increase in Heart Fire.

ZANG AND FU

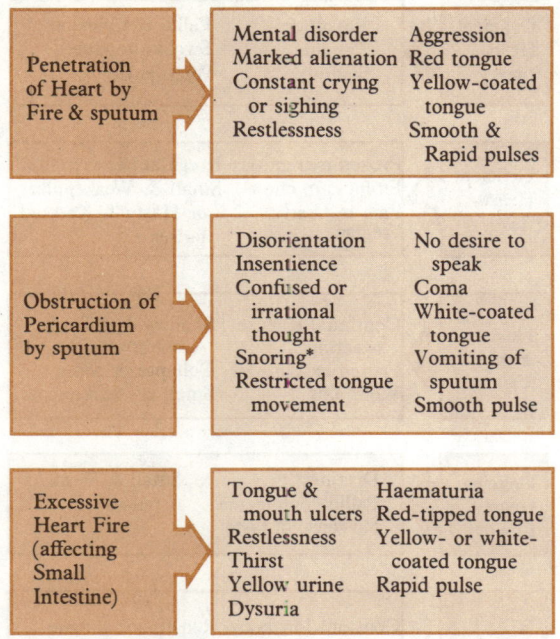

*This is caused by a build-up of sputum on the sides of the throat.

2. LIVER AND GALL BLADDER

Liver

The Liver is Zang, a Yin organ, one of the five viscera and belongs to the Wood element. Its Main Meridian is the Liver Meridian of Foot *Jue* (Absolute)-Yin and its Fu partner is the Gall Bladder.

The Liver regulates energy flow, stores and controls blood volume, nourishes the tendons, animates the eyes, directs the formation and secretion of bile, and governs the emotions.

The traditional Chinese perception of the Liver differs from the modern Western concept in that, although bile formation and secretion are recognized, the principal function of the Liver is more of a psychiatric and emotional one. Disorder of the Liver may be manifested in the central nervous system, blood, eyes or as a motor neuron disease.

Liver energy

Liver energy is very active, continually expanding and extending, and suffers when restrained. The ancient philosophers compared it to the 'growth of wood in Springtime' while contemporary Chinese acupuncturists classify Liver energy as another motivator of body resources, an agent which helps in the maturation of other body functions.

The most important function of Liver Yang is to regulate the flow of Liver blood directly to the:

- Stomach and Spleen to promote digestion;
- Heart (which in turn nourishes the Brain) to strengthen the *Shen* (Spirit);
- Uterus to balance the menses and support conception;
- tendons and extremities to assist physical activity;
- eyes to nourish and brighten them and clear the vision.

Liver Yang also sends blood and energy from the Twelve Main Meridians to the Lungs, completing the cycle initiated by the Lungs to nourish the entire body.

When Yang energy from the Lungs finally reaches the Liver, its energy content is so diminished that it provides little nourishment; but healthy Liver Yang is still able to direct Main Meridian energy back to the Lungs because it draws nourishment from Liver blood. If, however, the Liver is not healthy, there is obstruction of energy and stasis in the blood within the Twelve Main Meridians.

Disorders

Liver disorders generally arise from contraction of Liver Yang.

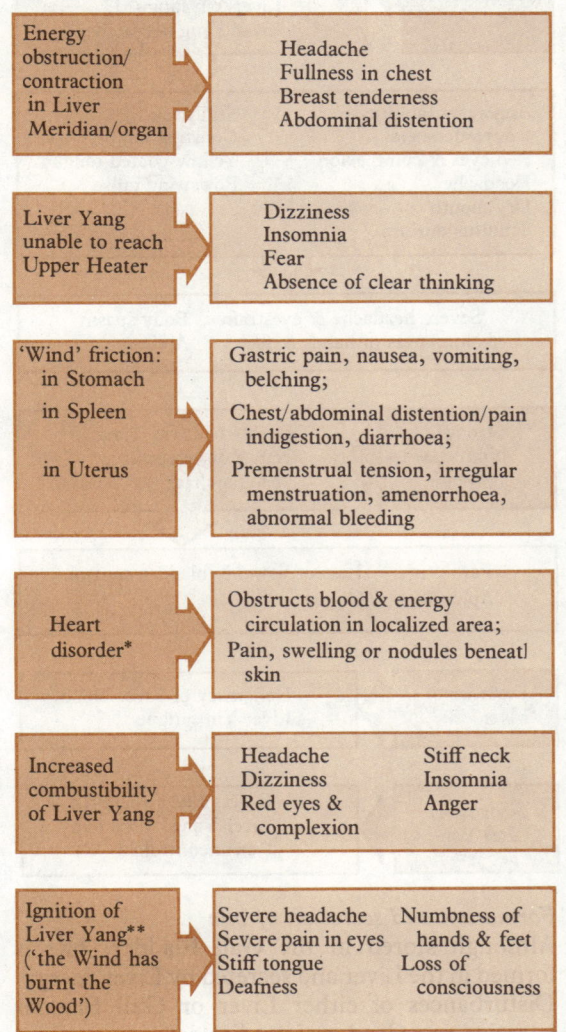

Energy obstruction/ contraction in Liver Meridian/organ	Headache Fullness in chest Breast tenderness Abdominal distention
Liver Yang unable to reach Upper Heater	Dizziness Insomnia Fear Absence of clear thinking
'Wind' friction: in Stomach	Gastric pain, nausea, vomiting, belching;
in Spleen	Chest/abdominal distention/pain indigestion, diarrhoea;
in Uterus	Premenstrual tension, irregular menstruation, amenorrhoea, abnormal bleeding
Heart disorder*	Obstructs blood & energy circulation in localized area; Pain, swelling or nodules beneath skin
Increased combustibility of Liver Yang	Headache Stiff neck Dizziness Insomnia Red eyes & Anger complexion
Ignition of Liver Yang** ('the Wind has burnt the Wood')	Severe headache Numbness of Severe pain in eyes hands & feet Stiff tongue Loss of Deafness consciousness

*Heat generated from contraction of Liver Yang inflames the Heart and, if severe, directs too much blood to the head, causing ocular or cerebral haemorrhage.

Emotion

Human nature expresses emotion through the various arts; music, writing, painting, dancing, all are extensions of the emotional lives of the artists. After expression of an emotionally artistic achievement, peace and awareness should follow: Yin balances Yang.

The Chinese, as already mentioned, recognize the five distinct emotions as being expressions of the workings of the five viscera. In moderation, the emotions and the physical body blend together harmoniously; however, in habitual distress, the emotions overwhelm, and often destroy, their respective organs. Overexpression of emotion spoils the 'Mind' and disturbs Zang functions, especially those of the Heart and Liver. Inhibited or restrained emotions can have similar or worse effects.

Although principally related to anger, the Liver is attuned to all emotional expression. The expansive nature of Liver Yang is an ideal medium for expressing, and maturing, the emotions. However, if Liver energy is restrained, Liver Yang activity is obstructed, resulting in anger, depression and emotional disturbance. Severe anger not only damages Liver Yang functions but also destroys Liver blood and Liver Yin, resulting in headache, vertigo, blurred vision, stiff neck and menstrual disorders.

Emotions must be cultivated as well as expressed. In Chinese medicine, mental exercises and emotional cultivation create harmonious communication between *Shen* and the physical body. Spring is considered the best time for cultivating the 'Will' and allowing it to grow freely. During this period the *NEI-JING* states that 'the body should be encouraged to live and not be "killed", that one should give to it freely and not take from it, and that one should reward it and not punish it.'

**Today this is called 'apoplexy'.

ZANG AND FU

Storage of Liver blood

In response to body stimuli, Liver Yang sends Liver blood to support body activity and nourish tissues and organs. When the body rests, Liver Yang rests and most of the blood then remains in the Liver. Blood storage is considered the most essential function of the Liver because, during storage, the blood is revitalized and made ready for use again by Liver Yang. An abundance of Liver blood nourishes Liver Yang and balances its functions, especially that of attuning emotional expression.

If blood does not return to the Liver (or if there is a blood deficiency), Liver Yang will drain the organ of its blood, exhausting the Liver Yin. Tendons then cramp through lack of nourishment; the *Chong* and Conception Vessel Meridians will both lose control of their blood, resulting in amenorrhoea or excessive menses; and the eyes (also undernourished) will tend towards dryness, night blindness and blurred vision.

Liver Yin and Yang

Functionally inseparable in a healthy body, Liver Yin and Yang are a good example of the solidarity that can exist between the Yin and Yang polarities. Working harmoniously together, they ensure the stability of a number of body functions but, when disturbed by emotional or physiological stress, these two forces become antagonistic, creating cycles of mutual defeat.

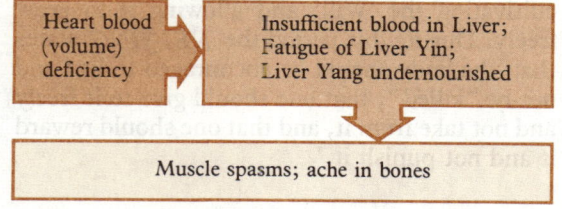

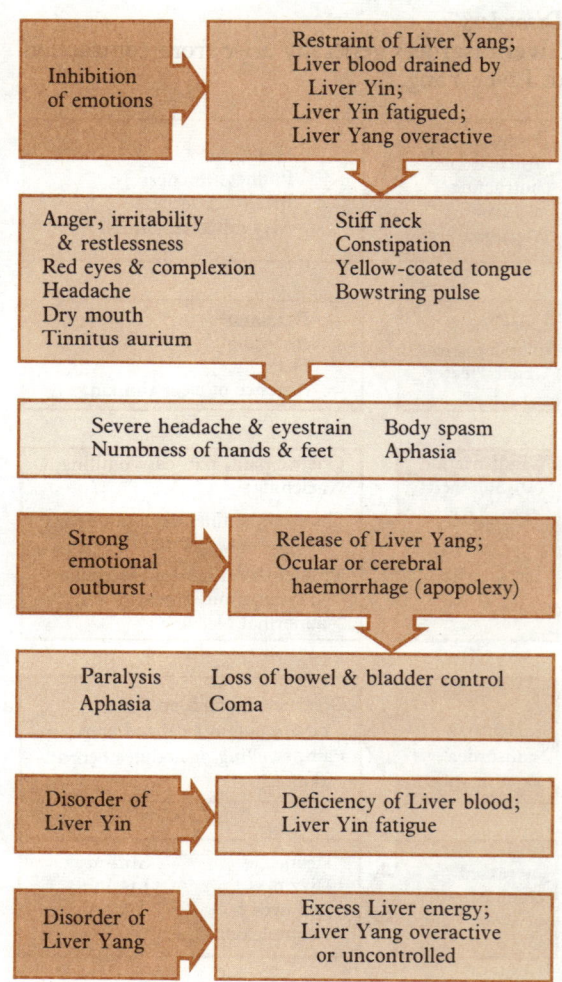

Formation and secretion of bile

Although stored in the Gall Bladder, bile is formed in the Liver and secreted by Liver energy. Disturbances of either Liver or Gall Bladder energies may lead to jaundice icterus, a bitter taste in the mouth, vomiting of yellowish fluids, fullness in the chest, abdominal distention and loss of appetite.

ZANG AND FU

Tendons

Liver Yang sends Liver blood to nourish and support the tendons and muscle functions. Strong healthy muscles which are supple in movement are an indication of good Liver (and Spleen) blood and energy. Muscular spasm, tremor or numbness of the limbs, opisthotonos and other signs of tendon malnutrition point to insufficient Liver blood and an imbalance of Liver Yang.

The ancient philosophers considered the nails to be extensions (or the ends) of the tendons. When Liver blood is healthy, the nails are strong and pink; a decrease in blood and energy is reflected in soft pale nails, and brittle nails are often a symptom of Liver disease. With age, nails invariably become brittle because of a proportional decrease in Liver blood and energy.

Eyes

The Chinese perceive the eyes to be unique in fulfilling dual functions, physiological and spiritual. The eyes, it is said, are windows of the soul; the Chinese also believe that they reflect the condition of the Liver.

Physiologically, the Yang, Heart and Liver Meridians, the Conception and Governor Vessel Meridians, and the Yin and Yang *Qiao* Meridians all pass through the eyes and help support and maintain their vital functions; but it is the Liver (organ) which provides them with nourishment.

Disorders in Meridian energy flows and body organs do, therefore, disturb the function of the eyes.

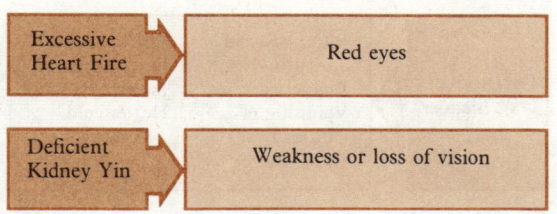

Gall Bladder

The Gall Bladder is Fu, a Yang organ, one of the six bowels and belongs to the Wood element. Its Main Meridian is the Gall Bladder Meridian of Foot *Shao* (Lesser)-Yang and its Zang partner is the Liver.

Unlike other Fu organs, the Gall Bladder tends to conserve, rather than expel, energy. It is a member of the Six Extra Fu (see page 33) and the only one of these unusual organs to have its own Meridian and complementary Zang organ.

The Gall Bladder stores bile, the only pure fluid stored (or formed) within the body. As with the Three Heater and Liver, the Gall Bladder holds a measure of 'Pure Fire' from Kidney Yang, *Ming Men Huo*. It is said that the purity of its energy and fluid gives the Gall Bladder the power to defend itself and the body both physically and emotionally. ('Its energy cuts through fear with bravery, counters hesitation with decisiveness, and delivers the body from discord and insult'). Fear readily affects any weakness in Gall Bladder energy, leaving the organ's function vulnerable to attack by disease. (A good Commander always has a healthy Gall Bladder!)

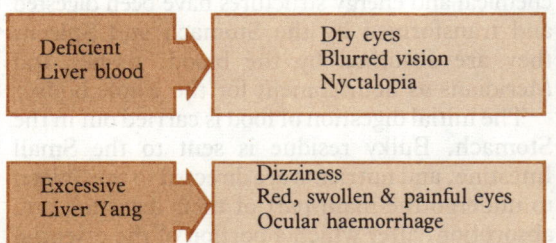

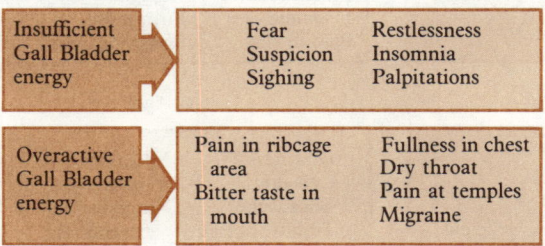

ZANG AND FU

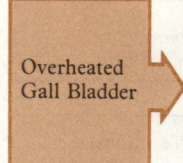

| Overheated Gall Bladder | Bitter taste in mouth / Fullness in chest / Vomiting of bitter fluids / Headache | Blurred vision / Deafness / Jaundice icterus / Hot & cold flushes |

| Liver Yin | Tendon & muscle spasms / Amenorrhoea / Excessive menses / Blurred vision / Dry tongue | Red tongue / Little or no tongue coating / Short, Rapid & Bowstring pulses |

Common disorders of the Liver and Gall Bladder

When Liver energy is disturbed, the emotions are heightened and the Liver's ability to store and revitalize blood is impaired. This is the most common disturbance of the Liver. The formation and secretion of bile and circulation of energies (the other important Liver function) are generally not affected in the initial stages of disorder.

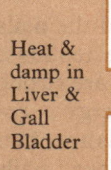

| Heat & damp in Liver & Gall Bladder | Pain in chest & ribs / Jaundice icterus / Bitter taste in mouth / Dry throat / Nausea / Vomiting | Indigestion / Abdominal pain / Alternating hot & cold body temperatures / Yellowish urine / Yellow-coated tongue / Red tongue / Bowstring pulse |

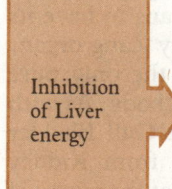

| Inhibition of Liver energy | Irritability / Anger / Depression / Dizziness / Abdominal pain / Diarrhoea / Fullness in chest / Loss of appetite | Bitter taste in mouth / Vomiting / Irregular menstruation / White-coated tongue / Bowstring pulse |

3. SPLEEN AND STOMACH
Spleen

The Spleen is Zang, a Yin organ, one of the five viscera and belongs to the Earth element. Its Main Meridian is the Spleen Meridian of Foot *Tai* (Greater)-Yin and its Fu partner is the Stomach.

Spleen energy penetrates all aspects of the digestive system; it forms the blood, protects its passage through the body and nourishes the muscles, extremities, mouth and lips.

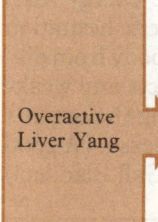

| Overactive Liver Yang | Anger / Restlessness / Palpitations / Stiff neck / Headache / Dry mouth / Tinnitus aurium / Dizziness / Bloodshot eyes / Insomnia / Pain in ribs | Bitter taste in mouth / Trembling hands / Numbness in hands & feet / Red-sided tongue / Yellow-coated tongue / Firm pulse / Bowstring pulse |

Digestion

Food in its raw state must undergo many changes before it can be used by the body. When its chemical and energy structures have been digested and transformed by the Stomach and Spleen, they are absorbed by the blood, tissues and Meridians as nourishment for the whole body.

The initial digestion of food is carried out in the Stomach. Bulky residue is sent to the Small Intestine, and nutrients are directed to the Spleen to undergo the main part of their digestion and absorption, after which a portion of the essential

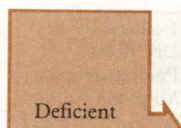

| Deficient | Dizziness / Constant headache / Tinnitus aurium | Nyctalopia / Insomnia / Numbness in extremities |

ZANG AND FU

substances is sent to the Lungs for distribution throughout the body. Liver and Kidney energies also contribute to food digestion and transportation. Kidney Yang warms the Stomach and Spleen, and Liver Yang supplies Liver blood.

When the Spleen enjoys a good supply of nutritious food, and its digestive, absorptive and transport functions are healthy, the nutrients produced are superfluous to the body's general needs; this excess of essential substances is stored in the Kidneys as postnatal energy.

When the Spleen is unable to absorb and transport food (or if, for other reasons, the essential substances are not circulating), there may be symptoms of indigestion, abdominal distention and pain, congested or gurgling stomach, fatigue, laziness and loss of appetite.

Formation of blood
Whilst some nutrients are directed to the Lungs for distribution throughout the body, a certain proportion is retained by the Spleen for further transformation into blood. As blood circulates it is protected by Spleen Yang which controls its flow to the blood vessels. Many disorders of the blood (including haemorrhage, melaena, bruises, aplastic anaemia and menstrual imbalance) indicate disorder within the Spleen.

Blood disorders require specialized treatment. Chinese herbs, together with a selection of acupuncture points from the (mainly) Liver, Spleen and Heart Meridians*, have been the first choice of traditional acupuncturists for centuries. Spleen 10 (Sea of Blood) is a specific point on the Spleen Meridian for blood disorders, but should not be thought of as a panacea for the blood.

*Blood is influenced and controlled by several different factors: it is formed within the Spleen and retained in the vessels by Spleen Yang; it is stored in the Liver during rest, guided by Liver Yang to support and nourish body activities, and controlled by the Liver when in the head region; its main circulation throughout the body is controlled by the Heart.

Water metabolism
Kidney Yang, and Spleen and Lung energies, direct the course of fluids through the body. A portion of the fluids absorbed by the Spleen is sent to the Lungs and the remainder is directed to the Kidneys. Through this system:

- the body is cleansed of toxins;
- the body is able to adjust to external and internal temperature changes;
- the movement of energies (including blood) is simplified.

If fluid is not absorbed by the Spleen but remains in the Stomach and Intestines, there is a watery faeces and oliguria. If retained in the Lungs there will be shortness of breath, cough, sputum, cradium and oedema beneath the skin.

If Kidney energy is low, there could be water retention in any part of the body. When Kidney Yang is deficient, the primary effect is oedema in the Spleen, Lungs and Bladder.

Emotion
Emotions and thoughts with a note of spontaneity are expressions of Heart energy; emotions and thoughts controlled through concentration and hindsight are expressions of Spleen energy. Reminiscence is the most recognized expression of Spleen function.

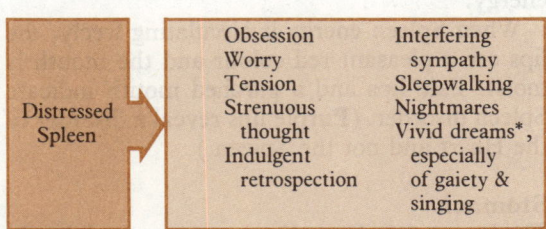

| Distressed Spleen | → | Obsession
Worry
Tension
Strenuous thought
Indulgent retrospection | Interfering sympathy
Sleepwalking
Nightmares
Vivid dreams*, especially of gaiety & singing |

*Meals before sleeping can induce dreams as Spleen energy tends towards excess.

ZANG AND FU

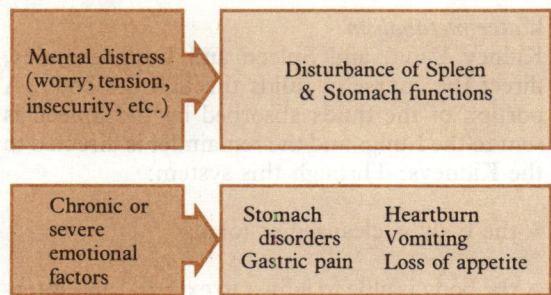

Relationship to muscles, extremities, mouth, tongue and lips

Blood, formed in the Spleen, nurtures the muscles and sustains their continual activity. A healthy Spleen together with correct exercise results in strong and firm body muscle. Insufficient Spleen energy or a Spleen disorder reduces muscle tone; weakness of the extremities, fatigue and laziness are apparent and, eventually, the body becomes wasted.

The Ancients said that the intelligence required to select the correct food is an expression of Spleen energy while the ability to taste it is a measure of Heart energy. This is based on the principle that Spleen energy extends to the root of the tongue while Heart energy passes through to the tip of the tongue.

Disorder in the Spleen results in a lack of appetite and a sweet or fatty taste in the mouth. In diagnoses of the tongue, its coating is based on Stomach energy and thus also relates to Spleen energy.

When Spleen energy is circulating freely, the lips are a pleasant red colour and the mouth is moist. Pale lips and a parched mouth indicate Spleen disorder. (Purple lips reveal a disorder of the Heart and not the Spleen.)

Stomach

The Stomach is Fu, a Yang organ, one of the six bowels and belongs to the Earth element. Its Main Meridian is the Stomach Meridian of Foot Yang-*Ming* (Sunlight) and its Zang partner is the Spleen.

The main function of the Stomach is to receive and digest food before directing nutrients to the Spleen and partially digested waste matter to the Small Intestine. When disorder of the Stomach results in undigested food, the various distress signals include upper abdominal pain, abdominal distention, nausea, vomiting and loss of appetite.

In the case of excess energy in the Stomach, there is halitosis, dry mouth, loss of appetite, epistaxis, tongue ulcers, toothache and bleeding gums.

Relationship to Spleen

Many activities of the Spleen and Stomach affect each other so subtly and closely that they cannot be spoken of separately. They are perfectly complementary although, in many cases, this is true only in potential. The Spleen needs a dry atmosphere, dislikes humidity and has an ascending circulation of energy. In contrast, the Stomach is naturally humid, dislikes dryness and has a descending circulation of energy. As moisture always gravitates downwards, the Spleen must be dry so that its energy circulation can rise. With a dry atmosphere this Zang organ is able to absorb and transform nutrients and body fluids before transporting them to the target organs.

As food is ingested, it passes down to the Stomach and then to the Small Intestine as partially digested waste matter. This downward motion follows the course of Stomach energy and, with its humid atmosphere, this Fu organ is able to receive and digest the food before passing on nutrients and waste to the respective organs.

Healthy Spleen and Stomach energy flows are able to support an abundance of nutrition (that is, basic vital energy), supplying all the organs, muscles and extremities. Energy deficiencies of these organs reduce that basic vital energy support and weaken all body functions. In particular, the body's defence mechanism is diminished, leaving it vulnerable to attack by disease.

In chronic disease the functions of the Spleen and Stomach must be protected because, when their energies are damaged, treatment becomes very difficult.

When there is a deficiency of Spleen energy, the organ becomes humid, rendering it incapable of efficiently absorbing and transforming food substances and body fluids and, ultimately, of forming blood.

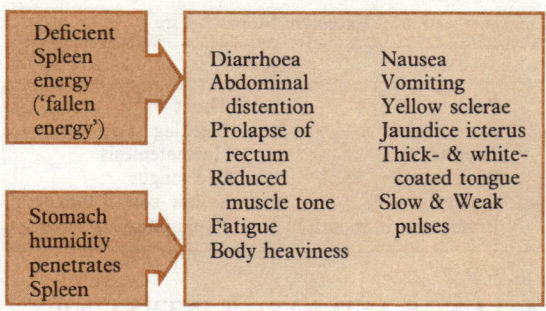

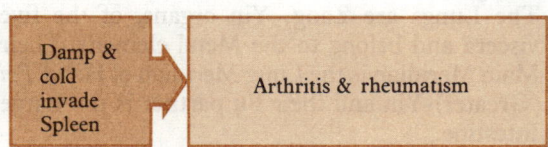

Causes of deficiency of Spleen energy:

- Mental distress;
- Irregular intake of food and drink;
- Overwork (mental and physical);
- Weak body condition following chronic illness with diminished appetite.

Causes of deficiency of Stomach energy:

- Irregular eating and drinking habits;
- Overeating of cold and raw foods;
- Too many cold drinks;
- Emotional distress;
- Excessive Liver Yang overwhelming the Stomach.

An accumulation of cold will cause upper abdominal pain which, if not relieved by food intake, can lead to:

Vomiting	White-coated tongue
Heartburn	Weak/Floating pulse
Pallid complexion	Bowstring pulse (with
Cold hands & feet	abdominal pain)
Swollen tongue	

Common disorders of the Spleen and Stomach

In the traditional Chinese perception of the Spleen, its main objectives are to digest, absorb and transport food, and to form and control the blood. These functions are affected by the most common of Spleen disorders: humidity.

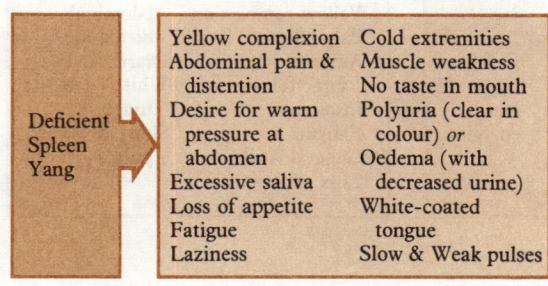

ZANG AND FU

Obstruction of Spleen Yang by excessive humidity →
- Loss of appetite
- Desire for hot fluids
- No taste in mouth
- Nausea or vomiting
- Excessive uterine discharge
- Heaviness in head
- Weak & heavy extremities
- Dislike of or difficulty in exercise
- No desire to talk
- Diarrhoea
- Thick-/white-coated tongue
- Weak pulse

Heat & damp in Spleen →
- Yellow sclerae
- Jaundice icterus
- Itching skin
- Fullness in chest
- Loss of appetite
- Fatigue
- Lassitude
- Thirst
- Bitter taste in mouth
- Fever
- Soft stools
- Yellow urine
- Yellow-coated tongue
- Rapid & Tight pulses

Deficient Spleen & Stomach energies →
- Yellow complexion
- Loss of appetite
- Stomach pain
- Desire for warm pressure on stomach
- Stomach distention
- Flatulence
- Lassitude
- Belching
- Diarrhoea
- Vomiting of acid
- Swollen tongue
- Serrated marks on tongue edges
- White-coated tongue
- Weak pulse

Deficient Spleen & Heart energies →
- Yellow complexion
- Palpitations
- Amnesia or forgetfulness
- Insomnia
- Fatigue
- General weakness
- Loss of appetite
- Abdominal distention
- Diarrhoea
- White-coated tongue
- Short & Weak pulses

Deficient Spleen & Kidney energies →
- Mental fatigue
- Lack of energy
- No desire to talk
- Excessive throat mucus
- Shortness of breath
- Wheezing cough
- Weak & cold extremities
- Morning diarrhoea
- Cold lumbar region
- Oedema, particularly ascites
- White-coated tongue
- Short & Weak pulses

The most common Stomach disorder is overactivity caused by too much heat:

Excessive Stomach Fire →
- Fever
- Constipation
- Toothache
- Restlessness
- Epistaxis
- Bitter taste in mouth
- Thirst
- Bleeding gums
- Haematemesis
- Red tongue
- Yellow-coated tongue
- Rapid pulse

4. LUNGS AND LARGE INTESTINE
Lungs

The Lungs are Zang, Yin organs, of the five viscera and belong to the Metal element. Their Main Meridian is the Lung Meridian of Hand *Tai* (Greater)-Yin and their Fu partner is the Large Intestine.

The Lungs are the principal components of the respiratory system. They synthesize all body energies, facilitate blood circulation, contribute to body fluids and metabolism, equalize internal temperature changes and balance body energy with external changes of temperature.

Synthesis of extrinsic energies
Air and the 'essence' of food (*Gu-Qi*) converge at the Lungs where, on shedding their individual qualities, they unite to become postnatal energy, *Zong-Qi*, which remains mostly in the Upper

ZANG AND FU

Heater, especially in the Lungs. *Yuan-Qi*, prenatal energy, remains for the most part in the Lower Heater, especially in the Kidneys. The fusion in the Lungs of these two energies (*Zong-Qi* and *Yuan-Qi*) creates the basic material of the Meridians, *Jing-Qi*. Hence, the Lungs are called the 'Centre of Energy'.

When energy has passed through the Twelve Main Meridians, it is returned to the Lungs by Liver energy. Both the Lungs and Liver need to be strong in order to circulate their energies freely. A deficiency of Lung energy is reflected in the quality and quantity of energy available to the body. Deficient Liver energy is an indication of obstruction of energy within the Meridians.

According to the Chinese, the Lungs consist of a series of air passages, including the nose, pharynx, larynx, trachea, bronchi and bronchioles. Their energies inhale clean external air (*Qing-Qi*) and exhale impure internal air (*Zhuo-Qi*). Inhalation and exhalation are well controlled by healthy Lung energy but, in cases of insufficient Lung energy, these two important functions are disturbed, resulting in symptoms such as coughing and fullness in the chest.

Blood and energy flows

'ENERGY is the master of blood.'
Without it, blood cannot circulate.

'BLOOD is the mother of energy.'
Its nutrients give birth to energy.

The natural interplay of Yin and Yang is exemplified in clinical practice by the relationship between the Lungs and Heart. Basically, the Lungs control energy and the Heart controls blood.

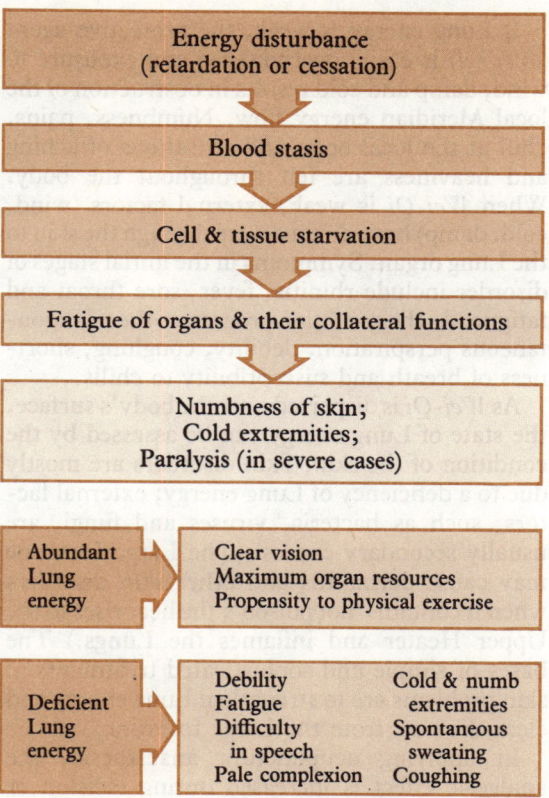

Skin and perspiration glands
('Gate of Energy')

The Lungs have two distinct energies: internal and external. Its primary power radiates from the Lung organ itself, while *Wei-Qi*, the derivative or secondary Yang energy of the Lungs, saturates the surface of the body. Using this distribution of energy, the Lungs are able to equalize changes of body temperature. If external factors overheat the body, Lung energy dilates the sweat glands and skin pores to induce sweating and release the heat. Conversely, during cold weather, Lung energy contracts the glands and pores to resist chilling.

ZANG AND FU

If Lung energy is weak, the protective agent (*Wei-Qi*) is easily overpowered and exposure to wind, damp and cold results in obstruction of the local Meridian energy flow. Numbness, pains, chill at the local area, and sensations of aching and heaviness are felt throughout the body. When *Wei-Qi* is weak, external factors (wind, cold, damp) have direct access through the skin to the Lung organ. Symptoms in the initial stages of disorder include rhinitis, fever, sore throat and fatigue. As the condition progresses there is spontaneous perspiration, debility, coughing, shortness of breath and susceptibility to chills.

As *Wei-Qi* is dispersed over the body's surface, the state of Lung energy can be assessed by the condition of the skin. Skin disorders are mostly due to a deficiency of Lung energy; external factors, such as bacteria, viruses and fungi, are usually secondary causes. (The Large Intestine may cause dermatitis and other skin disorders when it contains 'hot poison'; the heat rises to the Upper Heater and inflames the Lungs.) The bases of simple and sophisticated treatments of skin problems are to strengthen Lung energy and clear the heat from the Large Intestine.

In applying acupuncture anaesthesia, the analgesic effect is increased during incision or suture of the skin by appropriate selection and manipulation of points from the Lung Meridian.

Body hair

Lung energy, through *Wei-Qi*, saturates the surface of the body, including body hair. A good covering of body hair which is rich in colour indicates strong and freely circulating Lung energy. When hair colour fades and its growth rate is slower, it is a sign that Lung energy has decreased, usually through chronic illness.

Nose

As the nose and Lungs are contributors to the same process, the nose (which is external) can reflect the condition of the Lungs (which is internal). A test of the strength of Lung energy is whether the nose can distinguish the five odours: putrid, rotten, rancid, scorched, and fragrant.

The condition of the nose can also reveal whether an invasion by wind or cold has penetrated the Lungs. If such is the case, Lung energy is unable to extend to the nose, and nasal obstruction, loss of smell and a 'runny' nose are evident. If the Lungs are hot, symptoms then include epistaxis, dry cough and sore throat.

Body fluid metabolism

The Lungs and Spleen supplement Kidney energy to form the body fluid metabolism. The action of the Lungs in the Upper Heater is to balance the Kidneys in the Lower Heater so that body fluids can be evenly distributed throughout the body. The Lungs distribute body fluids over the skin by means of perspiration, thus contributing to balancing body fluid metabolism. The Spleen transports body fluids to the Lungs which, in turn, transform and distribute these substances to the organs and tissues.

An imbalance in Lung and Spleen energy flows leads to fluid retention in the Lungs, thus causing obstruction of respiratory air passages and formation of mucus. Symptoms include nasal obstruction, coughing, shortness of breath and fullness in the chest.

Voice

Lung Meridian energy flow passes through the pharynx and larynx, the 'Gates of the Lungs'. The Metal element, which is inherent in the Lungs, actuates the vocal chords.

- Healthy body energy promotes a well modulated voice;

- Deficient Lung energy causes soft or husky speech, or a low timbre;

ZANG AND FU

- A harsh loud voice indicates hyperactive Lungs;
- An inability or lack of desire to speak is symptomatic of severely disabled Lung power.

Emotion

Sadness and gloom, emotions identified with the Lungs, are the result of inadequate coping with stress and change. After an acute emotional attack (such as bad news in the family), a 'good cry' very often relieves the shock as well as the energy obstruction in the Lungs. Habitual sadness, however, produces a loss of Lung energy and disturbance of Spleen, Heart and Kidney functions. This leads to irregular breathing which obstructs the energy flow of the Upper Heater, especially the Heart function. Regular, deep and slow breathing calms Heart Fire and creates a quiet Mind; in this way joy will balance sadness.

When there is stasis of *Jing* blood and obstruction of *Wei* energy, Lung energy is damaged or lost. The ability to prevent invasion by external factors (wind, cold, damp) also declines, causing the body to 'feel the cold' more easily. Further symptoms may arise, such as fatigue, loss of interest in living, nasal obstruction, coughing, shortness of breath, fullness in the chest, and cold hands and feet.

Deficiency of Lung energy

A deficiency of Lung energy may be due to a chronic disorder in the Lungs or may result from deficient energy of the whole body. The Lungs, one of the gentle organs, are always vulnerable to attack by external factors (mostly winds, but also cold, damp, heat and dryness). However, only when Lung energy is disturbed internally is its protective mechanism lost and external factors able to penetrate.

Overwork, emotional distress, unhappiness, gloom, lack of mental discipline and physical exercise to balance the body, and environmental weather changes all drain Lung energy and weaken or obstruct its flow. Wind penetrates the skin (because of obstructed *Wei* energy and stasis of *Jing* blood) and passes through the nose and bronchi to the Lungs, thus damaging Lung functions. The many symptoms include:

Frequently 'feeling the cold'	Spontaneous sweating
Cold hands & feet	Coughing
Fear of cold	Shortness of breath
Pale complexion	Dyspnoea
Fatigue	Excessive white sputum
Debility	Swollen tongue
Lack of desire to speak	White-coated tongue
Soft & weak speech	Small & Weak pulses

Large Intestine

The Large Intestine is Fu, a Yang organ, one of the six bowels and belongs to the Metal element. Its Main Meridian is the Large Intestine Meridian of Hand Yang-*Ming* (Sunlight) and its Zang partner is the Lungs.

The principal activities of the Large Intestine are to process residual food matter and expel it from the body. Disturbance of these functions is usually caused by excessive heat and dryness in the Large Intestine. When water metabolism is out of balance, as it often is in clinical findings, the Zang organs are forced to draw water from the Fu. Whilst the former thus maintain adequate moisture, the Fu organs (Stomach, Small Intestine, Bladder and Large Intestine) are left hot and dry. In this condition, residual food matter is retained in the Large Intestine and the resultant heat and toxins rise directly to the Lungs and inflame the skin and nose. Symptoms include acne rosacea, dermatitis, eczema and other skin and nasal disorders.

The heat from the Large Intestine also inflames the Small Intestine and Stomach, and causes

ZANG AND FU

irritation to the mouth and throat. Symptoms include epistaxis, aptha, gingivitis, coughing and sore throat (for example, tonsillitis, pharyngitis, laryngitis, bronchitis). Appropriate treatment expels the heat from the Large Intestine; this includes treating the Lungs to relieve symptoms.

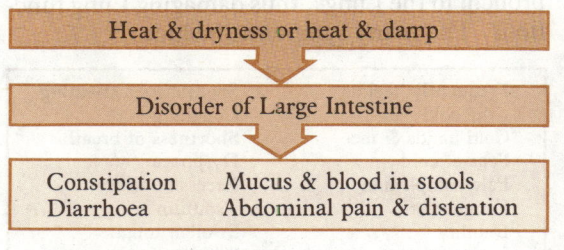

Common disorders of the Lungs and Large Intestine

Whilst water metabolism generally remains unaffected, the synthesis of extrinsic energies (the main function of the respiratory system) is the focus of most Lung disturbances. Common causes are a state of either deficiency or overactivity of the Lungs, or simply 'cold' Lungs.

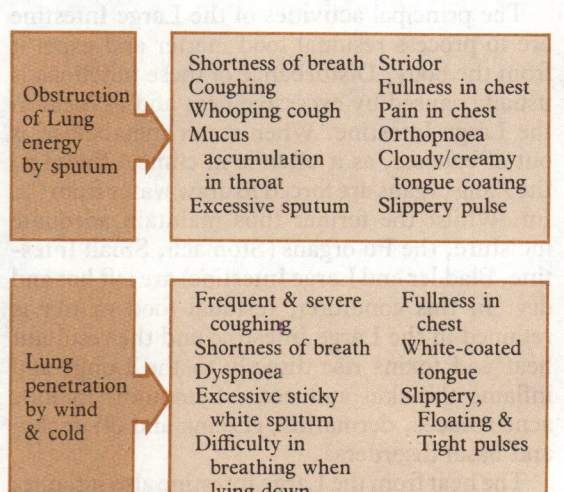

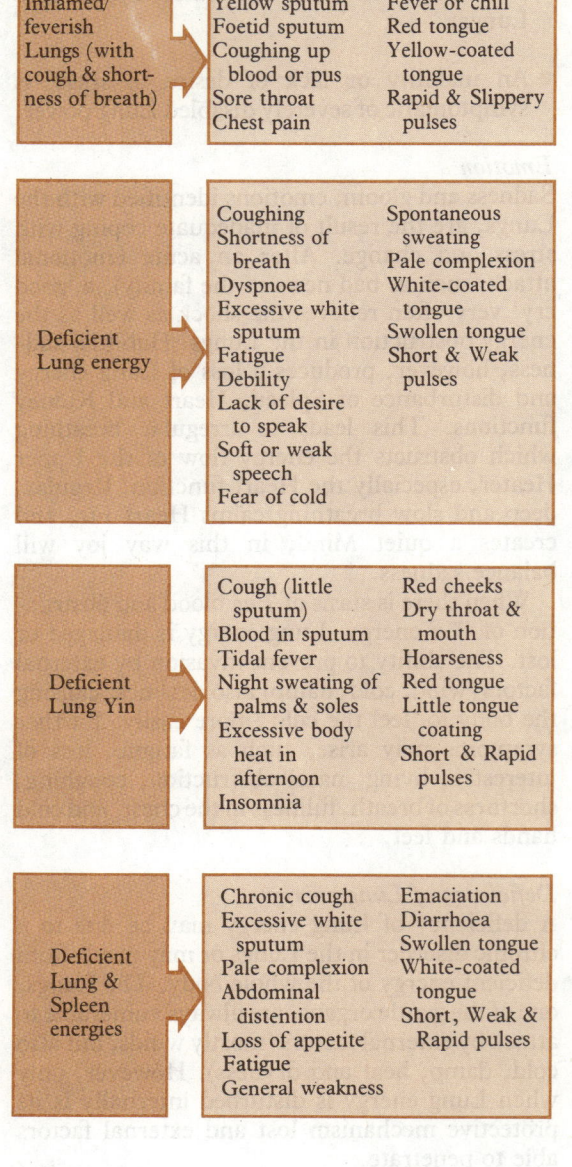

ZANG AND FU

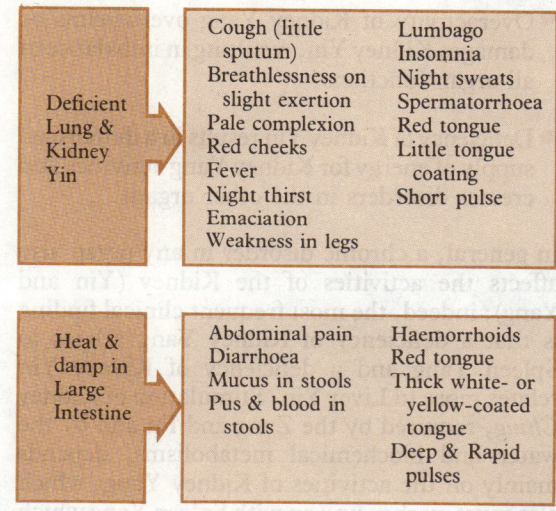

5. KIDNEYS AND BLADDER
Kidneys
The Kidneys are Zang, Yin organs, of the five viscera, and belong to the Water element. Their Main Meridian is the Kidney Meridian of Foot *Shao* (Lesser)-Yin and their Fu partner is the Bladder.

The Kidneys store *Shen Ching* (see below), govern *Ming Men Huo*, nourish bones and marrow, guide body fluids, assist inhalation and are responsible for the condition of the hair, ears, anus and urethra. The activities of the Kidneys also encompass the functions of the central nervous, endocrine (with special emphasis on the pituitary and adrenal glands) and urogenital systems.

Shen (Kidney) Ching
Shen Ching (often called *Shen* [Kidney] Yin) preserves in the Kidneys the essences of prenatal (intrinsic) and postnatal (extrinsic) energies. Body growth, development and reproductive functions depend upon *Shen Ching*.

Stored in the Kidneys as the postnatal (extrinsic) factor of *Shen Ching* is the surplus essence (initially derived from food and air) of the five Zang and six Fu. This reservoir of potential energy is constantly being drawn back into the system to support the physiological activity of the Zang and Fu.

The prenatal (intrinsic) quality of *Shen Ching* is called *Yuan-Qi* and is inherited from the parents. This nourishes the body, supports the physiological activity of the Zang and Fu and is the underlying essence of the reproductive system, particularly of sperm and ova. Constantly replenished by postnatal (extrinsic) *Shen Ching*, the strength of *Yuan-Qi* determines intelligence.

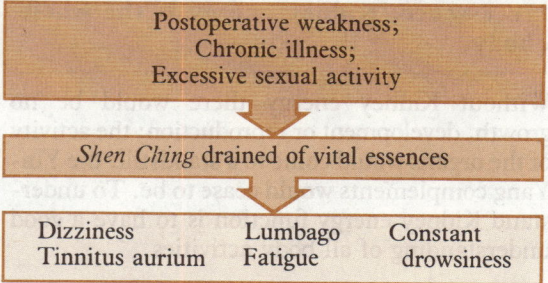

Ming Men Huo
Born out of *Yuan-Qi* and sustained by the Kidney *Ching*, *Ming Men Huo* is the most dynamic energy of the body. Also called 'Pure Fire' or Kidney Yang, it is the impetus behind all body activities.

- Through it, vital essences stored in Kidney Yin are released to support the physiological activity of the Zang and Fu;

- It assists digestion, absorption and transport of nutrients by inciting the functions of the Stomach and Spleen, and then circulates their essences throughout the body;

25

ZANG AND FU

- It stimulates the activities of the reproductive system (particularly sexual activity);
- It animates the energy flow of the Three Heater (sometimes described as the biochemical metabolism of the body);
- It augments the ability of the Lungs and nose to expand (inhale).

> Kidney Yin and Yang are the fundamental energies of the Zang and Fu;
>
> Kidney energy is the most active principle in the body;
>
> In essence, Kidney energy is the whole body.

Without Kidney energy there would be no growth, development or reproduction; the activity of the organs would come to a standstill; the Yin-Yang complements would cease to be. To understand Kidney energy function is to have a good understanding of all body activities.

- Kidney Yin controls Water (Pure Water = Pure Yin): it harvests and stores the basic source of energy for the creation of Kidney Yang; it stores *Yuan-Qi* (prenatal energy) and the essence of reproduction (*Ching-Qi*).

- Kidney Yang is Pure (Vital) Fire: it is the driving force (warmth) needed by *Shen Ching* (postnatal energy) in order to reach the Zang and Fu; indeed, it is the driving force of all activities of the Zang and Fu.

The balanced and mutually supportive relationship between Kidney Yin and Yang is necessary for the continual functioning of all the organs:

- Overactivity of Kidney Yang overwhelms or damages Kidney Yin, resulting in imbalance of all organ functions;

- Deficiency of Kidney Yin results in a diminished supply of energy for Kidney Yang activities and creates disorders in the other organs.

In general, a chronic disorder in any organ also affects the activities of the Kidney (Yin and Yang); indeed, the most frequent clinical finding is that a deficiency of Kidney Yang relates to Spleen Yang and a deficiency of Kidney Yin relates more to Liver Yin. Stimulation of Kidney *Ching*, required by the Zang and Fu and by the water and biochemical metabolisms, depends mainly on the activities of Kidney Yang, which also must work in unison with Spleen Yang which digests, absorbs, transports and supplies nutrients and water, especially to the Kidneys.

Deficient Kidney Yin (Water) causes

- Heat build-up in Zang and Fu with symptoms including vertigo, tinnitus aurium, dry mouth, dry throat, lumbago, nocturnal emissions, night sweats, sexual overactivity, weakness of feet, red tongue, Weak & Rapid pulses;

- Temporary upsurge of Kidney Yang (Fire), leading to increased Zang and Fu activity which eventually exhausts the already depleted Kidney *Ching*;

- Increase of Liver Yang and often of Liver Wind, producing anger and tension;

- Excess of Heart Fire, which leads to an imbalance of Heart/Kidney functions with insomnia as the most common symptom;

- Depletion of Lung energy with symptoms of

dry throat, dry cough and tidal fever; the heat generated may inflame the Upper Heater.

Deficiency Kidney Yang (Fire) causes
- Disruption of water metabolism;
- Inactivity of reproductive systems;
- Enfeebled Heart with symptoms including palpitations, sweating, shortness of breath and cold extremities;
- Deficient Yang state in Lungs, with typical symptoms of difficulty in inhalation, shortness of breath and spontaneous perspiration;
- Depleted Spleen energy with symptoms including indigestion, water retention and early morning diarrhoea;
- Inertia of essential essences within Kidneys, leading to weakness of the whole body.

Deficient Kidney Yang →	Darkened complexion Hair loss Fear of cold Cold hands & feet Shortness of breath Dyspnoea Fatigue Tinnitus aurium Lumbago Oedema	Nocturnal emissions Enuresis Morning diarrhoea Swollen tongue White-coated tongue Floating & Weak pulses *or* Deep, Slow & Weak pulses

The condition of the body influences Kidney Yin and Yang, often imperceptibly:

- When the Lungs are deficient of energy, they are unable to direct the essence of nutrients to the *Shen Ching*. The intrinsic essence of *Shen Ching* then has to compensate for the lack of extrinsic essence and it, too, becomes exhausted.

- A deficiency of Spleen Yang hinders the digestion, absorption and transport of nutrients and water, thus again draining the *Shen Ching* of its essences. The first sign is morning diarrhoea and, in time, the body becomes exhausted.

- Many disorders, including deficiency of Liver Yin, overactivity of Liver Yang and deficiency or excess of Heart energy, disrupt Kidney function by evaporating water and, eventually, the *Shen Ching*.

Cycles of growth
According to the *NEI-JING*, the physiological function of the Kidneys involves the processes of growth, development, reproduction and senility:

Female		Male	
Age (yrs)	Accompanying Features	Age (yrs)	Accompanying Features
7	Flourishing Kidney energy; growth of permanent teeth & hair	8	Developed testes (Kidney *Ching*); growth of permanent teeth & hair
14	Abundant energies of *Chong* & Conception Vessel Meridians; onset of menses (conception potential)	16	Abundant Kidney energy; onset of semen secretion (conception/union potential)

ZANG AND FU

21	Regular Kidney energy; wisdom teeth present; full maturation	24	Regular Kidney energy; wisdom teeth present; strong bones & muscles; full height; 'prime of life'
28	Full length of hair; strong bones & muscles; fertile body; 'prime of life'	32	Able-bodied & fertile; muscles & bones are flourishing
35	Decline of Yang Meridian energy (indicated by pulse); onset of facial wrinkling & hair loss	40	Smaller testicular emanations; onset of hair loss & tooth decay
42	Decreased Yang Meridian energy; complete facial wrinkling; greying hair	48	Reduced/exhausted muscular vigour; facial wrinkling; greying hair
49	Decreased Kidney energy; onset of body degeneration & cessation of reproductive functions	56	Decreased Liver energy; loss of muscle function, physical strength & semen secretion
56	Loss of conception potential & menses (decreased energies of *Chong* & Conception Vessel Meridians)	64	Decreased Kidney energy; loss of teeth & hair; onset of body degeneration & cessation of reproductive functions

Kidney (prenatal) energy is the basic essence of the Kidney and is continually nourished by postnatal energy. A combination of

- healthy prenatal energy inherited from the parents;
- careful attention to health and nutrition;
- an abundance of postnatal energy to nurture it;

produces a strong and healthy Kidney energy. This, in turn, ensures healthy growth, development and reproduction.

Location of Kidney energies
There are many conjectures concerning the location of Kidney Yin and Yang in the body. The ancient philosophers could agree on the principles of these two energies but were never unanimous as to their location. Their theories included:

- that Kidney Yin is found in both Kidneys and *Ming Men Huo* is at the periphery of these twin organs;
- that the left Kidney housed Kidney Yin and the right Kidney housed Kidney Yang;
- that Kidney Yin is in the left Kidney, but the right Kidney housed *Ming Men Huo*. (Presumably they believed that Kidney Yang and *Ming Men Huo* were the same energy. This is still a commonly held opinion.)

Although these theories have been widely adopted, they embrace one major contradiction: according to Chinese philosophy, life cannot continue without Kidney Yin, but it has been proved that life does continue without the left Kidney. Several explanations are given (one is that there is a nucleus of Kidney Yin in the Kidney Yang), but none is fully supported by clinical practice or observation.

One of the more acceptable theories suggests that Kidney Yin is housed in both Kidneys as it is, by definition, the basic substance of the organ itself. This leaves in doubt the location of Kidney Yang or *Ming Men Huo* ('Pure Fire'), the activities of which incorporate a range of functions throughout the entire body (as already noted, the Chinese perception of the Kidneys includes the endocrine system). Thus, it was considered impossible that *Ming Men Huo* be embodied in a single organ but rather that its energies, combined from all sources, could be tapped at one point: GV 4 (see Chapter 4).

Body fluid metabolism

It is essentially energy from the Kidneys, assisted by Spleen and Lung energies, which determines the distribution and expulsion of body fluids. When the Kidneys receive fluids from the Spleen and Lungs, Kidney Yang (through a biochemical function which warms body fluids) apportions a sufficient measure to the Zang and Fu as well as to other functions, and directs the remainder to the Bladder.

If Kidney Yang is strong and working in accord with Bladder energy, there is a surplus of fluids (for all needs of the body) and, more important, a balanced distribution of these fluids.

If Kidney Yang is weak, there is a deficiency of fluids and an imbalance in their allocation. The symptoms include dyspnoea, ascites, oedema, retention of urine, anuria, enuresis and polyuria.

Bone marrow* and teeth

With *Shen Ching* as a catalyst, Kidney energy in its totality nurtures the growth and development of the bones and marrow and, when necessary, aids in their reparation.

With healthy Kidney energy and an abundance of Kidney *Ching*, bone, marrow and teeth are sound, the physical body is strong, and the action

---

*It is an old Chinese precept that marrow passes through the spine to the Brain, the 'Centre of Marrow'; by 'marrow' the philosophers meant 'principal essence', and not the Western meaning of the word.

of the body is fast and accurate. However, if Kidney *Ching* is disturbed or insecure, the intellect decreases, there is forgetfulness and a lack of concentration, the bones ache, there is a tendency to dizziness, and the actions of the body are slow.

As the teeth are believed to be the 'ends of the bones', any imperfections are attributed to a deficiency of Kidney *Ching*. If the teeth develop poorly during the formative years or if adult teeth suddenly become loose, it is considered that the Kidney *Ching* is inadequate to nourish the bones and marrow.

Inhalation

The ability of the nose and Lungs to expand (to inhale) is augmented by Kidney energy. A deficiency of Kidney Yang renders respiration ineffectual, particularly if the Lungs are also impaired. Exhalation then becomes comparatively stronger than inhalation, often resulting in asthma which is characterized by short and shallow breathing.

Chronic coughing or bronchitis, both due to deficient Kidney energy, is often a precursor of emphysema in later life.

Hair

Hair is nourished by blood, but its growth and colouring are a result of Kidney energy. Good growth and richness of colour are indications of strong Kidney energy but, as Kidney energy weakens, the hair becomes thinner or falls out.

Ears, anus and urethra

Certain aspects of the ears (for example, their shape, condition and auditory strength) reflect the condition of Kidney energy. It is not surprising, therefore, that needle therapy for the ear (which comprises diagnosis and treatment of the whole body) is essentially treatment for balancing Kidney energy. Some ear disorders, such as tinnitus aurium and deafness, are often signs of Kidney energy deficiency.

The anus and urethra, elimination channels of the Lower Heater, also reflect the condition of Kidney energy. As problem areas, their symptoms include dysuria, retention or incontinence of urine, chronic diarrhoea and impotence.

Emotion

Fear is one of the symptoms of deficient Kidney energy. Its opposite, courage, comes from Liver blood (warmed by Kidney Yang when Kidney energy is abundant) and strong Gall Bladder energy.

True strength lies in an harmonious life, not an emotional one. Emotional problems disturb the mind and the physical body, resulting in great energy loss from which illness springs. We become slaves of our emotions when we burden ourselves with feelings such as aggression, apprehension, lack of confidence, fear, panic, self doubt and anxiety. These inner emotional conflicts drain Kidney energy and unbalance the whole body, in particular the Kidney, Heart and Liver. Waiting for inner peace to come is futile; it can only be created within oneself.

Other important symptoms of deficient Kidney energy are an increased or decreased sexual drive and decreased or absent sexual satisfaction. Since the reproductive system is one of the Kidney's functions, an emotion such as fear only makes the situation worse. Any imbalance of Kidney energy, either deficiency or excess, creates (mental) fear which disrupts Kidney function.

Bladder

The Bladder is Fu, a Yang organ, one of the six bowels and belongs to the Water element. Its Main Meridian is the Bladder Meridian of Foot *Tai* (Greater)-Yang and its Zang partner is the Kidney.

The function of the Bladder is relatively simple: by storage and excretion of waste body fluids, it assists Kidney energy in regulating water metabolism. Common disorders include dysuria, oliguria, anuria and haematuria.

However, the Bladder Meridian, by far the longest Meridian in the body, is more complex. It originates at the inner canthus (Bl 1), travels over the skull and down the neck, completes two laps of the back, descends over the buttocks to the back of the legs and terminates at the small toe (Bl 67). Along the Meridian are sixty-seven acupuncture points, a high percentage of which are useful for treatment.

With its protective Yang characteristics, the Meridian as a whole is able to safeguard its Yin counterpart, the Kidneys. In return, Kidney energy nourishes the Bladder Meridian which then distributes Kidney energy throughout its domain. This flow of energy penetrates many vital areas of the body, including the Brain, eyes, many muscular structures and the Back-*Shu* Points.

Similarly aligned to the sympathetic and parasympathetic nerves, the Back-*Shu* Points are a series of acupuncture points unique to the Bladder Meridian. They have a direct connection to the energy of the Zang and Fu as well as to other organs and strongly influence the condition of the internal body. (The Back-*Shu* Points are also useful in diagnosis.)

Feng-Men, Bl 12 ('Wind Gate') of the Bladder Meridian, *Feng-Chi*, GB 20 ('Wind Pool') of the Gall Bladder Meridian and *Feng-Fu*, GV 16 ('Wind House') of the Governor Vessel Meridian, are points particularly vulnerable to wind and cold. If weakened, Bl 12 gives wind and cold access to the internal body, causing chills, the common cold and kindred disorders. In Chinese medical diagnosis, they are known as '*Tai*-Yang disorders' (from the name of the Bladder Meridian).

Exercise strengthens the Bladder Meridian and

ZANG AND FU

Wei-Qi, and helps prevent attacks to and penetration of the body by external factors through the *Tai*-Yang Meridian. Moxibustion is often used to heat acupuncture point Bl 12 (see Chapter 4).

Common disorders of the Kidneys and Bladder

The Kidney is one of the most important organs in the body, housing Kidney *Ching*, the basic essence for growth, development and reproduction. Healthy Kidney energy produces strength and activity in the body whereas disorders in the Kidney cause problems throughout. ('It is vital to conserve Kidney energy and improve Kidney energy flow to prevent both disease attack and senility'.)

As the Kidneys support all body needs and activities, disturbances in any other organs drain Kidney energy and weaken their function. Thus, Kidney disorders are usually caused by deficient Kidney energy (including Kidney Yin and Yang) but, in some instances, may originate in the Kidney itself.

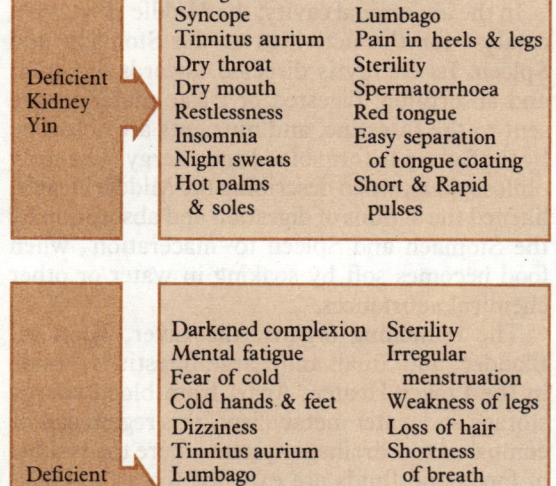

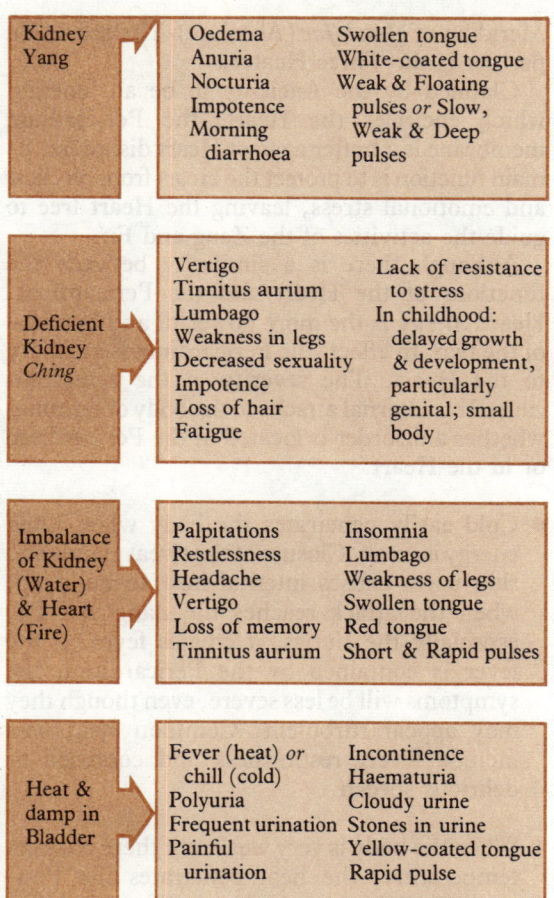

6. PERICARDIUM AND THREE HEATER

Pericardium

Although the Pericardium and Three Heater are not organs in the conventional sense, they are included in the Zang and Fu category because of their special qualities.

The Pericardium is Zang (not of the five viscera), Yin in character and belongs to the Fire element. Its Main Meridian is the Pericardium

ZANG AND FU

Meridian of Hand *Jue* (Absolute)-Yin and its Fu partner is the Three Heater.

Claimed by the Ancients to be an 'energy' which encircles the Heart, the Pericardium membrane is a buffer against Heart disorders. Its main function is to protect the Heart from physical and emotional stress, leaving the Heart free to guide the activities of the Zang and Fu.

Although there is a similarity between the functions of the Heart and the Pericardium, Heart energy is the more powerful and essential of the two. In effect, the Pericardium is auxiliary to the Heart. The severity of the symptoms caused by external attacks to the body determines whether a disorder is located in the Pericardium or in the Heart:

- Cold easily penetrates the body when Lung energy is weak. Closure of the sweat glands and skin pores causes internal heat to build up; when the attack reaches the Zang and Fu, especially the Lungs, it creates fever. If the fever is contained by the Pericardium, the symptoms will be less severe, even though they may appear turbulent. Common symptoms include fever, restlessness and confused or delirious speech.

- When the body is very weak or if there is a high temperature, the heat penetrates the Pericardium and enters the Heart. The symptoms are then severe and include high fever, coma or shock.

Three Heater

The Three Heater is Fu, one of the six bowels, Yang in character and belongs to the Fire Element. Its Main Meridian is the Three Heater Meridian of Hand *Shao* (Lesser)-Yang and its Zang partner is the Pericardium.

The exact function of the Three Heater was an enigma to the ancient Chinese; it is considerably more perplexing to contemporary researchers because it has no physical existence. While today's researchers consider it to have some bearing on the biochemical metabolism of the body, the ancient Chinese left as their legacy a number of often conflicting theories for appraisal.

The Three Heater may be described as ranging through three anatomical regions, the thoracic and abdominopelvic cavities, and as a synthesis of all the activities of the Zang and Fu. It is the impetus for the transportation of blood, energy and body fluids, and facilitates the elimination of waste materials.

In the thoracic cavity, the Heart, Lungs, Pericardium and activities of the Head represent the Upper Heater. It is here that the invisible energies of Mind, air and *Wei-Qi* are concentrated to assist the Lungs and Heart in distributing their fluids. Once blood, energy and fluids have accumulated in the Lungs and Heart, they are transformed through a biochemical reaction and then distributed by Lung energy to the rest of the body. It was this function of the Upper Heater which the ancient philosophers described as resembling 'mist'.

In the abdominal cavity, the Middle Heater is a catalyst for the activities of the Stomach and Spleen. Its energy is directed towards digestion and absorption: digested or waste materials are sent to the Intestine, and nutrients are absorbed by the Spleen to form blood and energy. The early philosophers, when describing the Middle Heater, likened the actions of digestion and absorption by the Stomach and Spleen to 'maceration', when food becomes soft by soaking in water or other chemical substances.

The remaining organs, the Liver, Kidneys, Bladder, and Small and Large Intestines, reside in the Lower Heater. Apart from blood/energy storage and water metabolism, this region can be compared to a drainage system where the residue of foods and fluids are expelled from the body.

ZANG AND FU

Indeed, the Ancients referred to the Lower Heater as a 'drain'.

The concept of the Three Heater is applicable in discussing attacks by external disease factors, the resultant symptoms and the progression of the disorder. For example, a deficiency of Lung energy reduces the protective function of the body (*Wei-Qi*), thus allowing external disease factors to easily penetrate the skin and gain direct access to the Lungs. In Chinese diagnosis this condition is known as a 'warm-hot disorder of the Upper Heater' and it is apparent almost at the outset when the body is being overwhelmed by the external disease factors. If the Upper Heater is overpowered, the disorder progresses to the Middle Heater and creates disturbances in the Spleen and Stomach energies.

When the activities of the Lower Heater are affected, the disturbance is severe and often dangerous. The Kidney Yin is exhausted, Liver blood becomes deficient or is lost, the Liver Yin is then incapable of balancing Liver Yang, and Liver 'Wind' is activated.

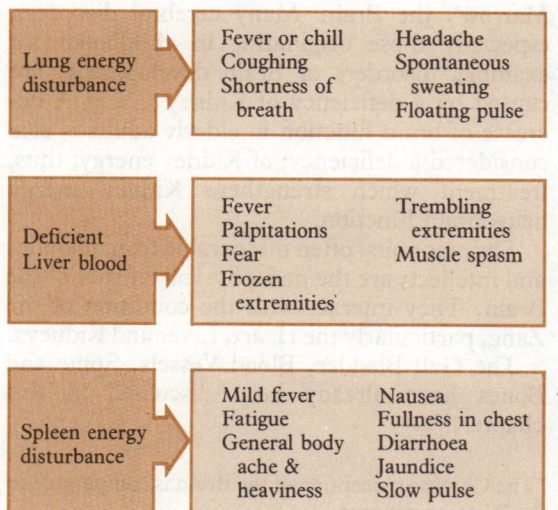

Inflamed Pericardium	Delirious speech / Stiffness of tongue	Red tongue / Frozen extremities
Stomach energy disturbance	Fever / Sweating / Thirst / Constipation	Oliguria / Yellow-coated tongue / Firm pulse
Deficient Kidney Yin	Fever / Red complexion / Restlessness	Insomnia / Dry lips & mouth / Hot palms & soles

7. THE EXTRA FU

'Form determines function' is a concept acknowledged by most branches of medicine; the ancient philosophers also expressed this but in their own terms. They conceived that organs could be categorized into two types: solid and hollow. The solid organs (Zang) conserve energy and the hollow organs (Fu) motivate energies.

All rules seem to have an exception, however; in this case, it is the Extra Fu, the collective name for a group of organs (Uterus, Brain, Gall Bladder, Blood Vessels, Spine and Bones) which have mixed Zang and Fu characteristics. As they tend to conserve energy, they resemble the Zang but, in shape, they are hollow, a Fu characteristic.

Each of the Extra Fu is dependent on Kidney *Ching* as is the rest of the body. However, the Uterus, Brain, Spine and Bones take energy directly from the Kidneys to support their own particular activities while the Gall Bladder and Blood Vessels take their energy from the Kidneys indirectly.

Uterus

Several energies contribute to the activities of the Uterus, but Kidney energy is its main source of nourishment, especially Kidney *Ching*. The *Chong* and Conception Vessel Meridians both support menstruation while energies of the Heart, Liver and Spleen provide the blood supply. As a whole, the nourishment and development of the Uterus is attributable to Kidney Yin while regular menstruation and the ability to conceive are indications of strong *Chong* and Conception Vessel Meridian energies. Menstruation relies on the quality of blood, and conception depends upon a healthy blood supply to the Uterus. The Heart, Spleen and Liver energies all control blood, their combined attributes determining the quality and quantity of blood, and regulating its transport throughout the body.

- A disturbance of Liver or Spleen energies, which regulate the blood circulation in the Uterus, leads to excessive menstrual flow, prolonged menstruation and greater frequency of periods;

- An emotional problem, such as depression, disturbs Liver function, and inhibition of Liver energy causes irregular and painful menstruation;

- An insufficiency of Heart and Spleen energies, caused by deficient blood supply to the Uterus, leads to a reduced menstrual flow and delayed or suppressed menstruation.

With their origins in the Uterus, the *Chong* and Conception Vessel Meridians ('Extra Meridians') influence menstruation. After leaving the Uterus, the Conception Vessel Meridian merges with the three lower Yin Meridians at CV 4. This meeting point balances the energies of the Liver, Spleen, Kidney and Conception Vessel and is called the 'Centre of Yin'.

The *Chong* Meridian emerges from the Uterus at the perineum with one branch joining the Kidney Meridian and another connecting to the Spine. In health, Kidney blood and energy are abundant and spill over into the *Chong* Meridian to enter the Uterus.

The *Chong* and Conception Vessel Meridians and Kidney *Ching* are the basic energies for Uterus development and regular menstruation. When these energies are not yet in abundance, as in a female under fourteen years of age, there is no menstruation; in women over fifty these energies are reduced and the menses cease. Any imbalance of these energies creates menstrual irregularities.

Brain*

Although some Chinese philosophers saw the Brain as an organ in its own right, the majority of the early medical practitioners (as well as the respected *NEI-JING*) considered the Brain to be an extension of Kidney *Ching*, by which it was physically nourished (just as the Heart ruled over the Spirit and emotions, and the Liver extended and explored the emotions).

The solid (physical) substance of the Brain is considered part of the skeleton. By nurturing Marrow, Kidney *Ching* is able to pass through the bones and Spine to replenish the 'Sea of Marrow', the Brain. Many cerebral disorders, especially those originating in childhood (for example, disorders of Brain development) are caused by a deficiency of Kidney *Ching*. A decrease of brain function in elderly adults is also considered a deficiency; of Kidney energy; thus, treatment which strengthens Kidney energy helps brain function.

The emotions, often inseparable from memory and intellect, are the non-physical entities of the Brain. They interact with the condition of the Zang, particularly the Heart, Liver and Kidneys.

The Gall Bladder, Blood Vessels, Spine and Bones have already been discussed in this chapter.

*The Chinese perception of the Brain is comparable to the Western concept.

3 PULSE DIAGNOSIS

GENERAL KNOWLEDGE

Pulse examination is an important aspect of Chinese medical diagnosis and is, in fact, the main method of diagnosis described in the *NEI-JING*. Modern scientific methods can detect, with remarkable precision, pathological changes in the internal organs as well as physical, mental and physiological changes; but these methods do not easily discern the mutations which have brought about these changes.

The Chinese, however, have tried and tested, over thousands of years, a system of diagnosis, the art of pulse reading, which clearly reveals these mutations. The method is effective because it is sensitive to the body which has formed the mutations. Pulse readings are perhaps the most valuable asset in the area of preventive medicine as, at their finest, they will detect the seeds of disorder often decades before manifestation of the disease.

In addition to a thorough knowledge of medicine, the practitioner must have a sympathetic understanding of human nature. He must fully comprehend all systems of diagnosis and, more importantly, follow them. Eastern and Western diagnostic systems, if used intelligently, will complement each other. Although their methods are fundamentally different, each is valid when followed systematically and independently of the other. Only the final results should be compared when selecting treatment. Although the names of organs and some functions may be identical in both systems, it must always be remembered that the scope or limitations of their activities are viewed from entirely different perspectives.

In simplified terms, a pulse is a point on a channel along which the basic 'matter' of the body (blood and energy) travels unimpeded. By examining this channel at various strategic points, the practitioner can assess the quality of blood and energy and thus quickly determine the condition, state of disease and recuperative powers of the body.

Pulses can be felt wherever an artery lies close to the body surface, whether over bone or soft tissue. The commonly probed areas are:

- radial artery at the wrist;

- common carotid artery along the anterior edge of sternocleidomastoid muscle at the level of the lower margin of the thyroid cartilage;

- facial artery at the lower margin of the mandible in line with the corners of the mouth (Point St 6);

- temporal artery lateral to the outer canthus or ear (Point *Tai*-Yang);

- superior mesenteric artery at the abdomen (near Points CV 12 and St 25 on the left side);

- femoral artery at the middle of the groin (Point Sp 12);

- dorsal artery of foot on the dorsum of the foot (Point St 41).

Each of these zones indicates the condition of the surrounding organs and tissue and of specific parts of the body. The pulse at *Tai*-Yang, for example, will reveal the quality of blood and energy in the Gall Bladder Meridian as it passes over the head. Usually, if a patient complains of migraine, this pulse will feel disturbed.

PULSE DIAGNOSIS

Pulse reading of radial arteries

Of all the above-mentioned arteries, the radial arteries at the wrists are the most frequently used for pulse reading. Being easily accessible, these arteries have become the basis of a self-contained system of diagnosis which is still the most popular method in use today.

The technique for reading the pulses of the radial arteries correctly is:

- The artery must always be approached from the lateral side of each wrist;

- The middle finger should first locate the styloid process, then slide over to the radial artery at the same level to locate the *Guan* pulse;

- Leaving the middle finger in the same position, the index and ring fingers should rest naturally on the artery, thus determining the *Cun* and *Chi* pulses respectively.

- The spacing of the three fingers will vary slightly according to the size of the patient's wrist; for children it may only be possible to apply the thumb for all three pulses.

These three radial pulses are divided into three levels: superficial, intermediate and deep. The first level is located by resting the three fingers superficially on the skin; pressure should then be increased almost to the bone to find the deeper pulse level, and in between these two is the intermediate level. The fingers must rest on the skin simultaneously, always at the same level and at the same pressure. (After these initial readings have been completed, the fingers may be applied separately to further compare each pulse). If the readings are to be professionally acceptable, this routine must be followed.

Collectively, the radial pulses depict the qualities of *Shen*, Stomach *Qi* and Root energies.

The superficial level reflects the strength of *Shen* (Spirit energy); ideally the pulse beats are regular, soft and clear but still with ample force. When Stomach *Qi* (energy) is healthy, the pulses at the intermediate level are regular, strong and forceful. With Root energy, revealed only at the deep level, the fundamental energy (Kidney energy) should be powerful.

In general, a healthy person has strong and regular pulse beats which do not 'float' on the surface but hold a distinct quality at each of the three levels. In addition, each of the *Cun*, *Guan* and *Chi* pulses displays individual characteristics which reflect the qualities of its parent organ. In this regard there are two widely held views, each of which is valid if followed systematically.

I. Dr. Pin Hoo Lee's pulse reading method

Pulse	Left Wrist	Right Wrist
Cun	Heart	Lung
Guan	Liver	Spleen
Chi	Kidney (Yin)	Kidney (Yang); *Ming Men Huo*

II. Twelve Main Meridian pulse reading method

Pulse	Left Wrist		Right Wrist	
	Superficial	Deep	Superficial	Deep
Cun	Small Intestine	Heart	Large Intestine	Lung
Guan	Gall Bladder	Liver	Stomach	Spleen
Chi	Bladder	Kidney	Three Heater	Pericardium

Dr. Lee's pulse reading method is used for diagnosing the energy flow of the internal organs while the Twelve Main Meridian method is diagnostic of the energy flow of those Meridians.

The philosophical basis of Dr. Lee's pulse reading method includes:

PULSE DIAGNOSIS

- The pulse of the Heart as the 'Centre of Blood' should be big, floating and scattered;

- The pulse of the Lungs, the 'Centre of Energy', should be floating but short (and definitely not smooth);

- The energy of the Stomach and Spleen which, in general, is reflected in all the pulses at the intermediate level, can be diagnosed in detail through the pulse at the right wrist (at *Guan*). This pulse should be full of power, revealing abundant energy;

- As the Kidneys store intrinsic energy, its pulse should be deep and full;

- The Liver pulse, revealing the quality and quantity of blood in this organ, should be deep and long with a slight 'bowstring' characteristic.

By looking at the relationship between the pulses of the Zang and Fu, and by contrasting them with the superficial, intermediate and deep levels, we find six distinct pulse characteristics:

1. On the left wrist the pulse that travels from *Chi* to *Cun* is basically Yang in nature and has been created by Yin. The Kidney pulse is located at *Chi*, the Liver pulse at *Guan* and the Heart pulse at *Cun*. According to the philosophy of the Five Elements, Water fosters Wood and Wood fosters Fire (Yin creates Yang).

2. On the right wrist the pulse that travels from *Chi* to *Cun* is basically Yin in nature and has been created by Yang. The pulse of *Ming Men Huo* is located at *Chi*, the Spleen/Stomach pulse at *Guan* and the Lung pulse at *Cun*. Again the philosophy of the Five Elements holds that Fire fosters Earth and Earth fosters Metal (Yang creates Yin).

3. As the pulse rises from the muscle and bone to the skin surface, it reflects distinct Yang characteristics and (if strong) abundant Yang energy.

4. After the pulse reaches its peak, it returns to the muscle and bone and in so doing reflects the quality of Yin energy.

5. The pulse is normal if it seems regular to the touch and corresponds with the patient's breathing.

6. The nature of a spasmodic pulse can be partly determined by the interval between the beats. When the pulse stops the condition is Yin, and when it re-emerges it becomes Yang. Into this category fall the Intermittent, Knotted and Rapid pulses, and the possibilities for diagnosis are manifold.

There are many vital factors (seasonal, environmental, emotional and occupational) which influence the pulses naturally and spontaneously. Some are discussed in detail later in this chapter; many others are encountered continually in clinical practice. It is particularly important to recognize these influences and to be aware of what constitutes the normal pulse; otherwise, any premature attempt at diagnosis could result in confusion.

- Heat weakens the pulses, but a cold environment fosters full and strong pulse beats.

- Long journeys, walking and alcohol each quicken the pulses to varying degrees.

- While fasting, the pulse rhythm appears weak and empty, but after food it should be strong and smooth.

37

PULSE DIAGNOSIS

- Obesity promotes slow and floating pulses whereas a slim or wiry build produces strong and deep pulse movements.

- A quiet temperament produces a Yin pulse with slow and small movements; three or four beats to the respiration (one act of inhaling and exhaling) is considered normal. Quickness and agility (in thought and movement) is associated with a Yang pulse, with five beats to the respiration considered normal.

PULSE DIAGNOSIS PROCEDURES

After entering the clinic, the patient should be allowed to relax before commencing diagnosis and treatment, as even the stress of rushing for an appointment can temporarily influence the tide of the pulses.

To prepare for pulse diagnosis, the patient may be either sitting up or lying down, but it is imperative that the position places blood and energy in equilibrium. This is easily achieved by following certain guidelines:

- The patient's arms must be outstretched and level with the heart;

- The wrists must be in line with the direction of the arms (often supported by a small cushion);

- The palms should face upwards.

Ideally the pulses should be read in the morning when Yin/Yang energies are near equilibrium, and social and environmental stresses are at their lowest. Certainly the time of day must be considered in the diagnosis.

1. Pulse rhythms

Before attempting to discern the idiosyncracies of a pulse, its overall rhythm must first be ascertained. A norman pulse has a regular beat with four or five movements to the respiration. A slow pulse, with less than four beats per respiration, shows Yin characteristics, indicating the possibility of a 'cold' syndrome. A pulse of only one or two beats per respiration indicates a severe disease characterized by an imbalance of Yin and Yang, for example, excess Yin energy and deficient Yang energy. Pulses with a fast rhythm, in excess of five beats per respiration, are Yang and denote excessive 'heat' in the body. A pulse with up to nine beats per respiration reveals excessive Yang energy at the expense of Yin; when the pulse goes beyond nine beats per respiration, the condition is recycling, signifying that Yang energy is nearly exhausted. Thus, from the rhythm of the pulse a disorder can be designated as 'hot' or 'cold', thereby determining the method of treatment: needle or moxa.

When reading the pulse, its rhythm should be carefully monitored by feeling the pulse beat fifty times or more. A regular fifty-beat pulse is an indication that the energy flows of the internal organs are in proper cycle. One beat missing in forty is a sign that the Kidney energy flow is not in equilibrium. As well as revealing specific ailments, an irregular pulse rhythm is an indication of a deteriorating condition.

2. Comparison of pulse levels

Disorder at the superficial pulse level is often expressed by a 'floating' quality and is indicative of an external ailment, a Yang condition. It may also indicate excessive Yang energy or an acute emotional disorder.

The intermediate pulse level reflects the source of pulse energy (Stomach *Qi*) and should always be full and strong. Any change within this level quickly manifests itself at every pulse level. Energy deficiency at the intermediate level always indicates severe disease.

Disturbance at the deeper pulse level suggests disorder of an internal organ, a Yin condition.

PULSE DIAGNOSIS

Tension at this level can mean severe pain in the internal organ.

Determining whether a condition is internal or external enables the choice of treatment and assessment of the rate of recovery to be made. Internal problems should be treated moderately to provide the time necessary to build up and balance the energy of the organs.

The depth of the disorder should suggest the needle technique. A superficial ailment requires only shallow needle insertion, otherwise a minor disorder may be given entry through the skin, muscle and Main Meridians into the internal organs. A chronic disorder requires very accurate needle treatment with the application of specific 'reinforcement' and 'reduction' techniques (see Chapter 5).

3. Three Heater pulses

Comparison of the three levels of pulses is followed by comparison of the *Cun*, *Guan* and *Chi* pulses. These three regions reveal the quality of energy in the Three Heater:

- The Lungs, Heart, Pericardium, upper extremities and head (all above the diaphragm) constitute the Upper Heater, whose energy is reflected by the pulses at *Cun*.

- The Middle Heater, whose energy is mirrored by the *Guan* pulse, constitutes the abdominal region, particularly the Stomach and Spleen, although the Large and Small Intestines are also influenced in this region. Heat and cold are the two common factors which affect the Middle Heater: adults accumulate heat within the Stomach and Intestines, but children tend to absorb the cold.

- The energy of the Lower Heater, reflected in the *Chi* pulse, is directed mostly through the Kidneys and Bladder to the other organs of the area, namely, the Liver, Gall Bladder, Small and Large Intestines, reproductive system and lower extremities. A disturbance in this pulse implies a chronic problem: a Yin disorder within the viscera.

It is imperative to compare the pulses at *Chi* and *Cun* as they tend to absorb any difficulties at *Guan*.

The pulses of the left and right wrists should always be compared. Variation in the overall level of energy between the pulses of both wrists implies an imbalance between the energies of each side of the body. Overactivity of energy at only one wrist refers to an external problem, possibly pain or obstruction of the Meridian energy flow. Underactivity of energy at only one wrist suggests a weakness of one side of an organ or may mirror the effects on the body (internally and externally) of an attack by cold. These evaluations determine whether the 'reduction' or the 'reinforcement' needle technique is used.

4. Floating and Sunken pulses

The Floating pulse is a Yang pulse whose excess energy is caught at the surface of the body. It is indicative (mostly) of an external problem caused by environmental influences such as wind and cold having attacked the body, or an excess of cold liquids or hot foods having inflamed the Stomach and Large Intestine, causing an obstruction of the Lung energy flow. An excess of sputum in the Lungs or an excess of Heart Fire will also create a Floating Pulse. It is clearly felt on a superficial reading but rapidly loses strength as finger pressure increases; it was described by the ancient philosophers as appearing to 'skim the surface of the skin as wood floats on water'.

To help ascertain the basic cause of the problem, the Floating pulse can be aligned with the theories of the Three Heater, the Zang and Fu, and the Eight Extra Meridians by reading *Cun*,

PULSE DIAGNOSIS

Guan and *Chi* pulses. Only by such thorough diagnosis can a complete picture of the disorder be established.

In clinical practice, the Floating pulse is always found with other pulse characteristics as it does not appear alone. In combination with the Rapid pulse, the Floating pulse conveys that wind and heat have attacked the body, and symptoms will include fever, a red complexion, moderate fear of wind, heat and cold, a dry cough and sore throat. A Floating right *Cun* pulse combined with a Firm and Tight pulse (extending to *Guan*) indicates the stress placed on the *Wei-Qi* by external attack by wind and cold. Accompanying symptoms then include fear of cold and heat, headache, runny nose, cough, a pale complexion, heaviness of the whole body, cold extremities, white-coated tongue and clear urine.

The Sunken pulse is a Yin pulse which relates to the internal organs deep within the body. Excess energy at this pulse coincides with pain in the internal organs, obstruction of energy or accumulation of cold within the muscles, bones and organs. It is found through deep pressure almost to the tendon and bone, and has soft, firm and regular beats. The ancient philosophers said it was 'like a stone thrown into water and one must go beneath the water to find it'.

The Sunken pulse indicates a 'heat' syndrome incubating within the internal organs when combined with the Rapid pulse; symptoms such as restlessness, abdominal and lower back pain, constipation and yellowish urine are apparent. A Sunken and Slow pulse combination reveals that the Yang energy is exhausted, disease has entered the viscera, and wind and cold are sealed within the body. A Sunken and Small pulse is a symptom of arthritis. Other common combinations include the Sunken and Full, Sunken and Weak, Sunken and Tight, and Sunken and Bowstring pulses.

5. Death pulses

As outlined by the ancient Chinese acupuncturists, there are some pulses which signify a great loss of *Yuan* energy within the organs. Their ominous nature has often led to their being referred to as the 'pulses of death'. They are:

- when the pulse of the Liver feels like the blade of a knife with short and bowstring pulse characteristics;

- when the pulse of the Heart feels to the touch like a knot moving in the artery and its beats are short, hard and hurried;

- when the pulse of the Spleen is extremely small and weak with beats that are irregular and fitful – suddenly fast, then slow;

- when the pulse of the Lung is big, soft and empty, feeling rather like wool;

- when the Kidney pulse is irregular: as it reaches its peak the beats are strong and hard but, after the peak, it is empty and blurred.

PULSES OF THE BODY

Although it is the pulses at the radial arteries that have been most clearly and effectively defined for day-to-day clinical use, it is also important to grasp the meaning of other body pulses, as they are very useful particularly in defining details in diagnosis. Often they are explained through the philosophy of 'Heaven, Man and Earth' but, in the following, their description is with reference to Meridian flow and body structure.

1. Pulses in the head

The head is the most active region of the body. It is fundamentally Yang in nature and its pulses express the quality of Yang energy. The Yang Meridians which pass through the head are numerous. They unite and balance their energies before circulating throughout the rest of the body. The most common symptom arising from a disturbance of Yang energies is headache.

The vitality of the Hand and Foot Yang-*Ming* Meridians (which are equal in high energy and high blood flows) is expressed by the pulses at Stomach (St) 6 and 3, which should be full and overflowing. However, any disturbance within these two Meridians can cause an overflowing of blood and energy, creating symptoms such as headache, red eyes, a red complexion, bleeding gums, epistaxis, sore throat, dry cough, toothache and constipation.

The Hand and Foot *Shao*-Yang Meridians (characterized by high energy and low blood flows) have one pulse at *Tai*-Yang and another at Gall Bladder (GB) 2. The paths of these two Meridians travel past the ears and eyes and over the head bilaterally, and their excess energies, plus that of the Liver, drive blood and energy through those areas, causing migraine, headache, ocular pain, red eyes, tinnitus aurium, and Full and Overflowing pulses at *Tai*-Yang and GB 2.

2. Pulses in the neck

The common carotid arteries are located in the neck bilaterally. Because it carries high blood and high energy flows, this region is basically Yang in nature.

The pulse located at St 9 is used mainly to determine the quality of energy within the three Yang Meridians, but it is also directly connected to the Heart and Lungs. The vitality of the Heart ('Centre of Blood') registers on the pulse of the left common carotid artery whereas the function of the Lungs ('Centre of Energy') is expressed through the same pulse on the right side. If these pulses are deficient or irregular, the disorder is severe.

The *NEI-JING* states that the pulses of the common carotid arteries should always be compared with the pulses of the radial arteries; the former pulses are Yang in nature and the latter are Yin. In Spring and Summer, the pulses of the common carotid arteries respond to the environment with full and strong pulse beats; but in Autumn and Winter the radial pulses seem stronger since, basically, they reflect the energy of the three Yin Meridians.

3. Pulses of the abdominal region

Most of the pulses in this region arise from the abdominal aorta and are found at the points of Conception Vessel (CV) 12, 9 and 6 and St 25. The Stomach is a source of postnatal energy, the root of all pulses and provides nourishment for the Lungs and rest of the body; it registers forcefully at its own pulse at CV 12, the *Mu* Point of the Stomach and its centre of energy. After meals, this pulse is particularly strong and forceful.

The energy of the Large Intestine is concentrated at its *Mu* Point, St 25. Excess energy of the Stomach and Large Intestine registers at CV 12 and St 25 respectively with full and powerful pulse beats. Such pulses are accompanied by symptoms of gastric pain, a red complexion, constipation, swollen gums, epistaxis, sore throat, dry cough, yellow urine, yellow-coated tongue and a Full pulse in the right-hand *Guan*.

Pulses at the points of CV 6 and 9 are located by deep pressure. More active in women, these pulses basically react to the quality of health in the urogenital area. When healthy, the pulse is soft and long. A Tight pulse at these two points, often accompanied by premenstrual tension, is caused by an imbalance of blood and energy flows within the uterus. The pulses at *Chi* will also feel Tight.

Since CV 6 is a centre of energy, care must be taken during *Tai Chi Chuan* (Chinese Energy Exercise) to conserve the energy flow at this important point.

PULSE DIAGNOSIS

4. Pulses at the Foot

In health, the pulses at the points of St 40, Kidney (K) 3 and Liver (Liv) 3 are soft and long. St 40 mirrors Earth/Stomach energy; K 3 reveals the *Yuan* energy of the Kidneys; and Liv 3 reflects that organ's capacity to store blood. When these three pulses are weak or absent, prenatal and postnatal energies are lost and Liver blood is deficient; death is imminent.

PULSE DIAGNOSIS OF CHILDREN

In children under three years of age, it is possible to assess the pulse rate (five to six beats per respiration) and to gauge the general health through the pulse characteristics; but assessment of the condition of the internal body in detail requires examination of the blood vessels on the ventral surface of the child's index finger.

The index finger is selected for diagnosis because its tissue is relatively thin, making the condition of the blood and energy readily apparent. Diagnosis is by inspection and touch. Traditionally the left index finger of boys is viewed and the right index finger of girls but, generally, readings are taken from both fingers and the results compared.

To simplify the process of diagnosis, the finger is considered in three parts:

The proximal phalanx or 'Wind Gate';

The middle phalanx of 'Energy Gate';

The distal phalanx or 'Vital Gate'.

In order that blood and energy be visible for inspection, the tip of the child's index finger is held and gently pressed between the distal and proximal phalanges on the medial, ventral and lateral aspects of the skin surface. The colour, number and distribution of blood vessels then become apparent. The finger of a healthy child is almost transparent when held up to the light, and the tissue and blood vessels at 'Wind Gate' will display a fresh red colour with a touch of violet.

When a surfeit of vessels replete with blood appears at 'Wind Gate' floating near the skin surface, it is an indication that external causes of disease (for example, wind and cold) have attacked the body. Treatment should be simple.

When a vessel abundant in blood diffuses into several channels deep within the tissue of 'Wind Gate' and 'Energy Gate', disease has entered the internal organs and disrupted the energy flow. The prognosis is poor and considerable thought must be given to the treatment.

When the vessels reach 'Vital Gate', Kidney energy has been diminished; recuperative powers are weak and the condition is fatal.

The colours of the three 'Gates' are also influenced by the aetiology of the disease. A pale colour denotes loss of Lung energy, a cold disorder. Deep red and violet tones are symptomatic of excessive heat. A greenish colour is associated with internal pain, particularly abdominal and chest pains, caused by wind and/or cold. Dark tones indicate stasis of blood or obstruction of energy flow caused by excessive sputum in the chest. Obstruction of Lung energy disrupts the circulation of Heart blood, making the disease potentially dangerous. Dark tones also indicate insufficient kinetic force of Kidney Yang caused by exhaustion of Kidney energy. Treatment is very difficult.

FEMALE PULSES

In women the Zang and Fu are continually modifying blood and energy to meet the needs of the reproductive system. These and other differences in physiological activity, adaptation of physique and even social pressures all contribute to the formation of the female pulses.

The female has a faster pulse than the male;

PULSE DIAGNOSIS

her *Cun* pulse is weaker than his, but her *Chi* pulse is considerably stronger. The vitality of Yin energy and *Ying* blood are critical in women: conception is contingent upon these factors. The strength of the Kidney pulse (substantial Yin energy) and the Heart pulse (Centre of Blood) helps to determine the condition of the reproductive system. By damaging Kidney energy and exhausting the blood, a combination of excessive Yang energy and deficient Yin blood can inhibit conception and impede the menses.

During the first three months of pregnancy, the Heart pulse should be full and smooth. An abundance of Heart blood may prevent spontaneous abortion by nourishing Kidney energy and balancing Kidney water.

After the third month of pregnancy, the Kidney pulse at *Chi* should feel rapid and smooth to the touch but, on deeper pressure, should be soft and scattered as the fetus is still gaining strength. After five months the energy of the fetus is abundant and the Kidney pulse is rapid, smooth and strong.

Many Chinese philosophers were able to determine the sex of a child by the characteristics of the pulses. Most agreed that the sex is discernible after the fourth month of pregnancy by comparing the *Chi* pulses of both wrists. A rapid and smooth Kidney Yin (left wrist) pulse indicated the birth of a boy, and a fast and smooth pulse at *Ming Men Huo* (right wrist) meant a girl. Rapid and smooth pulses on both wrists usually indicated twins.

The traditional acupuncturists developed two systems for reading pulses, one for women and another for men. The system for male pulses does not require explanation as it is widely used today (for both sexes). The system for reading female pulses is very different:

The philosophers always read female pulses on the right/Yin wrist before comparison with the pulses on the other side.

Pulse	Left Wrist	
	Superficial	Deep
Cun	Three Heater	*Ming Men Huo*
Guan	Stomach	Spleen
Chi	Large Intestine	Lungs

Pulse	Right Wrist	
	Superficial	Deep
Cun	Bladder	Kidney
Guan	Gall Bladder	Liver
Chi	Small Intestine	Heart

PULSES AND ENVIRONMENT
Influence of the Seasons

As the body responds to the pull of the Seasons and to the forces of night and day, blood and energy continually change their emphasis from organ to organ. These specific gradations of blood and energy were articulated by the philosophers in the form of a 'Chinese Clock'.

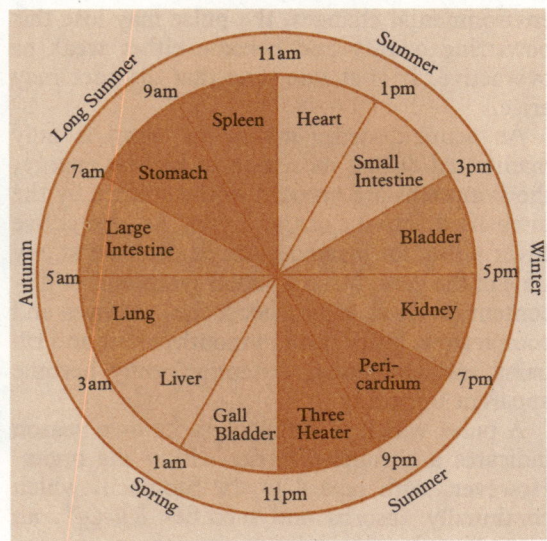

PULSE DIAGNOSIS

The Chinese Clock records the saturation point of blood and energy within each organ, thus illustrating the subtle changes in the pulses as they respond to the seasonal environment:

Season	Organ	Element	Pulse Characteristic
Spring	Liver	Wood	Bowstring
Summer	Heart	Fire	Strong & floating
Long Summer*	Spleen	Earth	Slow & full
Autumn	Lungs	Metal	Floats lightly on skin
Winter	Kidneys	Water	Deep & resolute like a stone

*end of Summer/beginning of Autumn

The Liver, for example, was equated by the Ancients with Springtime as both have energies which continually expand and reach outwards. In Spring a bowstring quality of the Liver pulse is considered normal but, if it cannot adjust to environmental changes, the pulse may lose this bowstring quality and become either weak or overactive. It is at this time that disorder may arise.

An acute disorder within an organ is only manifested during its season of highest energy; the symptoms are brought to the surface by the intensified activity of the organ. An overactive Liver pulse, for instance, can be detected at any time of the year, but the actual symptoms of discontent (such as anger, headache, red eyes and complexion, bitter taste in mouth, chest and rib pains and abdominal distention) only become apparent in Spring.

A pulse which is deficient in its own season indicates a chronic disorder within the organ. However, with regard to the Stomach, which continually absorbs and modifies *Ku-Qi**, an acute disorder may arise in any season.

During the diagnostic procedure, the seasonal pulse should be carefully monitored and, throughout every season, it is essential to contrast all pulses against the strength of the Stomach pulse. This pulse is the underlying strength of the blood and energy flows and has a direct and reciprocal communion with the Zang and Fu; hence, a substantial part of the energy which drives the pulses emanates from the Stomach. It is the pivot of the pulses, but not the instigator of all disorders.

In Spring, an overactive bowstring Liver pulse coupled with a weak Stomach pulse and a stomachache, is considered a Liver, rather than a Stomach, disorder. Liver symptoms, such as irritability, insomnia, headache, chest and rib pains, and a bitter taste in the mouth, are prominent. It is a case of the Wood (Liver) overwhelming the Earth (Stomach). Treatment should release Liver tension before balancing the Wood with the Earth.

Influence of the Climate

Climate also affects blood and energy flows in the body and is illustrated by the marked variances in pulses of populations living in different climates:

● Those living for a long period in hot regions where it is virtually always summer have soft pulses;

● Those living for a long period in places that are cold and windy the whole year have deep and strong pulses;

● Those who are mountain dwellers always have full and strong pulses as the conditions at higher altitudes are cold and dry;

*'*Ku*' means a grain of corn. *Ku-Qi* is the absorption of energy from the Stomach into the body, particularly to the Spleen and Lungs, which in turn produce other energies to combine with it.

PULSE DIAGNOSIS

- Those in regions where all the seasons are mild and spring-like have gentle and slow pulses.

However, there are instances where a person's character is not in accord with his climatic environment:

- A soft and slow pulse in spite of living in a cold region is a sign of a very gentle nature;

- A full and strong pulse in spite of living in a hot climate is a sign of a very strong and possibly aggressive personality.

PULSES AND EMOTION

Emotional disturbance is one of the most common causes of disease. Chinese medicine considers that all emotional expressions have an effect on the body and, more importantly, that a prolonged period of emotional disturbance eventually endangers organ function.

According to the *NEI-JING*, emotions are related to specific organs of the body (see page 6), a philosophy which acknowledges five spiritual resources as being controlled by the viscera:

- The Heart controls the Spirit;

- The Liver controls the Soul;

- The Spleen controls the Ideas;

- The Lungs control the Inferior or Animal Spirit;

- The Kidneys control the Will.

Normally the emotions have a natural response to daily and seasonal activities, but habitual emphasis on any one emotion interferes with the activities of its related Zang and, over a period of time, causes pathological disorder in that organ. (For example, habitual anger causes disorder in the Liver.) Conversely, a disease which disturbs the function of a Zang organ also interferes with its related emotional expression. (For example, a patient with asthma is very easily affected by gloom.)

Thus, on reading a patient's pulse, the possibility must be borne in mind that the disease of the organ is connected to the patient's emotions; then the original cause of the disorder must be established as being either the disease or the emotional disturbance.

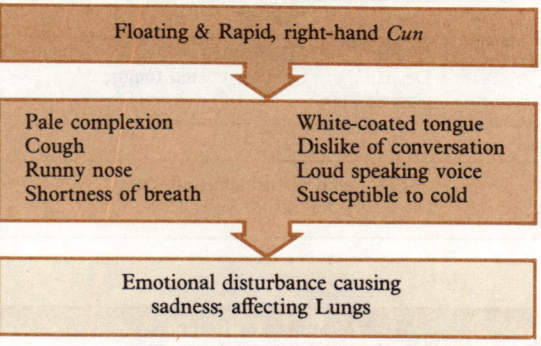

Floating & Rapid, right-hand *Cun*
↓
Pale complexion / White-coated tongue
Cough / Dislike of conversation
Runny nose / Loud speaking voice
Shortness of breath / Susceptible to cold
↓
Emotional disturbance causing sadness; affecting Lungs

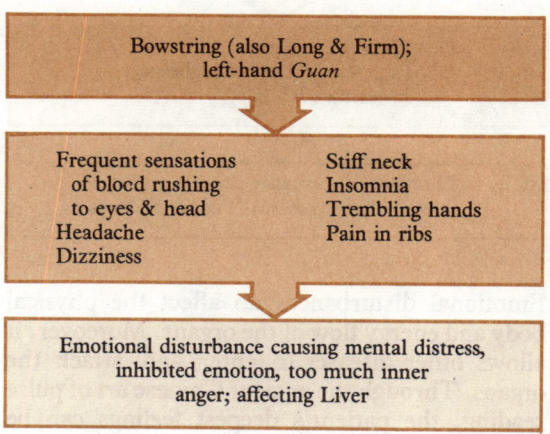

Bowstring (also Long & Firm); left-hand *Guan*
↓
Frequent sensations of blood rushing to eyes & head / Stiff neck
Headache / Insomnia
Dizziness / Trembling hands
/ Pain in ribs
↓
Emotional disturbance causing mental distress, inhibited emotion, too much inner anger; affecting Liver

PULSE DIAGNOSIS

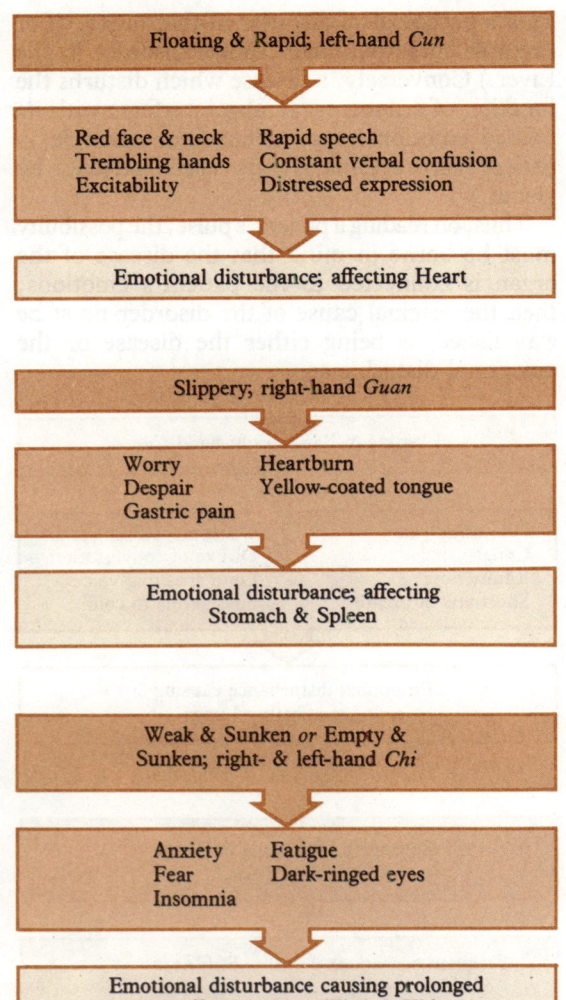

revealed. It is therefore important to establish the emotional state of the patient so that the mental stresses are treated before the organs are damaged.

INDIVIDUAL PULSES
1. Floating pulse

This pulse appears to 'skim the surface of the skin as wood floats on water'. It is felt clearly on a superficial reading but, as finger pressure increases, the pulse rapidly loses its strength. In general, a Floating pulse is a Yang pulse whose excess energy is caught at the surface of the body.

In Autumn a Floating pulse reveals that the body is healthy. In chronic disorders, such a pulse means that the disease is becoming worse (loss of Yang energy).

Clinically the Floating pulse most frequently indicates an external cause of disease in which environmental influences, such as wind and cold, have attacked the body, causing obstruction in Lung energy flow. Gloom and excessive Heart Fire also accompany this pulse.

Through the *Cun*, *Guan* and *Chi*, Floating pulses should be analyzed with the theories of the Zang and Fu, Three Heater and Eight Extra Meridians to help establish the basic cause or source of disorder. Only through such thorough diagnosis can there be a complete picture of the illness.

- A Floating *Cun* pulse coincides with the common cold (influenza);

- A Floating *Guan* pulse is associated with excessive Liver Fire or deficient Spleen energy;

- A Floating *Chi* pulse indicates wind and heat in the Lower Heater with accompanying symptoms, such as constipation and yellow urine.

Emotional disturbances do affect the physical body and energy flow of the organs. Moreover, it allows other diseases to enter and attack the organs. Through the ancient Chinese art of pulse reading, the patient's deepest feelings can be

This pulse in clinical practice is always found in combination with other pulse characteristics. For example, a Floating and Rapid pulse indicates that wind and heat have attacked the body. There are symptoms such as fever, a red complexion, a slight fear of wind, heat and cold, dry cough and sore throat.

A Floating right *Cun* pulse combined with a Firm and Tight pulse (extending to *Guan*) reveals the effects of an attack by external wind and cold on *Wei-Qi*. Symptoms include fear of cold and heat, headache, a runny nose, cough, pale complexion, heaviness of the body, cold extremities, white-coated tongue and clear urine.

2. Sunken or Deep pulse

According to the ancient philosophers, the Sunken or Deep pulse 'felt like a stone thrown into the water and one must go beneath the water to find it'. Through deep pressure almost to the tendon and bone, the Sunken pulse is found with its soft, firm and regular beats. This Yin pulse relates to the internal organs deep inside the body and, when found in the Winter of a cold region, it denotes a healthy condition.

Excess energy of this pulse is always accompanied by pain deep in the body (in the muscles, bones and internal organs).

- A Sunken *Cun* pulse is accompanied by shortness of breath and pain in the chest and ribs;

- A Sunken *Guan* pulse together with abdominal pain is symptomatic of an accumulation of cold within the Stomach and Spleen;

- A Sunken *Chi* pulse is found with back pain, lumbago and urogenital disorders.

A Sunken and Rapid pulse reveals heat within the internal organs associated with symptoms of restlessness, abdominal and lower back pain, constipation and yellow urine. A Sunken and Slow pulse indicates cold within the internal organs. Other combinations include the Sunken and Full, Sunken and Weak, and Sunken and Tight pulses.

3. Slow pulse

The pulse is said to be Slow when there are three pulse beats or less per respiration (inspiration and exhalation). This pulse indicates a Yin condition, a cold disorder in the viscera, the result of sluggish blood and energy flows initially due to a reduction of Yang energy.

A Slow pulse with only one beat per respiration signifies a complete loss of the Meridian blood and energy flows; one beat to two respirations indicates that the Kidney *Ching* is nearly lost; and one beat to three respirations, a 'pulse of death', is a sign that the blood and energy flows are coming to a halt.

Clinically a Slow pulse is evidenced by a loss of blood and energy flows, vulnerability to attack by external cold and, often, chronic disease.

- An habitually Slow *Cun* pulse reveals an imbalance in the Upper Heater. Generally there is cold in the chest and heart region characterized by cardiac pain;

- A Slow *Guan* pulse refers to cold in the Middle Heater, especially in the Spleen, which leads to fluid retention, excessive sputum in the Lungs and disturbances of water metabolism;

- A Slow *Chi* pulse signifies that the Lower Heater, particularly the Kidneys, is deficient in energy. Supporting indications are lower back pain, heaviness in the legs, and pain and disorder in the urogenital area.

A Slow and Weak *Chi* pulse found together with

PULSE DIAGNOSIS

chronic illness means the disorder is becoming worse. Other combinations include the Full and Slow, Empty and Slow, Floating and Slow, and Sunken and Slow pulses.

4. Rapid pulse

The Rapid pulse has six or more beats to a respiration, a pace due to blood and energy flows being driven by an excess of Yang energy (Heart or Kidney Fire [*Ming Men Huo*]) which, by consuming blood and other fluids, drains Yin energy and upsets the balance within the body. Symptoms such as restlessness, syncope and acute delirium are usual.

Whilst four (sometimes five) beats per respiration are considered normal, a Rapid pulse of three beats in excess indicates loss of restraint of the blood and energy flows within the Meridians. A pulse of four beats in excess (nine beats to one respiration) signifies loss of Kidney *Ching*, and five extra beats is a sign that the life force is fading.

In children, five or six beats per respiration are considered normal because they are still growing and developing and are full of Yang energy. These childhood pulses must not be misinterpreted as fever or heat in the body.

- A Rapid left *Cun* pulse reflects excessive Heart Fire, often with symptoms such as tongue and mouth ulcers and a sore throat. Such a pulse at the right *Cun* refers to heat in the Lungs with symptoms of coughing and blood in the sputum;

- A Rapid left *Guan* pulse accompanied by anger, irritation, migraine, headache, red eyes and a bitter taste in the mouth is symptomatic of excess Fire in the Liver and Gall Bladder. At the right *Guan* a Rapid pulse reveals surplus heat within the Stomach;

- A Rapid *Chi* pulse indicates a threat to the Kidneys by excessive heat in the Lower Heater.

Clinically the Rapid pulse is usually combined with other pulses:

- A Rapid and Floating pulse suggests a superficial disturbance (heat); the disorder has not yet attacked the internal organs;

- A Rapid and Sunken/Deep pulse reveals heat in the internal organs;

- A Rapid and Full pulse indicates a general excess of heat in the body;

- A Rapid and Weak pulse typifies loss of Yin and Yang energies, but still shows a heat symptom (often called 'heat beneath the deficiency of Yin energy') which always accompanies chronic disease or a disorder which is getting worse.

In a patient with chronic Lung weakness, the Rapid pulse (always the result of excessive Heart Fire and *Ming Men Huo* draining Yin fluids) is particularly ominous if found in Autumn. An important aspect of treatment is to increase or strengthen Lung energy and reduce the Heart and Kidney Fires. However, treatment is difficult and improvement in the patient is always very slow.

5. Slippery pulse

The Slippery pulse, which almost always coincides with an excess of Yang energy, is very forceful and moves smoothly and continuously 'as a pearl gliding through the artery and the water flowing further and further'. Replete with blood, it is found in athletes and is also a sign of a healthy pregnancy. In all other cases, however, this pulse indicates disorder: an overexpansion of blood flow. The most common causes are attacks by wind, cold and food or a lack of restraint in Kidney and Liver Fires (Fire heats the blood) arising from increased Yang energy. In a child a Slippery and Floating pulse indicates a chill (the common cold).

- A Slippery *Cun* pulse reveals congestion of sputum in the chest which affects Heart Yang and Lung energy flow. Symptoms include vomiting, 'heartburn', stiff tongue and coughing;

- A Slippery *Guan* pulse indicates heat within the Liver and Spleen caused by indigestion;

- A Slippery *Chi* pulse denotes disorder in the urogenital tract, Kidneys and Lower Heater, characterized by diarrhoea, diabetic urine and gonorrhoeal urethritis.

6. Choppy pulse

The Choppy pulse (Yin) is rough and uneven with small and short movements described by the ancient philosophers as 'raindrops plopping into sand'. This pulse arises from a deficiency of *Jing* blood or loss of Kidney *Ching*, and initial symptoms include profuse sweating, continual vomiting and other forms of severe fluid loss. Established symptoms may be menstrual distress, sterility, secondary amenorrhoea or retardation of the fetus due to insufficient blood.

- A Choppy *Cun* pulse with chest pain is symptomatic of insufficient Heart blood;

- A Choppy *Guan* pulse is evidence of weakness of the Stomach and Spleen energies; there may be a fullness in the chest and ribs;

- A Choppy *Chi* pulse suggests disorders of Kidney *Ching* and Liver blood, and symptoms of constipation, cystitis and intestinal haemorrhage are apparent.

PULSE DIAGNOSIS

7. Empty pulse

An Empty pulse appears big and slow superficially but lacks substance at the deeper levels. This Yin pulse was called '*Xu-Mai*' by the Chinese, the word '*Xu*' meaning 'deficiency' or 'weakness'; thus, '*Xu-Mai*' describes a pulse which is deficient in energy due to weakness in the physical body. However, in a different context it can be translated literally as 'empty pulse'.

This pulse, found only when the body is weak, is actually caused by a loss of *Yuan* energy. Associated symptoms include spontaneous perspiration, fear, timidity and palpitations.

- An Empty *Cun* pulse suggests a condition with insufficient blood to nourish the Heart;

- An Empty *Guan* pulse signifies deficient energy of the Stomach and Spleen and, particularly, a disturbance within the digestive and absorptive processes;

- An Empty *Chi* pulse indicates a loss of Kidney *Ching* and blood, exemplified in clinical practice by disorder in the bones and lower extremities.

Generally, *Xu-Mai* is found together with the other pulses of deficiency:

- Floating: blood deficient (*Shieh-Xu*)

- Deep: energy deficient (*Qi-Xu*)

- Rapid: Yang deficient (*Yang-Xu*)

- Slow: Yin deficient (*Yin-Xu*)

Clinically the *Xu-Mai* pulse always appears in a *Yuan* energy-deficient condition. Therefore, when blood is deficient, treatment should nourish *Jing*

PULSE DIAGNOSIS

blood; when energy is deficient, treatment should reinforce energy.

If the pulse is *Yin-Xu*, the patient has a heat disorder caused by insufficient Yin energy to balance Yang. In this case, treatment should reinforce Yin energy to relieve heat in the body.

8. Full pulse
The Full pulse is abundant, forceful and long; it is a Yang pulse. It registers more clearly at the superficial and deep levels and its qualities are most evident immediately before and after the pulse peak. This pulse suggests a state in which powerful external causes of disease (cold, wind, damp) have invaded the body and are being counterattacked by a strong and healthy body energy. It may also indicate a heat-dominated Three Heater.

- A Full *Cun* pulse, caused by excessive wind and heat in the Upper Heater, is associated with headache, fever, sore throat, a stiff tongue, red complexion and fullness in the chest;

- A Full *Guan* pulse, together with abdominal pain or related symptoms, is a sign of surplus heat in the Stomach and Spleen;

- A Full *Chi* pulse is due to excess heat in the Lower Heater, causing lumbago, abdominal pain and constipation.

9. Long pulse
Full of *Yuan* energy, the Long pulse (Yang) appears soft and steady. The movements are slightly elongated just before the pulse reaches its peak but, overall, the beats are of uniform length. This pulse is always an indication of good health; only when it is long and tense does it suggest disorder.

- A Long left *Cun* pulse is displayed by a healthy energetic person with a strong *Shen*;

- A Long *Guan* pulse in Spring signifies that Liver energy is in equilibrium;

- A Long *Chi* pulse indicates that Kidney energy, particularly the prenatal, is strong.

A Long and Tense pulse at Yang-*Ming* is symptomatic of Stomach and Large Intestine disorders arising from an excess of heat. Epilepsy is also synonymous with a Long and Tense pulse.

10. Short pulse
In contrast to the Long pulse, the Short pulse is so short and small that it barely registers on the radial artery. At *Cun* and *Chi* it is particularly short, virtually gone before it has arrived. It is a Yin pulse caused by a deficiency of blood and energy because the energy flow has not enough (kinetic) force to move the blood flow.

- A Short *Cun* pulse always denotes a deficiency of Heart and Lung energies. The main symptoms are anxiety and headache;

- A Short *Guan* pulse is a sign that Liver energy is not in equilibrium and apparent symptoms include rib and chest pains;

- A Short *Chi* pulse appears when Kidney Fire is deficient. Lower abdominal pain is a common symptom.

Clinically, alcoholism is revealed by a Short and Smooth pulse, and chest and abdominal pain by a Short and Deep pulse.

11. Overflowing pulse
The Overflowing pulse responds to the touch 'like a wave rising from the ocean full of strength, and

PULSE DIAGNOSIS

then – with ease – departing slowly'. It is often referred to as the 'majestically flowing' pulse.

Although it is the normal Yang pulse of Summer, in any other season its presence heralds disorder. The Overflowing pulse becomes apparent when much Yin blood and body fluid have been drained by excessive internal heat. Excessive Heart Fire (accompanied by a sore throat and ulcers on the tongue and mouth) is a common instigator. The prognosis is serious when this pulse develops in a patient already suffering from acute haemorrhage, chronic diarrhoea or chronic cough, or who has been bedridden for a long time.

- An Overflowing right *Cun* pulse reveals excessive Fire in the Lungs with symptoms including coughing, shortness of breath, chest pain and blood in the sputum;

- An Overflowing left *Guan* pulse indicates only one condition, overactive Liver Fire; if found at the right *Guan*, the diagnosis is more complicated. If symptoms include Stomach distention and frequent vomiting, it is a sign of excessive heat in the Stomach*. If there is diarrhoea (chronic or dysenteric) or dysentery, it signifies loss of body fluid and surplus Yang energy*;

- An Overflowing *Chi* pulse reveals a loss of Kidney *Ching*.

12. Minute pulse

The Minute pulse, although extremely soft and small, can be found through careful examination. It is apparent when the finger rests lightly on the surface of the artery but, on deeper pressure, it gradually fades away.

This pulse is inauspicious. It materializes with chronic disorder, deficient Yang energy and severe loss of *Jing* blood. Related symptoms may include cold extremities, fever, spontaneous perspiration and fear of cold.

- A Minute *Cun* pulse reveals deficient Lung or Heart energy accompanied by shortness of breath and palpitations;

- A Minute *Guan* pulse indicates deficiency of Spleen and Stomach energies. Symptoms include indigestion and abdominal pain;

- A Minute *Chi* pulse is a sign of loss of Kidney *Ching* and *Jing* blood, and loss of prenatal energy. Chills, lower abdominal pain, thirst, hunger and polyuria are accompanying symptoms.

13. Tight pulse

The Tight pulse is forceful with a movement likened to a taut rope. Its pulsating motion clearly impregnates all levels of *Cun*, *Guan* and *Chi*, appearing almost as just one movement.

The Tight pulse may be due to an attack by external cold, severe stasis of blood and energy flows (leading to abdominal pain) or by obstruction of Meridian energy flow (leading to aches and pains throughout the whole body).

- A Tight left *Cun* pulse suggests damage to the internal organs by excessive cold; at the right *Cun* it is an indication of external attack by cold;

- A Tight *Guan* pulse signifies abdominal pain caused by obstruction of Spleen and Stomach energies due to cold and humidity;

---

*Treatment for these two conditions (with the same pulse) is different. In chronic diarrhoea, body fluids are increased in order to balance Yang; to eliminate heat from the Stomach, bowel movements are induced by acupuncture or herbs.

PULSE DIAGNOSIS

- A Tight *Chi* pulse coincides with cold within the hip joint, pain in and around the perineum, acute lower abdominal pain, chest and throat symptoms, palpitations and headache.

A Tight and Floating pulse indicates an external attack by cold which has not yet penetrated the internal organs. A Tight and Deep pulse, however, is evidence that external cold has entered the internal organs.

14. Unhurried pulse

The Unhurried pulse moves regularly and gently 'like a willow dancing under the Spring breeze'. At about four beats to the respiration, it should not be confused with the Slow pulse. The Unhurried pulse is a normal pulse. It has *Shen*, showing vitality, and an abundance of both Stomach energy and prenatal Kidney *Ching*. Only when combined with other characteristics does it convey disorder.

- An Unhurried *Cun* pulse which also appears to be floating means that the body is experiencing an external attack by wind, resulting in deficient *Jing* blood. A corresponding increase of *Wei-Qi* then fights against the attack;

- An Unhurried and Deep left *Guan* pulse signifies obstruction of Liver and Gall Bladder energies accompanied by headache and dizziness. When Stomach energy is deficient, the right *Guan* pulse is always Unhurried and Slow;

- An Unhurried and Slow *Chi* pulse reveals cooling of Spleen Yang due to diminution of Kidney Yang. A common symptom is morning diarrhoea. An Unhurried and Full *Chi* pulse suggests that wind and damp have obstructed the energy flow of the lower Yang Meridians, thus creating residual humidity in the lower extremities and weakness in both legs, making walking difficult.

15. Hollow pulse

At the surface of the artery the Hollow pulse feels soft and large; on deeper pressure it appears to be firm at the sides but with an empty centre. The Chinese called this pulse '*Akung*' (onion stalk) as it refers to an artery with insufficient blood.

Because this pulse is only found after massive blood loss, no truly preventive treatment is applicable. If the haemorrhage is the result of attack of the three Yang Meridians by a 'hot' syndrome (excessive heat), there may be vomiting or coughing up of blood or epistaxis. If symptoms include melaena or menorrhagia, the cause is then an attack by heat of the three Yin *Luo* Meridians.

- A Hollow *Cun* pulse indicates a lack of nourishment (insufficient blood in the Heart due to haemorrhage). Common symptoms are tension and palpitations;

- A Hollow *Guan* pulse follows upon excessive vomiting of blood;

- A Hollow *Chi* pulse is associated with bleeding from the uterus, rectum or bladder.

16. Bowstring pulse

The Bowstring pulse can be compared to the string of a lute. It is the natural pulse of Springtime with movements that are long, steady and resilient. In other seasons this pulse is associated with Liver disorder (always caused by an excess of Liver energy, especially Liver Yang), headache, dizziness, irritability and a temperamental disposition, chest, rib and abdominal pains, indigestion, sighing (to release the tension in the chest) and bloodshot eyes.

- A Bowstring *Cun* pulse is evidence of a disturbance in the Upper Heater accompanied by headache and obstruction of sputum in the chest;

- A Bowstring left *Guan* pulse indicates that external causes of disease have entered the *Shao*-Yang Meridian *via* the *Tai*-Yang Meridian. Common symptoms are hot and cold flushes;

- A Bowstring right *Guan* pulse appears when the Liver (Wood) is overpowering the Spleen/Stomach (Earth), leading to symptoms such as abdominal pain and excessive Stomach acid;

- A Bowstring *Chi* pulse is a reflection of the effects of an attack by cold on weak Liver and Kidney energies. Symptoms include lower abdominal pain and muscular spasm of the lower extremities.

The Bowstring pulse is always found with other pulse characteristics:

- A Bowstring and Floating pulse is accompanied by symptoms of coughing, dyspnoea, asthma and oedema;

- A Bowstring and Deep pulse appears with symptoms of coughing, pain in the chest and ribs, and fluid retention;

- A Bowstring and Rapid pulse suggests an excess of heat;

- A Bowstring and Slow pulse reveals an excess of cold.

17. Leather pulse

The Leather pulse is apparently large and bowstring at the surface of the artery but, on deeper pressure, resembles a drum – taut on the outside and empty inside. It is a combination of the Bowstring and Hollow pulses, and indicates a deficiency of Kidney *Ching* and loss of *Jing* blood (a Hollow pulse condition) and a 'cold' syndrome attack (a Bowstring pulse condition).

- A Leather left *Cun* pulse is a sign of Heart blood deficiency with cardiac pain. At the right *Cun*, this pulse indicates a deficiency of Lung energy with shortness of breath and spontaneous perspiration;

- A Leather left *Guan* pulse is accompanied by pain in the groin and, at the right *Guan*, by a Stomach disorder in the form of indigestion or abdominal distention;

- A Leather pulse at the left *Chi* is often found in men and at the right *Chi* in women. For a man it signifies severe loss of Kidney *Ching* and loss of *Jing* blood with spermatorrhoea as a common symptom. A woman can expect a miscarriage or menorrhagia as a result of Kidney *Ching* loss.

18. Firm pulse

The Firm pulse, by description, is complex. Its depth exceeds that of the Deep pulse but not that of the Hidden pulse. It is not palpable at the superficial or intermediate levels, but is captured at the deep level with bowstring, long, full and hard characteristics.

This pulse is caused by an overwhelming reaction of *Qi* to a consolidated attack by external causes of disease, particularly when there is already an accumulation of external cold in the internal organs. Over a period of time the cold-affected organs may inhibit Liver energy, disrupt the activities of Spleen function (including nutritional absorption and transportation), and create pain in the Heart and abdominal regions.

PULSE DIAGNOSIS

In general, where there is a loss of Kidney *Ching* and *Jing* blood, there is a Leather pulse. Finding a Firm pulse instead, however, indicates that the disorder has become dangerous. When there is a deficiency of Yin energy and loss of *Jing* blood, the symptoms are then represented by a pulse with characteristics opposite to the Leather pulse. If external cold has taken a firm hold of the internal body, it will damage both *Yuan* and postnatal energies, leaving the patient unprotected. The condition is dangerous and the prognosis very poor.

19. Weak/Floating pulse

The Weak/Floating pulse is extremely soft and fine, 'floating like cottonwool' on the surface of the artery. The pulse has no Root energy and, with little pressure, vanishes. This pulse is a result of loss of *Jing* blood and deficient Spleen energy.

The Weak/Floating pulse is found in elderly persons with chronic illness or in women after childbirth. There has been loss of blood and energy but, although the body is weak, there is room for recovery. If this no-Root pulse appears without evidence of severe disease, it is an indication of loss of Spleen and Kidney energies; the prognosis is not favourable.

- A Weak/Floating *Cun* pulse is found with symptoms of spontaneous perspiration, night sweats and body weakness caused by deficient Yang energy and loss of the protective *Wei-Qi*;

- A Weak/Floating *Guan* pulse reveals a lack of Spleen/Stomach energy. There may be accompanying diarrhoea, a husky or weak voice, no energy for conversation and extreme body weakness;

- A Weak/Floating *Chi* pulse is a sign that Yin cold has entered the Lower Heater and disorder has drained *Jing* blood and Kidney *Ching*.

20. Weak pulse

The Weak pulse is extremely fine and soft. Heavy pressure may find it but it is completely lacking in force. It is not found at either the superficial or intermediate levels of the radial artery.

This pulse indicates a deficiency of *Qi*, an insufficiency of power to fully motivate blood circulation, low blood quantity and depleted Kidney *Ching*. The Weak pulse is commonplace in the aged but alarming when found in a younger person.

When Yang energy is deficient, *Jing* and *Wei* are decreased in energy proportionately and the unprotected body becomes vulnerable to attack by external causes of disease, with symptoms of fever and fear of cold. Although these hot and cold symptoms are usually characterized by a Floating pulse, in these particular cases (where Yang energy is deficient and the body is defenceless) the pulse is Weak. If cold accumulates within the body, thus precipitating additional cycles of discord, blood and energy are further drained and life is endangered. Nourishing the *Jing* blood and strengthening Yang energy are the most important aspects of treatment for this condition.

- A Weak left *Cun* pulse tells of a deficient Heart energy and may include palpitations and loss of memory. The same pulse at right *Cun* reveals Lung energy weakness with symptoms such as spontaneous perspiration and dyspnoea;

- A Weak *Guan* pulse always indicates a deficiency of Stomach and Spleen energies accompanied by physical and mental fatigue;

- A Weak *Chi* pulse reveals that Lower Heater Yang energy is extremely weak and Yin energy is diminished. The patient will have muscle spasms in both legs.

21. Scattered pulse
The Scattered pulse is large and floating with an erratic rhythm. Although clearly palpable at the superficial level, it loses approximately twenty-five percent of its force at the intermediate level and is nonexistent at the deeper level.

This pulse indicates damage to pre- and postnatal energies and severe disruption to Kidney and Spleen Yang energies. The condition is serious. During pregnancy the Scattered pulse proclaims the onset of labour; in the early months it is a warning of miscarriage.

- A Scattered *Cun* pulse reflects deficiency of Heart Yang and loss of Lung *Wei* energy. Common symptoms are palpitations, dyspnoea and spontaneous perspiration;

- A Scattered *Guan* pulse indicates deficiency of Spleen Yang energy in the Middle Heater, from where the accumulation of humidity begins to 'fall', causing the feet to swell;

- A Scattered *Chi* pulse, if found together with a chronic disorder, suggests that Kidney *Yuan* energy has been damaged; the condition is dangerous. Treatment must be given with the utmost care.

22. Fine pulse
The Fine pulse is soft and fine with little force, but is larger than the Minute pulse. It is clear at all three levels and responds to the touch 'like a soft thread of silk'. This pulse is evidence of diminution of blood and energy flows.

In Autumn and Winter, a Fine pulse in an elderly person shows successful adjustment to environmental changes as, in both these seasons, older people are naturally short of Yang energy.

On the other hand, a Fine pulse in Spring or Summer in a younger person reveals discord in health as the pulses of youth in these two seasons should be Full or Bowstring.

Mental fatigue, emotional imbalance, overwork and loss of Kidney *Ching* all produce a Fine pulse.

- A Fine *Cun* pulse is the result of frequent vomiting which drains body energy;

- A Fine *Guan* pulse indicates weak Spleen and Stomach energies, often in the form of abdominal distention in a patient who is otherwise usually thin;

- A Fine *Chi* pulse is symptomatic of a severe loss of *Yuan* energy. With additional symptoms of spermatorrhoea, diarrhoea and cold in point CV 4, depletion of Kidney *Ching* will occur.

After massive loss of blood and draining of body fluids the Fine pulse appears, indicating loss of Yin energy.

23. Hidden pulse
The Hidden pulse is the innermost of all the pulses, found only by pushing aside muscle and tendon and exerting pressure almost to the bone.

Cold disorders residing internally obstruct the blood and energy flows of the Meridians and restrain energy to the organs; this is the primary cause of the Hidden pulse. If Yang energy is able to penetrate the obstruction, the body perspires and the course of the disease changes, possibly to an attack of the muscle Meridians by external cold. If a cold disorder has blocked the blood and energy flows, treatment should not include induced sweating but should warm the internal organs with herbal medicines to increase Yang energy and re-establish its normal flow.

PULSE DIAGNOSIS

- A Hidden *Cun* pulse is found when a cold disorder attacks the Upper Heater, causing retention of food in the Stomach and inhibition of energy flow within the chest. Efforts to vomit fail because the chest has insufficient energy to expel the food, and both Stomach and chest feel uncomfortable;

- A Hidden *Guan* pulse reveals retention of cold and humidity in the Middle Heater with consequent abdominal pain and body heaviness;

- A Hidden *Chi* pulse with severe pain in the hips and groin is the result of either cold or obstruction of energy in the Lower Heater.

24. Moving pulse
The Moving pulse combines into one movement the characteristics of the Rapid, Smooth, Tight and Short pulses, the total effect feeling like a 'blow' to the artery. The overall 'shape' of the pulse is 'like a bean, with no head or tail'.

This pulse indicates antagonism between the Yin and Yang energies; the losing energy is constantly agitated while the healthy energy remains unobtrusive. As expressed by the Ancients, 'Yang movements represent deficient Yang energy; Yin movements represent deficient Yin energy'.

- A Moving *Cun* pulse is produced by perspiration, a Yang movement (deficient Yang energy). The left *Cun* is controlled by the Heart which has perspiration as one of its fluids. The right *Cun* represents the Lungs, which control and balance the skin and body hair as well as perspiration;

- A Moving *Guan* pulse indicates that heat and cold have created an imbalance in the Stomach and Spleen. Symptoms include abdominal pain, diarrhoea, muscular spasm and indigestion;

- A Moving *Chi* pulse is produced by fever, a Yin movement (deficient Yin energy), brought about by Kidney Yin and Yang imbalance. Water cannot balance Fire and the result is fever.

25. Hasty pulse
The Hasty pulse is similar to the Rapid pulse (see page 48); its movement comes and goes rapidly, missing a beat at irregular intervals. This pulse reveals an accumulation of Fire in the Three Heater. Excessive Yang Fire overwhelms Yin fluid, thus disturbing blood and energy flows. If the interval between the missing pulse beats increases, the disorder has become worse; a decrease signifies improvement.

- A Hasty *Cun* pulse indicates excessive Heart or Lung Fire with symptoms of severe coughing, dyspnoea, palpitations and delirium;

- A Hasty *Guan* pulse is a sign of excessive Fire in the Liver and Spleen evidenced by indigestion and blood stasis in the Liver;

- A Hasty *Chi* pulse reveals excessive Fire in the Kidney due to either loss of *Yuan* energy or severe imbalance of Yin and Yang energies. This condition is dangerous and the prognosis is poor.

26. Knotted pulse
The Knotted pulse also misses beats at irregular intervals but, unlike the Hasty pulse, the movements are slow. This pulse indicates an excess of Yin and cold in the internal organs caused by a deficiency of Yang energy, thus disturbing blood and energy flows. A Knotted pulse is always found with a chronic condition resulting from long periods of illness in which Yang energy and Kidney *Ching* are lost, and blood and energy flows disturbed.

PULSE DIAGNOSIS

- A Knotted *Cun* pulse reveals congestion in the Lungs with symptoms of cardiac pain;

- A Knotted *Guan* pulse indicates the presence of cold in the Spleen, abdominal pain, indigestion and diarrhoea;

- A Knotted *Chi* pulse implies an excess of Yin and cold in the Kidneys, causing aches and pain in the lower back and weakness of the lower extremities.

27. Intermittent pulse

The Intermittent pulse has missing beats separated by regular and rather long intervals of rhythmic beating. Two beats following in quick succession after an interval indicate restitution of a lost pulse beat, but there is no restitution if a missing beat is followed by the normal rhythmic beating. This pulse arises from an absence of Zang blood and energy, and from a deficiency of *Yuan* energy due to chronic disorder. The prognosis is poor but may be improved with treatment. An Intermittent pulse during the third month of pregnancy indicates an urgent need to tone the body as *Yuan* energy is insufficient. Severe diarrhoea and vomiting accompanying the Intermittent pulse indicate loss of *Yuan* energy and deficiency of Spleen and Stomach energies.

The Intermittent, Knotted and Hasty pulses have distinctly irregular rhythms revealing internal disorder. (In Western medicine it is considered a cardiac disorder.) There are some instances, however, when an irregular pulse is only a reflection of an individual's intrinsic nature. Such individuals during disorder react differently to those with regular pulses. In the latter group, once the disease is cured, the irregular pulse reverts to its normal regularity. In those with naturally irregular pulses the disorder is severe and, because of the lack of a defence system, continuous attack by the disease quickly penetrates the internal organs. The condition is dangerous and the prognosis is poor.

Through careful observation, the ancient Chinese philosophers discovered that the length of the intervals between missing pulse beats identified specific disorders:

Missing Pulse Beats	Condition
1 in 50	Healthy
1 in 40	Disorder in Kidneys
1 in 30	Disorder in Liver
1 in 20	Disorder in Spleen
1 in 10	Disorder in Heart
1 in 4–5	Disorder in Lungs
1 in 3	Dangerous: Life Force is nearly spent

28. Hurried pulse

The Hurried pulse is similar to the Rapid pulse (see page 48). A pulse of eight beats per respiration is considered a Hurried pulse; clinically the condition is dangerous, and diagnosis and treatment are urgently required.

The Hurried pulse reveals an extreme imbalance of Yin and Yang energies. In such a condition the pulse is 'out of Meridian' and 'the Soul about to depart'. If the pulse continues to increase, reflecting an extremely high level of Yang and extremely low level of Yin energies, the prognosis is then very grave. The simultaneous existence of both extremes of energy will destroy the Yin and Yang relationship and bring about the next change: death.

- A Hurried left *Cun* pulse is a sign that Heart Fire is consuming itself. This pulse at right *Cun* suggests that Lung Metal has been burnt by Heart Fire;

PULSE DIAGNOSIS

- A Hurried left *Guan* pulse signifies diminished Liver Yin, at right *Guan* that Spleen Yin is exhausted;

- A Hurried *Chi* pulse implies that Water has been drained and Kidney *Ching* is nearly gone.

A Hurried pulse is felt in chronic or Heart diseases and treatment is very difficult. A combination of Eastern and Western methods of treatment should be applied in an effort to save the patient's life.

4 FOURTEEN MERIDIANS AND ACUPUNCTURE POINTS

THE MERIDIAN COMPLEX

The *'NEI-JING'* describes a Meridian as a pathway for 'body energy flow', that is, the system of energy circulation throughout the body. The Chinese call it the *Jing-Luo* System or Meridian Complex. There have been many attempts to explain the system and these theories are still being researched today.

The principal network, the 'Twelve Main Meridians', is the main pathway for body energy circulation and connects the internal organs with the energy flow at the body surface. There are two Meridians for each organ, one on each side of the body in a mirror-image arrangement. Beginning at the Lungs, the network traces a pathway wherein each Meridian completes its part of the course (as in a relay), passing in turn through each organ. Terminating with the Liver Meridian, the cycle begins again at the Lungs.

There are small energy circulations or minor branches called the Governor Vessel (GV) and Conception Vessel (CV) Meridians, the latter running down the middle of the front of the body and the other running down the middle of the back. These are connected to the Twelve Main Meridians and together they form the Fourteen Meridians along which the acupuncture points are found

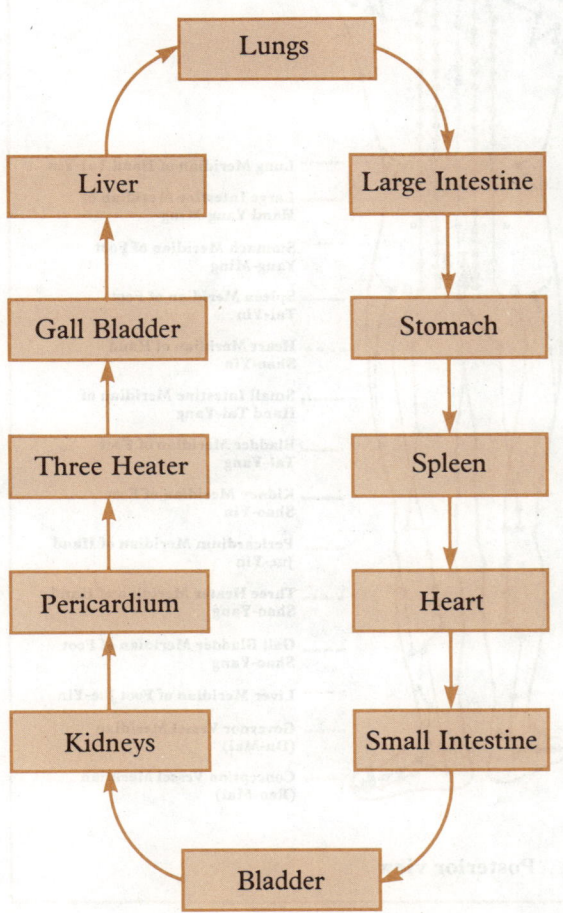

FOURTEEN MERIDIANS AND ACUPUNCTURE POINTS

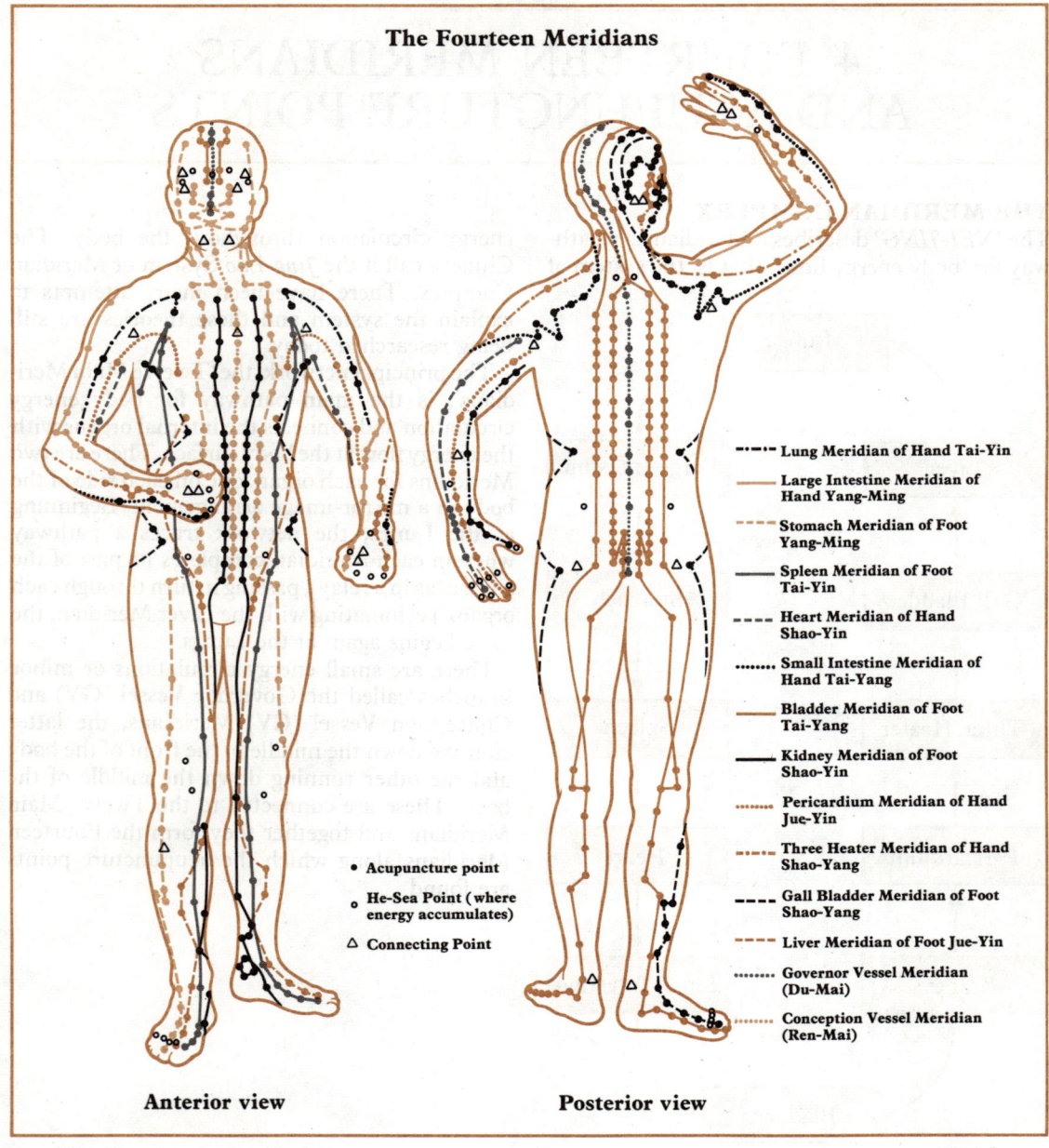

FOURTEEN MERIDIANS AND ACUPUNCTURE POINTS

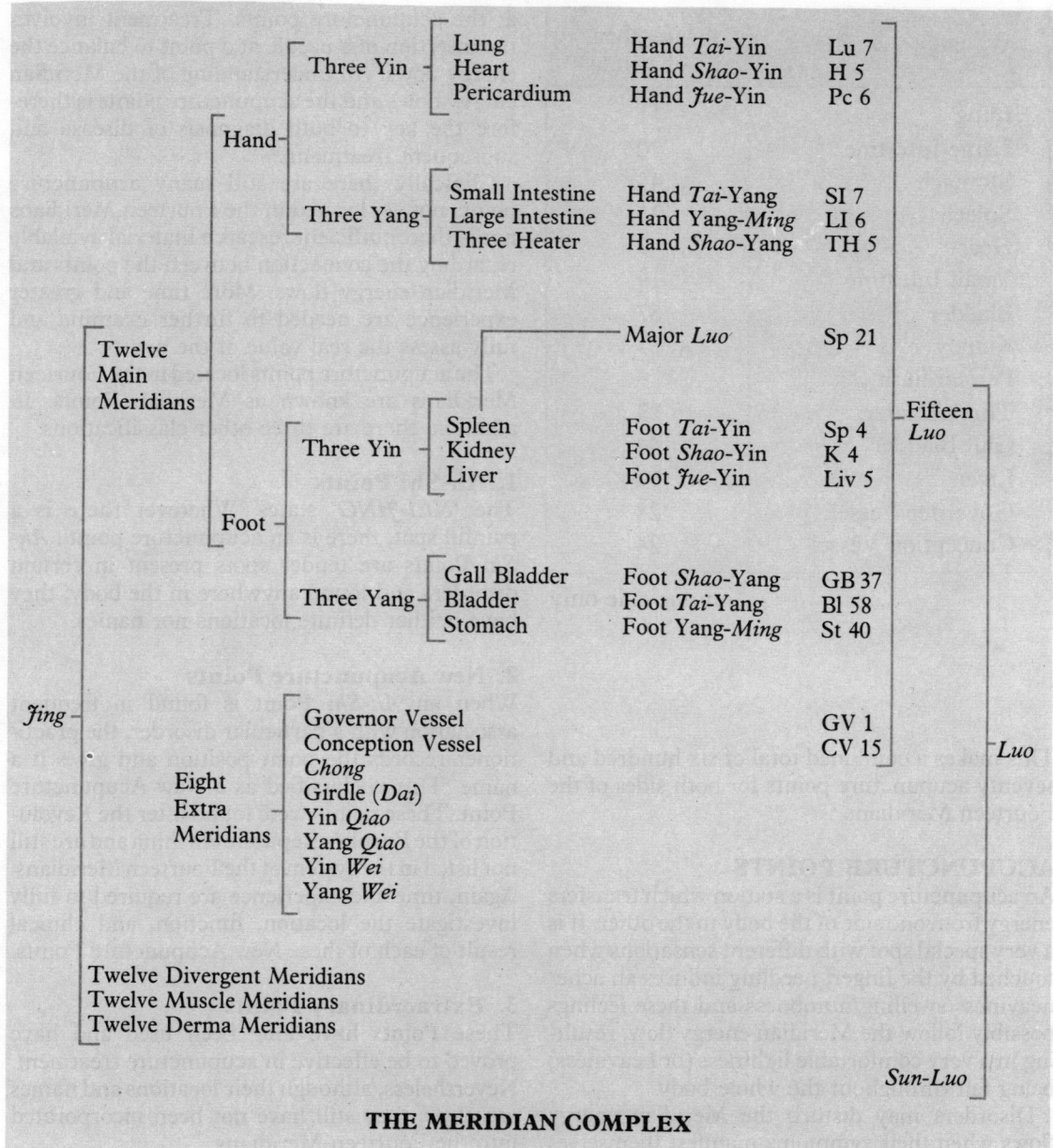

THE MERIDIAN COMPLEX

FOURTEEN MERIDIANS AND ACUPUNCTURE POINTS

Meridian	Number of points*
Lung	11
Large Intestine	20
Stomach	45
Spleen	21
Heart	9
Small Intestine	19
Bladder	67
Kidney	27
Pericardium	9
Three Heater	23
Gall Bladder	44
Liver	14
Governor Vessel	28
Conception Vessel	24

*on one side only

This makes a combined total of six hundred and seventy acupuncture points for both sides of the Fourteen Meridians.

ACUPUNCTURE POINTS

An acupuncture point is a station which transfers energy from one side of the body to the other. It is a very special spot with different sensations when touched by the finger; needling induces an ache/heaviness/swelling/numbness and these feelings possibly follow the Meridian energy flow, resulting in a very comfortable lightness (or heaviness) being felt throughout the whole body.

Disorders may disturb the Meridian energy flows when their symptoms manifest themselves at the acupuncture points. Treatment involves the insertion of a needle at a point to balance the energy flows. An understanding of the Meridian energy flows and the acupuncture points is therefore the key to both diagnosis of disease and subsequent treatment.

Clinically there are still many acupuncture points not yet located in the Fourteen Meridians nor is there sufficient research material available regarding the connection between the points and Meridian energy flows. More time and greater experience are needed to further examine and fully assess the real value of the points.

The acupuncture points located in the Fourteen Meridians are known as Meridian Points. In addition, there are three other classifications:

1. Ah-Shi Points

The *'NEI-JING'* states 'Wherever there is a painful spot, there is an acupuncture point'. *Ah-Shi* Points are tender spots present in certain disorders and found anywhere in the body; they have neither definite locations nor names.

2. New Acupuncture Points

When an *Ah-Shi* Point is found in frequent association with a particular disorder, the practitioner records the point position and gives it a name. This is classified as a New Acupuncture Point. These points were found after the Revolution of the People's Republic of China and are still not listed in the system of the Fourteen Meridians. Again, time and experience are required to fully investigate the location, function, and clinical result of each of these New Acupuncture Points.

3. Extraordinary Points

These Points have long been used and have proved to be effective in acupuncture treatment. Nevertheless, although their locations and names are clear, they still have not been incorporated into the Fourteen Meridians.

FOURTEEN MERIDIANS AND ACUPUNCTURE POINTS

The Meridian, *Ah-Shi*, New Acupuncture and Extraordinary Points are all widely used in clinical practice today. The selection of points, and therefore the results, depend largely on the disease, the structure of the body and the experience of the practitioner.

Naming of points

Except for the *Ah-Shi*, all acupuncture points have a specific name with a special meaning which always attempts to convey the anatomical location, physiological function and treatment result. Because of the difficulty in combining these three concepts into one word, the ancient Chinese used words from nature, such as mountain, hill, valley, well, fountain or rivulet, to describe a point located in a high or low region.

Name	Description/Meaning
GB 34, 'Yang Hill Rivulet'	In the leg, external (Yang), between the Hill (tibia) and Rivulet (fibula).
Sp 9, 'Yin Hill Rivulet'	In the leg, internal (Yin), between the Hill (tibia) and Rivulet (gastrocnemius muscle).
St 36, 'Three Mile Leg'	In the leg, a very good point for reinforcing the physical body. (Walking three miles without tiring will make the body strong.)
GV 23, 'Superior Star'	On the top of the head.

Architectural terms, such as door, room, house or palace, were used to express the energy level (either big or small). Cosmic terms, like universe, stars, heaven or celestial, were appropriate for points at the top of the body, or for the sensations of points. Animal names, for example, fish, hare or calf, were used for point locations. Finally, there was frequent use of the Chinese words for anatomy and for physiological functions, such as bone, blood, energy, *Ching* and *Shen*.

Point location

The most practical way to find a point is to use finger pressure on certain areas, such as in a depression of the bone or muscle, which will produce a specific acupuncture sensation. ('Puncture wherever there is tenderness'.)

Each acupuncture point has a definite location which must be determined with great accuracy for effective treatment. There are several different methods for accomplishing this:

1. Following body structure

Almost all points are located on or at a prominence or depression of the bone, joint or muscle, at a skin crease or hairline, at the side of the nail, nipple, umbilicus, eye, mouth and so on. Using these guides, points can be located easily.

2. Proportional measurement

The length or width of various sections of the body is divided into a specific number of equal parts, each part being termed one *cun*. Obviously, the length of the *cun* depends on the structure of the individual, whether fat or thin, tall or short, and will vary accordingly.

FOURTEEN MERIDIANS AND ACUPUNCTURE POINTS

STANDARD PROPORTIONAL MEASUREMENTS

DISTANCE	CUN	REMARKS
HEAD		
Anterior hairline to posterior hairline	12	If the hairlines are indistinguishable, the distance from the glabella to the process of the seventh cervical vertebra is 18 *cun*.
Anterior hairline to glabella	3	
Posterior hairline to the process of the seventh cervical vertebra	3	
Hairline between the two temporal regions	9	Between the tips of the two mastoid processes is also measured as 9 *cun*.
THORAX & ABDOMEN		
Between the nipples	8	
Lower end of sternum to centre of umbilicus	8	The anterior aspect of the chest is measured according to the intercostal spaces. The width of every rib is 1.6 *cun*.
Centre of umbilicus to upper border of pubic symphysis	5	
Axillary crease to tip of eleventh rib	12	

DISTANCE	CUN	REMARKS
BACK		
Medial border of scapula to midline of back	3	To locate points vertically on the back, the intervertebral spaces may be used as landmarks.
UPPER EXTREMITIES		
Transverse axillary fold to cubital crease	9	The distances are identical for the anterior, lateral and medial aspects.
Cubital crease to transverse wrist crease	12	
LOWER EXTREMITIES		
Upper level of the greater trochanter to middle of patella	19	The distances are identical for the anterior, posterior and lateral aspects.
Middle of patella to top of lateral malleolus	16	
Upper border of pubic symphysis to upper border of femoral epicondyle	16	The distances are identical for the medial aspect.
Medial tibial condyle to tip of medial malleolus	13	

FOURTEEN MERIDIANS AND ACUPUNCTURE POINTS

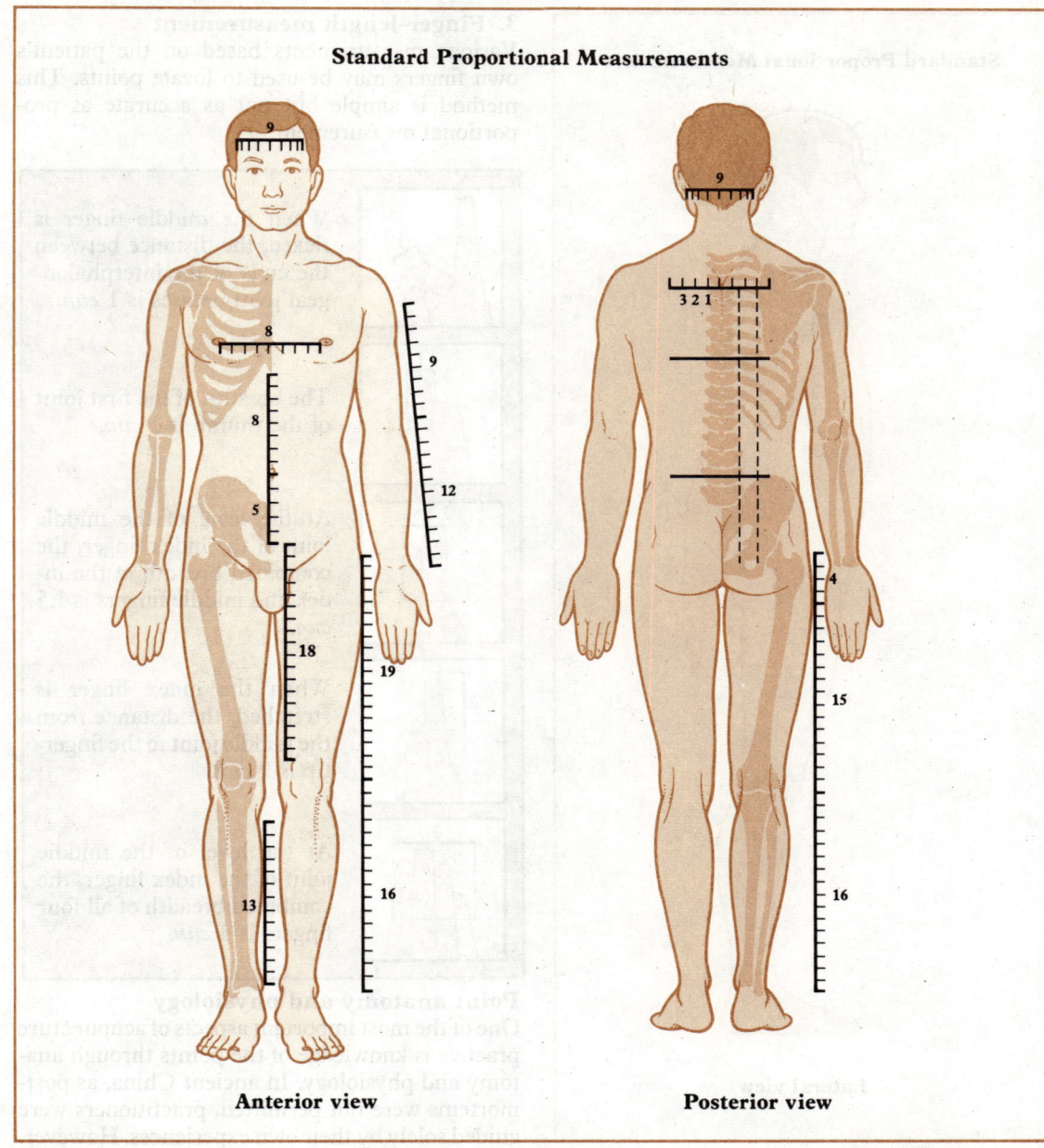

FOURTEEN MERIDIANS AND ACUPUNCTURE POINTS

Standard Proportional Measurements

Lateral view

3. Finger-length measurement

Various measurements based on the patient's own fingers may be used to locate points. This method is simple but not as accurate as proportional measurement.

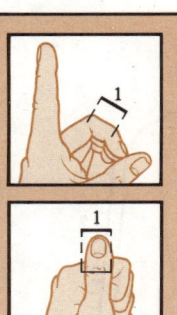
When the middle finger is flexed, the distance between the ends of the interphalangeal joint creases is 1 *cun*.

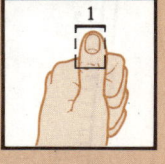
The breadth of the first joint of the thumb is 1 *cun*.

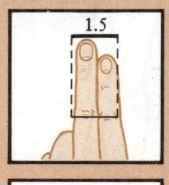
At the level of the middle joint of the index finger, the combined breadth of the index and middle fingers is 1.5 *cun*.

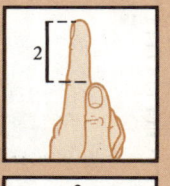
When the index finger is stretched, the distance from the middle joint to the fingertip is 2 *cun*.

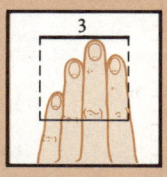
At the level of the middle joint of the index finger, the combined breadth of all four fingers is 3 *cun*.

Point anatomy and physiology

One of the most important aspects of acupuncture practice is knowledge of the points through anatomy and physiology. In ancient China, as postmortems were not permitted, practitioners were guided solely by their own experiences. However, comparative studies of animal body structure did provide some understanding of how to avoid damaging the vital organs of the human body. The 'NEI-JING' gave the following warning for needling:

- Into the Brain, death is immediate (Points GV 15, GV 16, GV 17);
- Into the Heart, death occurs in 1 day;
- Into the Lung, death occurs in 3 days;
- Into the Liver, death occurs in 5 days;
- Into the Kidney, death occurs in 6 days;
- Into the Spleen, death occurs in 10 days;
- Into an artery (for example, St 30) causes swelling in the groin.
- The needle should not be used on anyone who has been poisoned, who is very angry or overtired, who has just eaten a large meal, who is hungry or very thirsty or who has a phobia about needles.

In those early days, many acupuncture points were clearly marked as forbidden for needling or moxibustion; even today, with our knowledge of anatomy and physiology, it is still difficult to give an explanation as to why this was so. For example, the needle was forbidden at Point LI 13; obviously it must have been one of the points used when an accident had occurred.

The practitioners of ancient China followed specific rules and beliefs when treating patients:

'On inserting a needle into an acupuncture point, one had to think clearly, concentrate one's energy on manipulating the needle, watch the patient, and be aware of one's own feelings about the actual treatment. In believing acupuncture to be the optimum treatment, one first had to fully understand it in order to give of one's best to patients.'

Functions and symptoms

The functions and symptoms of the Meridian points have long been known; in particular, in Dr. Yang's book, *Compendium of Acupuncture and Moxibustion* (AD 1600), the subject had been revised, corrected, then carefully chronicled. The functions of the points were described in terms of Chinese medicine and the points for use in acupuncture were designated according to the symptoms presented.

There is no one acupuncture point nor one needle capable of treating every disorder. Each point has its own character and specific function, and can only contribute in its own particular way towards balancing the energy disorder in certain diseases. An unfamiliar point may perhaps play an important part in treatment when the body has a particular need; in practice, however, there are certain points in good positions which are recognized as being important (see **'Specific points'**). Often it may be necessary for several points to be used together to complete treatment.

Specific points

Some of the acupuncture points in the Main Meridians have specific functions and produce particular results in acupuncture treatment. They are grouped into ten categories.

1. Shu (Five Element Acupuncture) Points
These points lie between the tips of the fingers and the elbow, and between the tips of the toes and the knee. Traditional Chinese belief was that the energy flow in a Meridian was similar to the motion of water and was expressed as:

- Where energy starts to bubble, *Jing*-Well Points;
- Where energy flow begins to flourish, *Ying*-Spring Points;
- Where energy movement increases, *Shu*-Stream Points;

YIN AND YANG MERIDIANS, FIVE SHU POINTS AND FIVE ELEMENTS

Yang Meridian	Metal	Water	Wood	Fire	Earth
Five Shu Points	*Jing*-Well	*Ying*-Spring	*Shu*-Stream	*Jing*-River	*He*-Sea
Yin Meridian	Wood	Fire	Earth	Metal	Water

YIN MERIDIANS, FIVE SHU POINTS AND FIVE ELEMENTS

Five Shu Points	*Jing*-Well	*Ying*-Spring	*Shu*-Stream	*Jing*-River	*He*-Sea
Five Elements	Wood	Fire	Earth	Metal	Water
Five Zang					
Three Yin Meridians of Hand					
Lung	Lu 11	Lu 10	Lu 9	Lu 8	Lu 5
Pericardium	Pc 9	Pc 8	Pc 7	Pc 5	Pc 3
Heart	H 9	H 8	H 7	H 4	H 3
Three Yin Meridians of Foot					
Spleen	Sp 1	Sp 2	Sp 3	SP 5	Sp 9
Liver	Liv 1	Liv 2	Liv 3	Liv 4	Liv 8
Kidney	K 1	K 2	K 3	K 7	K 10

YANG MERIDIANS, FIVE SHU POINTS AND FIVE ELEMENTS

Five Shu Points	*Jing*-Well	*Ying*-Spring	*Shu*-Stream	*Jing*-River	*He*-Sea
Five Elements	Metal	Water	Wood	Fire	Earth
Six Fu					
Three Yang Meridians of Hand					
Large Intestine	LI 1	LI 2	LI 3	LI 5	LI 11
Three Heater	TH 1	TH 2	TH 3	TH 6	TH 10
Small Intestine	SI 1	SI 2	SI 3	SI 5	SI 8

Three Yang Meridians of Foot					
Stomach	St 45	St 44	St 43	St 41	St 36
Gall Bladder	GB 44	GB 43	GB 41	GB 38	GB 34
Bladder	Bl 67	Bl 66	Bl 65	Bl 60	Bl 40

- Where energy flow is abundant, *Jing*-River Points;
- Where all the energy accumulates, *He*-Sea Points.

Clinically, there are two different ideas surrounding the understanding and the use of the five *Shu* Points or the Five Element Acupuncture Points:

- Following the Five Element Theory to select points for acupuncture treatment.
- Following the energy flow concept to select the points.
- *Jing*-Well Points are very sensitive; they strongly influence energy flow and can, in fact, initiate the energy flow. They are always used for reviving from unconsciousness and for bringing mental and physical energies together. In clinical practice, they are used for treating mental illness and for the feeling of fullness in the chest.
- *Ying*-Spring Points are used for treating fever.
- *Shu*-Stream Points are used for pain relief and the feeling of heaviness in the body.
- *Jing*-River Points are often used for dyspnoea, coughing and throat disorders.
- *He*-Sea Points are always used to treat disorders of the Fu organs (Stomach, Small and Large Intestines, Bladder and Gall Bladder).

2. Yuan (Source) Points

These points are located where *Yuan* energy passes through or accumulates. There is a *Yuan* (Source) Point for each of the Twelve Main Meridians and all are in the extremities. A specific sensation is always felt at the associated points when disease attacks the body's internal (Zang/Fu) organs. The *Yuan* (Source) Points are, therefore, significant in the diagnosis and treatment of some of the disorders affecting the Zang and Fu organs.

TWELVE YUAN (SOURCE) POINTS		
Meridian		*Yuan* (Source) Point
Three Yin Meridians of Hand	Lung Pericardium Heart	Lu 9 Pc 7 H 7
Three Yin Meridians of Foot	Spleen Liver Kidney	Sp 3 Liv 3 K 3
Three Yang Meridians of Hand	Large Intestine Three Heater Small Intestine	LI 4 TH 4 SI 4
Three Yang Meridians of Foot	Stomach Gall Bladder Bladder	St 42 GB 40 Bl 64

3. Luo Points

Each of the Fourteen Meridians has a *Luo* Point and the Spleen Meridian has an extra point called 'Major *Luo*' (Sp 21),* making fifteen in all. The main function of these points is to connect the energy flows of the Yin and Yang Meridians. For example, Lu 7 is a *Luo* Point which connects the energy flow of the Lung to that of the Large Intestine. A *Luo* Point, therefore, is used for treating diseases which involve two (external and internal) related Meridians as well as for treating disorders in the regions served by them.

FIFTEEN LUO POINTS

Yang Meridian	Luo Point
Large Intestine	LI 6
Three Heater	TH 5
Small Intestine	SI 7
Stomach	St 40
Gall Bladder	GB 37
Bladder	Bl 58
Governor Vessel	GV 1
Lung	Lu 7
Pericardium	Pc 6
Heart	H 5
Spleen	Sp 4*
Liver	Liv 5
Kidney	K 4
Conception Vessel	CV 15

*Major *Luo* (Sp 21)

4. Xi (Cleft) Points

A *Xi* (Cleft) Point is located deep between two separate body tissues where Meridian energy is concentrated. Altogether there are sixteen *Xi* Points in the body's extremities: one in each of the Twelve Main Meridians; and one in each of the Four Extra Meridians (Yin *Wei*, Yang *Wei*, Yin *Qiao* and Yang *Qiao*).

The *Xi* Points are often used for treating acute disorders. When massaged, the points can feel painful because of disorders in their respective Meridians and in their connecting organs. Hence, *Xi* Points can be used for diagnosing disorders in those organs.

SIXTEEN XI (CLEFT) POINTS

Meridian		Xi (Cleft) Point
Three Yin Meridians of Hand	Lung	Lu 6
	Pericardium	Pc 4
	Heart	H 6
Three Yin Meridians of Foot	Spleen	Sp 8
	Liver	Liv 6
	Kidney	K 5
Three Yang Meridians of Hand	Large Intestine	LI 7
	Three Heater	TH 7
	Small Intestine	SI 6
Three Yang Meridians of Foot	Stomach	St 34
	Gall Bladder	GB 36
	Bladder	Bl 63
Four Extra Meridians	Yin *Wei*	K 9
	Yang *Wei*	GB 35
	Yin *Qiao*	K 8
	Yang *Qiao*	Bl 59

FOURTEEN MERIDIANS AND ACUPUNCTURE POINTS

5. Eight Confluent Points of the Eight Extra Meridians

Within the Twelve Main Meridians are Eight Confluent Points in the extremities which communicate with the Eight Extra Meridians. Although the latter do not directly circulate in the extremities, their energies are connected to the energy flows of the Twelve Main Meridians. These points, therefore, are used for treating disorders related to the Twelve Main Meridians and to the Eight Extra Meridians.

In clinical practice, combinations of the Eight Confluent Points are necessary for total treatment, for example, combining points of the upper extremities (Pc 6) with those of the lower (Sp 4) in order to treat disorders of the heart, chest or stomach region.

6. Eight Influential Points

These Eight Influential Points in the Fourteen Meridians have special functions in connection with certain related organs and their functions. These functions are always described in terms of Chinese medicine.

Clinically, Liv 13 can be used for treating disorders of the five Zang (Lungs, Heart, Liver,

EIGHT CONFLUENT POINTS

Organ/Function	Influential Point
Zang	Liv 13
Fu	CV 12
Energy (*Qi*)	CV 17
Blood	Bl 17
Tendon	GB 34
Blood Vessel (Pulse)	Lu 9
Bone	Bl 11
Marrow	GB 39

EIGHT INFLUENTIAL POINTS

Main Meridians	Eight Confluent Points	Eight Extra Meridians	Principal Areas of Treatment
Spleen Pericardium	Sp 4 Pc 6	*Chong* Yin *Wei*	Heart, chest, stomach
Small Intestine Bladder	SI 3 Bl 62	Governor Vessel Yang *Qiao*	Eyes, neck, ear, bladder, shoulder, small intestine
Three Heater Gall Bladder	TH 5 GB 41	Yang *Wei* Girdle Vessel	Eyes, ear, cheek, neck, shoulder
Lung Kidney	Lu 7 K 6	Conception Vessel Yin *Qiao*	Lungs, throat, chest

FOURTEEN MERIDIANS AND ACUPUNCTURE POINTS

Spleen and Kidneys). Point CV 17, a centre of energy, can be treated with moxa to balance and increase body energy level.

7. Back-Shu Points

These points are at the back of the body in the Bladder Meridian and 1.5 *cun* lateral to the Governor Vessel. Their special function is in relation to the internal organs (Zang and Fu) whose energies accumulate in some of the Back-*Shu* Points.

In clinical practice, any disorders of the Zang and Fu manifest themselves in the corresponding Back-*Shu* Points through symptoms such as tenderness, lumps, swelling and aches. Thus, these points play an important role in disease diagnosis, and needling gives good results in treatment.

In practical terms as well as following the philosophy of Yang balancing Yin, the Back-*Shu* Points (Yang) are used mostly for treatment of disorders of the Zang organs (Yin) whereas in disorders of the Fu organs (Yang), the Front-*Mu* Points (Yin) are more frequently used.

8. Front-Mu Points

These points are at the front of the body in the chest and abdomen and serve the same functions as the Back-*Shu* Points. Correspondingly, it is in some of these Front-*Mu* Points that the energies of the related Zang and Fu accumulate. Disorders in the Zang and Fu also reveal themselves in these points so that they, too, are useful for diagnosis as well as treatment.

TWELVE BACK-SHU POINTS

Organ	Back-*Shu* Point
Lung	Bl 13
Pericardium	Bl 14
Heart	Bl 15
Liver	Bl 18
Gall Bladder	Bl 19
Spleen	Bl 20
Stomach	Bl 21
Three Heater	Bl 22
Kidney	Bl 23
Large Intestine	Bl 25
Small Intestine	Bl 27
Bladder	Bl 28

TWELVE FRONT-MU POINTS

Lateral Aspects of Chest and Abdomen	
Internal Organ	Point
Lung	Lu 1
Liver	Liv 14
Gall Bladder	GB 24
Spleen	Liv 13
Kidney	GB 25
Large Intestine	St 25

Midline of Chest and Abdomen	
Internal Organ	Point
Pericardium	CV 17
Heart	CV 14
Stomach	CV 12
Three Heater	CV 5
Small Intestine	CV 4
Bladder	CV 3

FOURTEEN MERIDIANS AND ACUPUNCTURE POINTS

Likewise, following the philosophy of Yin balancing Yang, the Front-*Mu* Points (Yin) are preferred in treating disorders of the *Fu* organs (Yang) whereas, for disorders of the Zang organs (Yin), the Back-*Shu* Points (Yang) are more frequently used.

The general rules for selecting Back-*Shu* and Front-*Mu* Points are:

Disorders of the Zang organs, Back-*Shu* Points;
Disorders of the Fu organs, Front-*Mu* Points;

Acute diseases, Back-*Shu* Points;
Chronic diseases, Front-*Mu* Points;

Shi (excess) syndromes, Back-*Shu* Points;
Xu (deficiency) syndromes, Front-*Mu* Points.

9. Meeting (or Crossing) Points

The point of intersection of two or more Meridians is known as a Meeting or Crossing Point. Such points are used to treat not only its own Meridian disorder but also disorders of the other Meridians crossing through it. For example:

- CV 4 is the Meeting Point of three Yin Meridians of the Foot; thus, it is used to treat disorders of the Conception Vessel Meridian as well as those of the Spleen, Liver and Kidney Meridians.

- Sp 6 is where the Kidney and Liver Meridians cross. Thus, it is used for treating disorders of the Spleen Meridian as well as those of the Kidney and Liver Meridians.

10. He-Sea Points

These points, part of the Five *Shu* Points, are important for treating disorders of the Fu organs; for example, Bl 39 is used for treatment of urine retention, St 37 for treatment of colitis and St 39 for treatment of spasm of the Small Intestine. Each of the six Fu has a *He*-Sea Point in the three Yang Meridians of Foot. (The three Yang Meridians of Hand have three inferior *He*-Sea Points in the Yang Meridians of Foot.)

SIX HE-SEA POINTS

Fu Organ	Point
Stomach	St 36
Large Intestine	St 37
Small Intestine	St 39
Three Heater	Bl 39
Bladder	Bl 40
Gall Bladder	GB 34

POINTS OF THE FOURTEEN MERIDIANS

1. Lung Meridian of Hand Tai-Yin

This Meridian is characterized by high energy flow and low blood flow. Lung Meridian energy flow originates in the Stomach deep at CV 12, descends to connect with the Large Intestine, returns to the Stomach and passes through the diaphragm to enter the Lung, its home. From there, it rises to the larynx and changes direction at Lu 1 to travel along the medial aspect of the upper arm. Passing in front of the Heart and Pericardium Meridians to reach the cubital fossa, the energy flows down the forearm and arrives at the styloid process of the radius above the wrist at Lu 7. From this point the flow branches: it continues along the radial border of the hand to end at Lu 11 and the tip of the thumb; and it flows directly to the tip of the index finger where it joins the Large Intestine Meridian at LI 1.

There are eleven acupuncture points on each side of the Lung Meridian.

Associated organs
- Belongs to Lungs;
- Related to Large Intestine;

FOURTEEN MERIDIANS AND ACUPUNCTURE POINTS

- Directly connected to Stomach and Kidney.

Symptomatology
- Disorders along Meridian course
  - Fever
  - Nasal obstruction
  - Headache
  - Pain in supraclavicular fossa, chest, shoulder, back, arm & hand

- Disorders in organ
  - Coughing
  - Dyspnoea
  - Shortness of breath
  - Restlessness
  - Fullness in chest
  - Dry throat
  - Haemoptysis
  - Diarrhoea

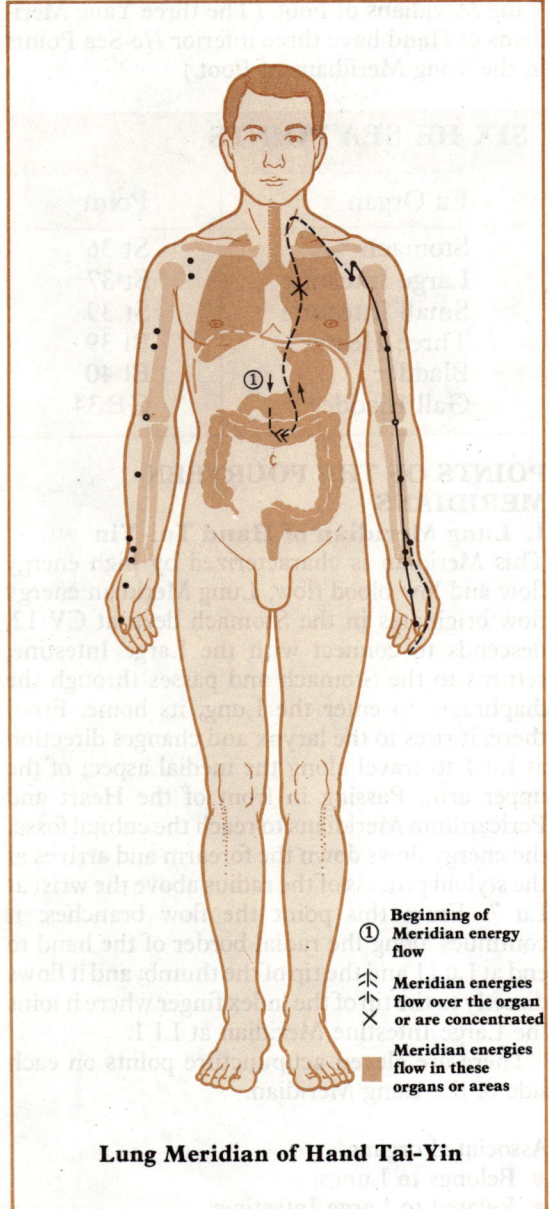

① Beginning of Meridian energy flow

⇈ Meridian energies flow over the organ or are concentrated

✕ Meridian energies flow in these organs or areas

Lung Meridian of Hand Tai-Yin

Acupuncture Points of Lung Meridian

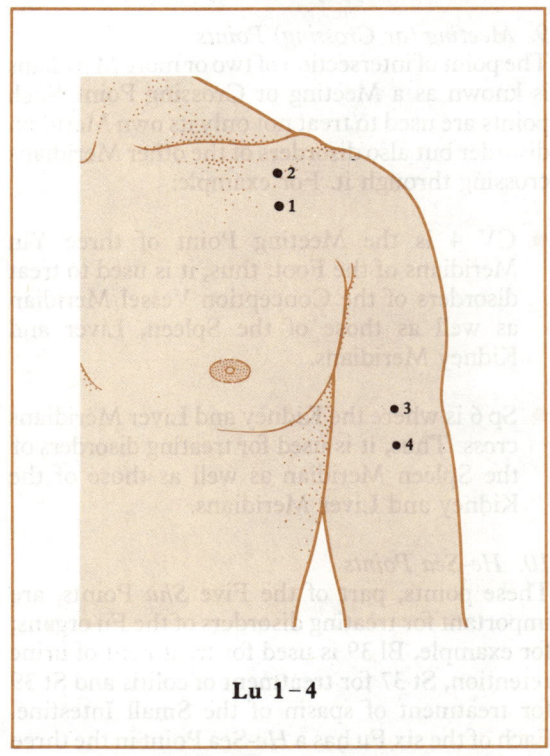

Lu 1–4

FOURTEEN MERIDIANS AND ACUPUNCTURE POINTS

Lu 1; *Zhong-Fu*; 'Central Palace'

Location
  Below acromial extremity of clavicle, 1 *cun* directly below Lu 2.

Regional anatomy
  Greater & smaller pectoral muscles;
  Axillary artery & vein;
  Thoracoacromial artery & vein;
  Intermediate supraclavicular nerve;
  Branches of anterior thoracic nerve;
  Lateral cutaneous branch of intercostal nerve;
  Suprapleural membrane;
  Apex of lung.

Connecting points
  Front-*Mu* Point of Lung;
  Meeting point of Hand & Foot *Tai*-Yin Meridians;
  Main connecting points Sp 21 & CV 12.

Functions
  Regulates Lung energy flow;
  Expels heat from Upper Heater.

Symptoms
  Swelling of upper limbs
  Pain in chest, shoulder & back
  Fullness in chest
  Coughing
  Dyspnoea
  Shortness of breath
  Perspiration

Clinical formula
  Lu 1 + Lu 6 + Bl 13 = Chronic bronchitis

Method of treatment
  Needle: 0.3 inch obliquely towards the lateral aspect of the chest.
  Moxa: Warm heating, 3 minutes.
  Feeling: Ache and/or swelling.
  Warning: Puncturing perpendicularly and too deeply affects function of the Lungs.

Lu 2; *Yun-Men*; 'Gate of the Cloud'

Location
  In depression below acromial extremity of clavicle.

Regional anatomy
  Cephalic vein;
  Thoracoacromial artery & vein;
  Axillary artery;
  Intermediate & lateral supraclavicular nerves;
  Branches of anterior thoracic nerve;
  Lateral cord of brachial plexus;
  Suprapleural membrane.

Symptoms
  Pain in chest, shoulder & arm
  Fullness in chest
  Coughing
  Shortness of breath

Clinical formula
  Lu 2 + K 27 = Coughing

Method of treatment
  Needle: 0.3 inch perpendicularly.
  Moxa: Warm heating, 2 minutes.
  Feeling: Heaviness and/or numbness.
  Warning: Puncturing too deeply affects breathing.

Lu 3; *Tian-Fu*; 'Celestial Palace'

Location
  On medial aspect of upper arm, 3 *cun* below end

FOURTEEN MERIDIANS AND ACUPUNCTURE POINTS

of axillary fold; on radial side of biceps muscle of arm, 6 *cun* above Lu 5.

Regional anatomy
  Biceps muscle of arm;
  Cephalic vein;
  Muscular branches of brachial artery & vein;
  Lateral cutaneous nerve of arm.

Symptoms
  Epistaxis
  Shortness of breath
  Pain in medial aspect of arm

Clinical formula
  Lu 3 + LI 4 = Epistaxis

Method of treatment
  Needle: 0.4 inch perpendicularly.
  Moxa: **Forbidden.**
  Feeling: Swelling and/or numbness.

Lu 4; *Xia-Bai*; **'White of the Canyon'**

Location
  On medial aspect of upper arm, 1 *cun* below Lu 3 on radial side of biceps muscle of arm.

Regional anatomy
  Biceps muscle of arm;
  Cephalic vein;
  Muscular branches of brachial artery & vein;
  Lateral cutaneous nerve of arm.

Connecting point
  Divergent Meridian of Hand *Tai*-Yin Meridian.

Symptoms
  Shortness of breath
  Pain in cardiac region
  Fullness in chest

Clinical formula
  Lu 4 + Bl 64 = Pain in cardiac region

Method of treatment
  Needle: 0.3 inch perpendicularly.
  Moxa: Warm heating, 2 minutes.
  Feeling: Ache and/or numbness.

Lu 5–11

Lu 5; *Chi-Ze*; **'Ulna Marsh'**

Location
  At crease of cubital fossa on radial side of tendon of biceps muscle of arm, located with elbow slightly flexed.

FOURTEEN MERIDIANS AND ACUPUNCTURE POINTS

Regional anatomy
  Origin of brachioradial muscle;
  Branches of radial recurrent artery & vein;
  Cephalic vein;
  Lateral cutaneous nerve of forearm;
  Radial nerve;
  Elbow joint.

Connecting point
  He-Sea Point.

Functions
  Expels heat from Lungs & Upper Heater;
  Draws down pathogenic energy in Lungs.

Symptoms
  Spasmodic pain in elbow & arm
  Fullness in chest
  Coughing
  Palpitations
  Shortness of breath

Clinical formula
  Lu 5 + SI 1 = Palpitations

Method of treatment
  Needle: 0.3 inch perpendicularly.
  Moxa: **Forbidden.**
  Feeling: Ache and/or numbness.
  Warning: Puncturing too deeply affects movement of elbow.

Lu 6; *Kong-Zui*; 'Supreme Hole'

Location
  On anterior aspect of forearm on line joining Lu 5 and Lu 9, 5 *cun* below Lu 5.

Regional anatomy
  Brachioradial muscle;
  Cephalic vein;
  Radial artery & vein;
  Lateral cutaneous nerve of forearm;
  Superficial branch of radial nerve.

Connecting point
  Xi-Cleft Point.

Functions
  Moistens respiratory tract;
  Expels heat from Upper Heater.

Symptoms
  Haemoptysis
  Sore throat
  Pain in elbow & arm
  Headache

Clinical formula
  Lu 6 + H 3 + Bl 13 = Haemoptysis

Method of treatment
  Needle: 0.3 inch perpendicularly.
  Moxa: Warm heating, 2 minutes.
  Feeling: Ache and/or numbness.

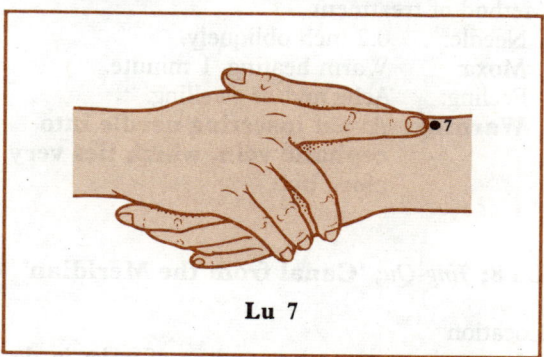
Lu 7

FOURTEEN MERIDIANS AND ACUPUNCTURE POINTS

Regional anatomy
  Cephalic vein;
  Branches of radial artery & vein;
  Lateral cutaneous nerve of forearm;
  Superficial branch of radial nerve.

Connecting points
  Luo-Connecting point;
  One of Eight Confluent Points connecting to Conception Vessel Meridian.

Functions
  Expels wind from Lungs;
  Releases energy obstruction in Lung Meridian.

Symptoms
  Facial paralysis
  Swelling of upper limbs
  Weakness & pain in wrist
  Headache at back of skull
  Stiff neck
  Shortness of breath
  Coughing

Clinical formula
  Lu 7 + SI 3 = Headache at back of skull

Method of treatment
  Needle: 0.2 inch obliquely.
  Moxa: Warm heating, 1 minute.
  Feeling: Ache and/or swelling.
  Warning: Avoid inserting needle into cephalic vein, which lies very close by.

Lu 8; *Jing-Qu*; 'Canal from the Meridian'

Location
  1 *cun* above transverse crease of wrist in depression on radial side of radial artery.

Regional anatomy
  Quadrate pronator muscle;
  Radial artery & vein;
  Lateral cutaneous nerve of forearm;
  Superficial branch of radial nerve.

Connecting point
  Jing-Well Point.

Symptoms
  Chest & back pains
  Fever
  Shortness of breath
  Coughing

Clinical formula
  Lu 8 + Liv 2 = Coughing

Method of treatment
  Needle: 0.2 inch perpendicularly or 0.3 inch obliquely.
  Moxa: **Forbidden.**
  Feeling: Ache and/or numbness.
  Warning: Application of moxa cone at this point affects Shen (Spirit).

Symptoms
  Feverish headache
  Sore throat
  Dry cough
  Abdominal pain
  Haemoptysis

Clinical formula
  Lu 10 + H 7 + Liv 8 = Haemoptysis

Method of treatment
  Needle: 0.2 inch perpendicularly.
  Moxa: **Forbidden.**
  Feeling: Ache and/or pain.

Lu 9; *Tai-Yuan*; 'Supreme Abyss'

Location
At transverse crease of wrist, in depression on radial side of radial artery.

Regional anatomy
Radial flexor muscle of wrist;
Long flexor muscle of thumb;
Radial artery & vein;
Lateral cutaneous nerve of forearm;
Superficial branch of radial nerve.

Connecting points
Shu-Stream and *Yuan*-Source Points;
One of Eight Influential Points, being a special meeting point at the pulse (blood vessel).

Functions
Eliminates wind;
Dispels phlegm in Lungs;
Regulates Lung energy and stops coughing;
Clears energy obstruction in Lungs.

Symptoms
Pain in chest
Pain in medial aspect of forearm
Haemoptysis
Ophthalmalgia
Coughing
Dry throat

Clinical formula
Lu 9 + Lu 8 + K 3 = Coughing and insomnia

Method of treatment
Needle: 0.2 inch perpendicularly.
Moxa: Warm heating, 1 minute.
Feeling: Ache and/or numbness.

Lu 10; *Yu-Ji*; 'Border of the Fish Body'

Location
On radial aspect at midpoint of first metacarpal bone, at junction of dorsum and palm of hand.

Regional anatomy
Short abductor muscle of thumb;
Opposing muscle of thumb;
Venules of thumb draining to cephalic vein;
Superficial branch of radial nerve.

Connecting point
Ying-Spring Point.

Functions
Balances Lung and Stomach energies;
Dispels heat from larynx and pharynx;
Eliminates heat in blood.

Symptoms
Feverish headache
Sore throat
Dry cough
Abdominal pain
Haemoptysis

Clinical formula
Lu 10 + H 7 + Liv 8 = Haemoptysis

Method of treatment
Needle: 0.2 inch perpendicularly.
Moxa: **Forbidden.**
Feeling: Ache and/or pain.

FOURTEEN MERIDIANS AND ACUPUNCTURE POINTS

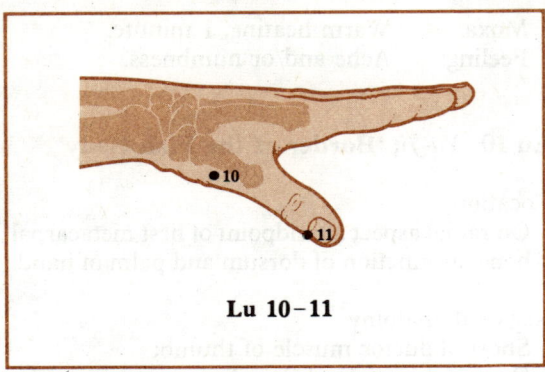
Lu 10-11

Lu 11; *Shao-Shang;* **'Young Merchant'**

Location
  On radial side of thumb about 0.1 *cun* posterior to corner of nail.

Regional anatomy
  Palmar digital arteries & veins;
  Terminal network formed by branches of lateral cutaneous nerve of forearm & superficial branch of radial nerve;
  Palmar (anterior) digital branch of median nerve.

Connecting point
  Jing-Well Point.

Functions
  Regulates Lung Meridian energy flow;
  Revives from unconsciousness;
  Clears energy obstruction in Lungs;
  Dispels heat from larynx & pharynx;
  Expels excess heat from Twelve Main Meridians.

Symptoms
  Loss of consciousness
  Fever
  Common cold
  Restlessness
  Sore throat
  Swelling in throat
  Swelling, numbness & pain in thumb

Clinical formula
  Lu 11 + CV 22 + LI 4 = Sore throat

Method of treatment
  Needle: 0.1 inch obliquely upwards or prick with three-edged needle to cause bleeding.
  Moxa: Not suitable; apply moxa cones for treating mental illness only.
  Feeling: Painful.
  Warning: Moxa is forbidden during pregnancy.

2. Large Intestine Meridian of Hand Yang-Ming

This Meridian is characterized by high energy and high blood flows. Its energy flow originates at LI 1 at the tip of the index finger, where it links with and receives energy from the Lung Meridian, and travels up the posterolateral surface of the arm to reach the shoulder point, LI 15. From there it continues to LI 16 just short of the acromion, ascends to points SI 12 and GV 14, and returns to the supraclavicular fossa. It then descends to connect with the Lung and, finally, passes through the diaphragm to enter the Large Intestine. (The Meridian has an inferior *He*-Sea point, St 37, which links the Large Intestine energy flow to the Stomach Meridian.)

From the supraclavicular fossa the Main Meridian ascends into the neck, passes over the cheek and enters the lower gum, at which point it curves around the upper lip, St 4. At the philtrum, GV 26, the two Large Intestine Meridians cross, the left Meridian to the right side of the nose, and

FOURTEEN MERIDIANS AND ACUPUNCTURE POINTS

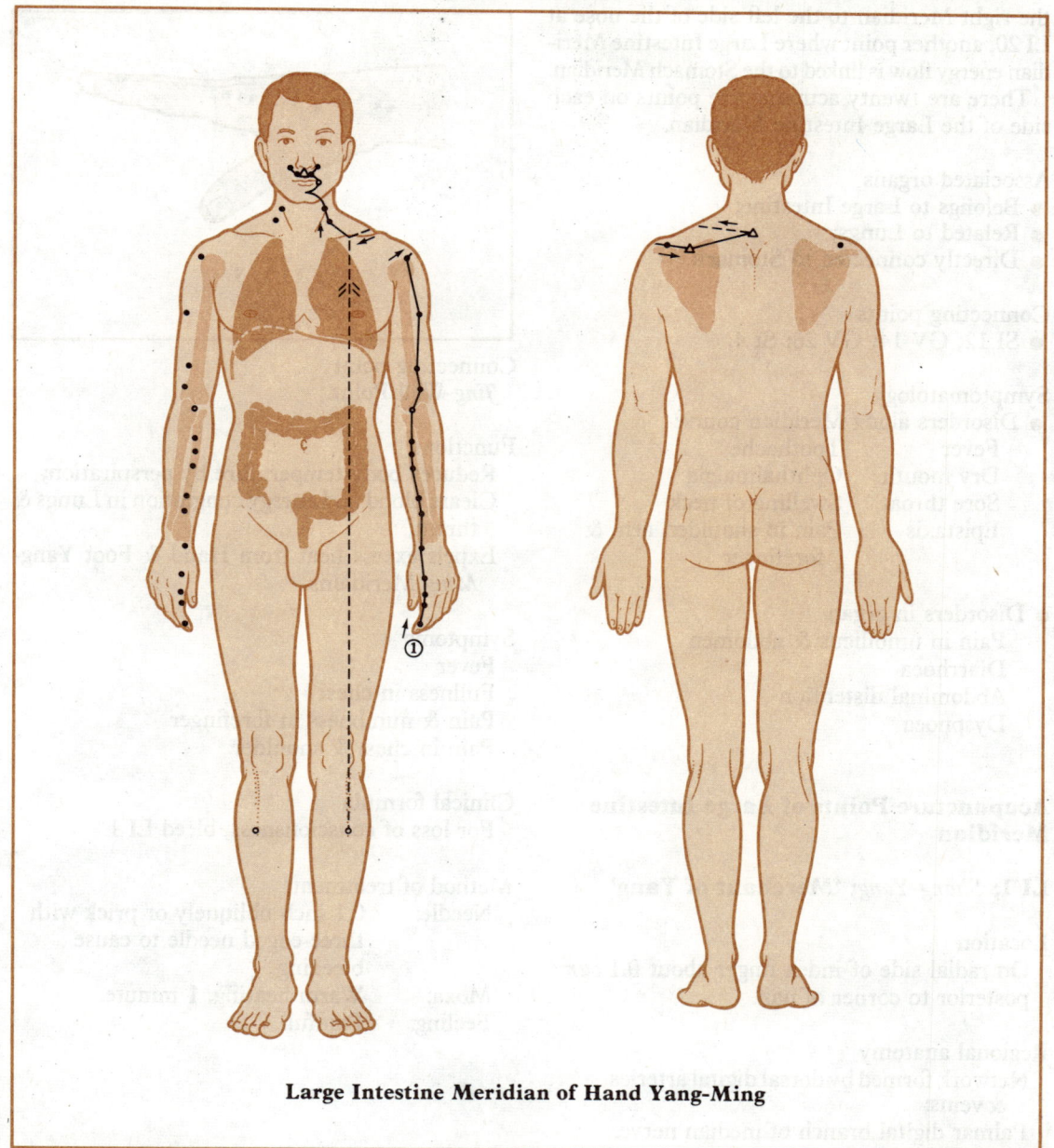

Large Intestine Meridian of Hand Yang-Ming

FOURTEEN MERIDIANS AND ACUPUNCTURE POINTS

the right Meridian to the left side of the nose at LI 20, another point where Large Intestine Meridian energy flow is linked to the Stomach Meridian.

There are twenty acupuncture points on each side of the Large Intestine Meridian.

Associated organs
- Belongs to Large Intestine;
- Related to Lungs;
- Directly connected to Stomach.

Connecting points
- SI 12; GV 14; GV 26; St 4.

Symptomatology
- Disorders along Meridian course
    Fever   Toothache
    Dry mouth   Ophthalmalgia
    Sore throat   Swelling of neck
    Epistaxis   Pain in shoulder, arm & forefinger

- Disorders in organ
    Pain in umbilicus & abdomen
    Diarrhoea
    Abdominal distention
    Dyspnoea

Acupuncture Points of Large Intestine Meridian

LI 1; *Shang-Yang*; 'Merchant of Yang'

Location
  On radial side of index finger about 0.1 *cun* posterior to corner of nail.

Regional anatomy
  Network formed by dorsal digital arteries & veins;
  Palmar digital branch of median nerve.

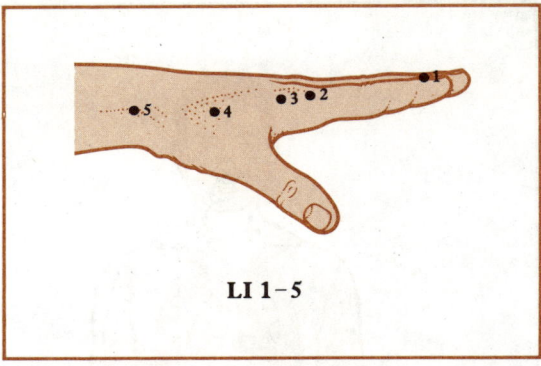

LI 1–5

Connecting point
  Jing-Well Point.

Functions
  Reduces body temperature by perspiration;
  Clears blood and energy congestion in Lungs & throat;
  Expels excess heat from Hand & Foot Yang-*Ming* Meridians.

Symptoms
  Fever
  Fullness in chest
  Pain & numbness in forefinger
  Pain in chest & shoulder

Clinical formula
  For loss of consciousness, bleed LI 1.

Method of treatment
  Needle: 0.1 inch obliquely or prick with three-edged needle to cause bleeding.
  Moxa: Warm heating, 1 minute.
  Feeling: Painful.

FOURTEEN MERIDIANS AND ACUPUNCTURE POINTS

LI 2; *Er-Jian*; 'Second Section'

Location
On radial side of index finger distal to metacarpophalangeal joint, located with finger slightly flexed.

Regional anatomy
Deep & superficial flexor muscles of fingers;
Dorsal & palmar digital arteries, veins & nerves.

Connecting point
Ying-Spring Point.

Functions
Expels excess body heat;
Clears blood and energy obstructions in throat.

Symptoms
Sore throat
Fever
Toothache
Pain in shoulder & back
Epistaxis
Fear

Method of treatment
Needle: 0.2 inch perpendicularly.
Moxa: Warm heating, 1 minute.
Feeling: Ache and/or swelling.

LI 3; *San-Jian*; 'Third Section'

Location
On radial side of index finger in depression superolateral to head of second metacarpal bone.

Regional anatomy
First dorsal interosseous muscle of hand;
Dorsal venous network of hand;
Branch of first dorsal metacarpal artery;
Superficial branch of radial nerve.

Connecting point
Shu-Stream Point.

Functions
Expels excess body heat;
Clears blood & energy obstructions in throat;
Regulates Fu energy flow.

Symptoms
Sore throat
Toothache in lower gum
Ophthalmalgia
Fullness in chest
Pain & swelling in index finger
Drowsiness

Clinical formulae
LI 3 + LI 2 = Drowsiness
LI 3 + SI 2 = Ophthalmalgia

Method of treatment
Needle: 0.3 inch perpendicularly towards ulna.
Moxa: Warm heating, 2 minutes.
Feeling: Ache and/or swelling.

LI 4; *He-Gu*; 'Joining of the Valleys'

Location
On dorsum of hand midway along second metacarpal bone on radial side.

Regional anatomy
First dorsal interosseous muscle of hand;
Adductor muscle of thumb;
Venous network of dorsum of hand;
Superficial branch of radial nerve;
Palmar digital nerve.

FOURTEEN MERIDIANS AND ACUPUNCTURE POINTS

Connecting point
  Yuan-Source Point.

Functions
  Reduces body temperature depending on perspiration;
  Eliminates body wind;
  Clears energy obstruction in Lungs;
  Draws down pathogenic energy in Stomach & Large Intestine.

Symptoms
  Common cold (influenza)   Deafness
  Headache   Facial paralysis
  Migraine   Facial swelling
  Stiff neck   Amenorrhoea
  Toothache   Delayed labour
  Sore throat   Abdominal pain
  Epistaxis   Hidrosis

Clinical formulae
  LI 4 + K 7 = Hidrosis
  LI 4 + St 36 + St 6 + St 7 = Toothache

Method of treatment
  Needle: 0.3 inch perpendicularly.
  Moxa: Warm heating, 2 minutes.
  Feeling: Ache/swelling/heaviness.
  Warning: Experience in needle manipulation is essential to prevent the patient from fainting. No needle or moxa cone is to be used during pregnancy (LI 4 + Sp 6 = miscarriage). Avoid puncturing vein and artery with needle.

Note
This is a major acupuncture point for problems of the face and head, and relieves pain in this region. This is also a sensitive point. The needle sensation not only follows its Meridian energy flow but also spreads in the direction of other Meridians.

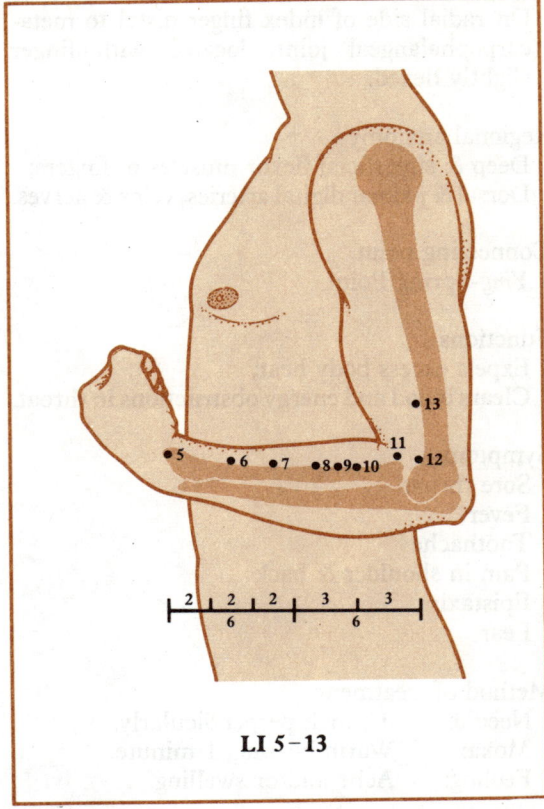

LI 5–13

LI 5; *Yang-Xi*; 'Rivulet of Yang'

Location
  With thumb pointing upwards, point lies in depression between tendons of long and short extensor muscles of thumb.

Regional anatomy
  Tendons of long & short extensor muscles of thumb;
  Cephalic vein;

FOURTEEN MERIDIANS AND ACUPUNCTURE POINTS

Radial artery & dorsal carpal branch;
Superficial branch of radial nerve.

Connecting point
  Jing-River Point.

Functions
  Eliminates body wind & heat;
  Expels excess heat from Yang-*Ming* Meridians.

Symptoms
  Headache   Deafness
  Swelling & pain in eyes Tinnitus aurium
  Sore throat   Wrist pain

Clinical formula
  LI 5 + SI 5 = Swelling & pain in eyes

Method of treatment
  Needle: 0.3 inch perpendicularly.
  Moxa: Warm heating, 2 minutes.
  Feeling: Ache and/or numbness.

LI 6; *Pain-Li*; 'Inclined Passage'

Location
  3 *cun* above LI 5 (The distance from LI 5 to LI 11 is 12 *cun*.)

Regional anatomy
  Tendon of short radial extensor muscle of wrist;
  Long abductor muscle of thumb;
  Cephalic vein;
  Lateral cutaneous nerve of forearm;
  Superficial branch of radial nerve;
  Posterior cutaneous nerve of forearm;
  Posterior interosseous nerve of forearm.

Connecting point
  Luo-Connecting Point transverse to *Tai*-Yin Meridian.

Functions
  Clears Lung energy flow;
  Regulates water metabolism;
  Frees *Luo* Meridian energy flow.

Symptoms
  Pain in shoulder, arm,   Epistaxis
    forearm & wrist   Dry throat
  Toothache   Restlessness

Method of treatment
  Needle: 0.3 inch obliquely.
  Moxa: Warm heating, 2 minutes.
  Feeling: Ache and/or swelling.

LI 7; *Wen-Liu*; 'Warm Current'

Location
  5 *cun* above LI 5.

Regional anatomy
  Short radial extensor muscle of wrist;
  Long abductor muscle of thumb;
  Radial artery;
  Cephalic vein;
  Posterior cutaneous nerve of forearm;
  Radial nerve.

Connecting point
  Xi-Cleft Point.

Functions
  Expels excess body heat;
  Balances function of Stomach & Large Intestine.

Symptoms
  Abdominal pain   Ache & pain in upper limbs
  Headache   Mania

Method of treatment
  Needle: 0.3 inch obliquely.

Moxa: Warm heating, 2 minutes.
Feeling: Ache and/or swelling.

LI 8; *Xia-Lian*; 'Inferior Region'

Location
4 *cun* below LI 11.

Regional anatomy
Short radial extensor muscle of wrist;
Long abductor muscle of thumb;
Radial artery;
Cephalic vein;
Posterior cutaneous nerve of forearm;
Radial nerve.

Symptoms
Abdominal pain
Pain in elbow & forearm
Restlessness
Shortness of breath

Method of treatment
Needle: 0.5 inch obliquely.
Moxa: Warm heating, 3 minutes.
Feeling: Ache and/or needle sensation towards index finger.

LI 9; *Shang-Lian*; 'Superior Region'

Location
3 *cun* below to LI 11.

Regional anatomy
Short radial extensor muscle of wrist;
Long abductor muscle of thumb;
Radial artery;
Cephalic vein;
Posterior cutaneous nerve of forearm;
Radial nerve.

Symptoms
Hemiplegia
Headache
Shortness of breath
Ache & pain in arm, elbow & forearm

Method of treatment
Needle: 0.5 inch obliquely.
Moxa: Warm heating, 3 minutes.
Feeling: Ache and/or needle sensation towards both elbow and index finger.

LI 10; *Shou-San-Li*; 'Three Mile Arm'

Location
2 *cun* below LI 11.

Regional anatomy
Short radial extensor muscle of wrist;
Long abductor muscle of thumb;
Cephalic vein;
Branches of radial recurrent artery & vein;
Radial artery;
Posterior cutaneous nerve of forearm;
Radial nerve.

Functions
Eliminates body wind;
Frees *Luo* Meridian energy flow;
Balances Stomach & Large Intestine functions.

Symptoms
Hemiplegia
Muscle spasm in elbow
Pain in shoulder, arm & finger
Toothache

Method of treatment
Needle: 0.2 inch perpendicularly.
Moxa: Warm heating, 3 minutes.
Feeling: Ache/heaviness/numbness;

FOURTEEN MERIDIANS AND ACUPUNCTURE POINTS

needle sensation moves towards forearm and finger, and also upwards towards elbow.

Note
This is the major acupuncture point for relieving pain in the shoulder, arm, elbow, forearm and fingers.

LI 11; *Qu-Chi*; 'Crooked Pond'

Location
With arm bent at 90°, point lies at lateral end of transverse cubital crease midway between Lu 5 and lateral epicondyle of humerus.

Regional anatomy
Elbow joint;
Long radial extensor muscle of wrist;
Brachioradial muscle;
Branches of radial recurrent artery & vein;
Posterior cutaneous nerve of forearm;
Radial nerve.

Connecting point
He-Sea Point.

Functions
Expels excess body heat;
Eliminates body wind & damp;
Frees blood & energy circulation in joints;
Balances blood & energy flows.

Symptoms
Pain in shoulder, arm, forearm & fingers	Dry skin
Fever	Eczema
Fullness in chest	Urticaria
Hemiplegia	Abdominal pain
	Amenorrhoea

Clinical formulae
LI 11 + St 36 + GV 10 = Urticaria
LI 11 + St 36 + K 7 = Fever

Method of treatment
Needle: 0.5 inch perpendicularly with arm bent to 90° before insertion.
Moxa: Warm heating, 3 minutes.
Feeling: Ache/heaviness/numbness; needle sensation moves towards forearm and index finger.
Warning: Arm movement must be avoided after insertion.

LI 12; *Zhou-Liao*; 'Elbow Bone'

Location
With elbow flexed, point lies 1 *cun* superolateral to LI 11 on medial border of humerus.

Regional anatomy
Brachial muscle;
Triceps muscle of arm;
Radial collateral artery & vein;
Posterior cutaneous nerve of forearm;
Radial nerve.

Symptoms
Pain in arm & elbow
Drowsiness

Method of treatment
Needle: 0.3 inch obliquely towards LI 13.
Moxa: Warm heating, 3 minutes.
Feeling: Ache and/or swelling.

LI 13; *Shou-Wu-Li*; 'Five Mile Arm'

Location
3 *cun* above LI 11 on line connecting LI 11

FOURTEEN MERIDIANS AND ACUPUNCTURE POINTS

& LI 15.

Regional anatomy
Brachioradial muscle;
Triceps muscle of arm;
Radial collateral artery & vein;
Posterior cutaneous nerve of forearm;
Radial nerve.

Symptoms
Pain in arm & elbow   Fear
Drowsiness   Fullness in chest

Method of treatment
Needle: **Forbidden.**
Moxa: Warm heating, 3 minutes.
Warning: Only moxibustion or massage is to be used.

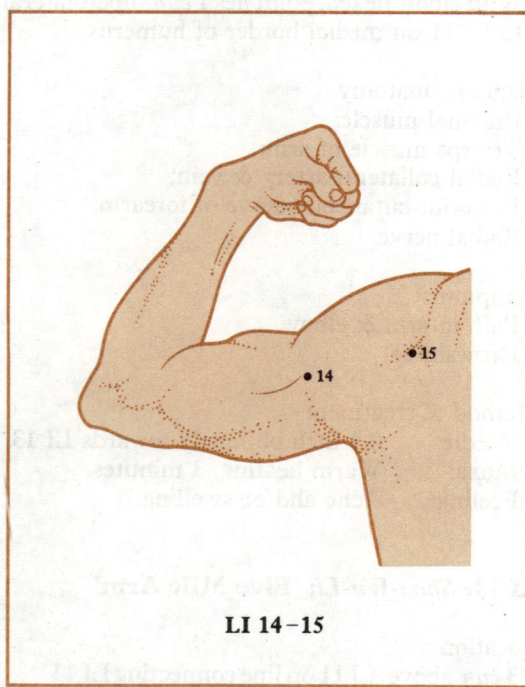

LI 14–15

LI 14; *Bi-Nao*; 'Hollow of the Arm'

Location
7 *cun* above LI 11.

Regional anatomy
Deltoid muscle;
Triceps muscle of arm;
Branches of posterior circumflex humeral artery & vein;
Deep brachial artery & vein;
Posterior cutaneous nerve of arm;
Radial nerve.

Connecting points
Meeting Point of Hand Yang-*Ming* & *Luo* Meridians;
Meeting Point of Hand & Foot *Tai*-Yang & Yang-*Wei* Meridians.

Symptoms
Pain in shoulder & arm

Method of treatment
Needle: 0.3 inch perpendicularly.
Moxa: Warm heating, 3 minutes.
Feeling: Ache and/or swelling.
Warning: As it is dangerous to insert a needle perpendicularly more than 0.3 inch at this point, it is mainly suitable for moxa. However, if a needle is used, experience in needle manipulation is essential for correct depth and direction.

Note
This point has been used for lung operations under acupuncture anaesthesia.

FOURTEEN MERIDIANS AND ACUPUNCTURE POINTS

LI 15; *Jian-Yu*; 'Depression of Shoulder'

Location
With arm in passive abduction, two depressions appear at anterior border of acromioclavicular joint; point lies in anterior depression in middle of upper part of deltoid muscle.

Regional anatomy
Deltoid muscle;
Posterior circumflex artery & vein;
Lateral supraclavicular nerve & axillary nerve.

Connecting point
Meeting Point of Hand Yang-*Ming* & Yang-*Qiao* Meridians.

Functions
Eliminates wind & damp in *Jing-Luo*;
Expels excess heat in Yang-*Ming* Meridians;
Frees energy obstruction in shoulder joints.

Symptoms
Pain in shoulder & arm
Hemiplegia

Clinical formula
LI 15 + LI 11 + GB 21 + SI 11 = Frozen shoulder

Method of treatment
Needle: 0.6 inch obliquely.
Moxa: Warm heating, 3 minutes.
Feeling: Ache.

LI 16; *Ju-Gu*; 'Large Bone'

Location
On upper posterior aspect of shoulder, in depression between acromial extremity of clavicle and scapular spine.

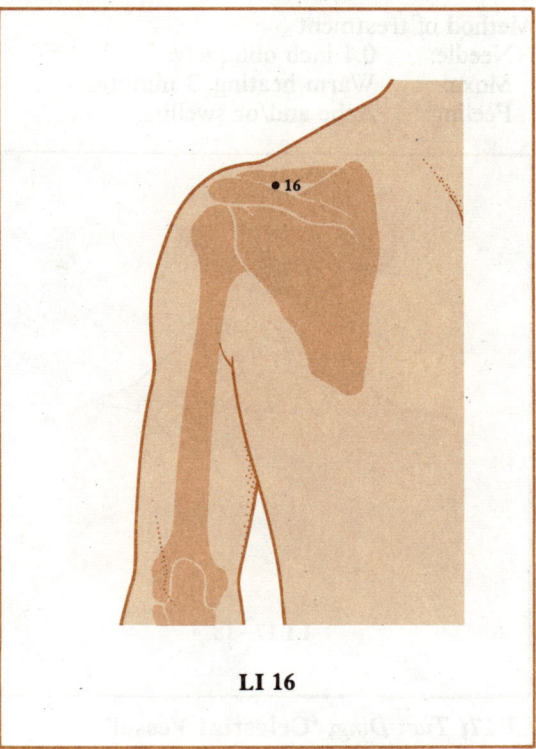

LI 16

Regional anatomy
Trapezius muscle;
Supraspinous muscle;
Suprascapular artery & vein;
Lateral supraclavicular nerve;
Branch of accessory nerve;
Suprascapular nerve.

Connecting point
Meeting Point of Hand Yang-*Ming* & Yang-*Qiao* Meridians.

Symptoms
Pain in shoulder & arm
Blood congestion in chest
Fear

FOURTEEN MERIDIANS AND ACUPUNCTURE POINTS

Method of treatment
  Needle: 0.4 inch obliquely.
  Moxa: Warm heating, 3 minutes.
  Feeling: Ache and/or swelling.

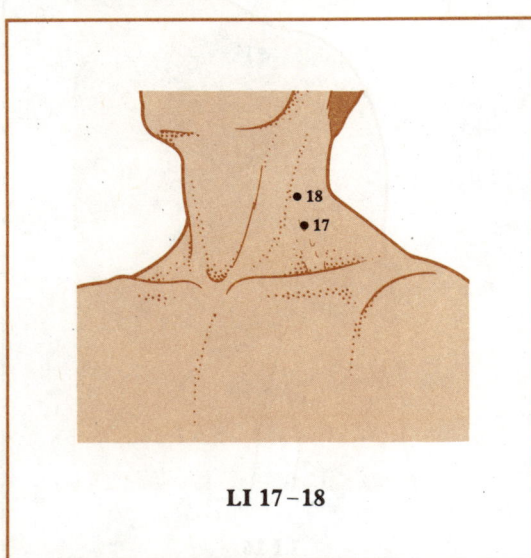

LI 17−18

LI 17; *Tian-Ding*; 'Celestial Vessel'

Location
  1 *cun* inferior to LI 18 on posterior border of sternocleidomastoid muscle.

Regional anatomy
  Sternocleidomastoid muscle;
  Platysma muscle;
  Middle scalene muscle;
  External jugular vein;
  Supraclavicular nerve;
  Cutaneous cervical nerve;
  Phrenic nerve.

Functions
  Frees blood & energy obstructions in throat;
  Clears Lung energy flow.

Symptoms
  Sore throat
  Hoarse voice

Clinical formula
  LI 17 + LI 4 + CV 24 + K 3 = Loss of voice

Method of treatment
  Needle: 0.3 inch perpendicularly.
  Moxa: Warm heating, 2 minutes.
  Feeling: Ache and/or swelling.
  Warning: Do not insert needle too deeply. Experience in needle technique is essential.

LI 18; *Shui-Xue (Fu-Tu)*; 'Water Point'

Location
  On lateral side of neck at level of tip of thyroid cartilage (Adam's apple) between sternal and clavicular heads of sternocleidomastoid muscle.

Regional anatomy
  Sternocleidomastoid muscle;
  Platysma muscle;
  Levator muscle of scapula;
  Ascending cervical artery & vein;
  Great auricular nerve;
  Cutaneous cervical nerve;
  Lesser occipital nerve;
  Accessory nerve.

Symptoms
  Coughing   Sore throat
  Shortness of breath   Hoarse voice

Method of treatment
  Needle: 0.3 inch perpendicularly.
  Moxa: Warm heating, 2 minutes.
  Feeling: Ache and/or heaviness.
  Warning: Do not insert needle too deeply.

FOURTEEN MERIDIANS AND ACUPUNCTURE POINTS

Experience in needle technique is essential.

Note
This point has been used for thyroidectomies under acupuncture anaesthesia.

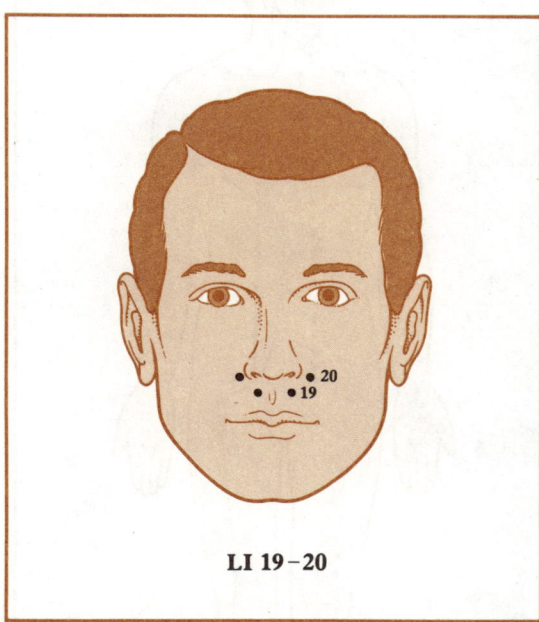

LI 19–20

LI 19; *He-Liao*; 'Small Bone'

Location
  Directly inferior to lateral margin of nostril.

Regional anatomy
  Levator muscle of upper lip;
  Superior labial branches of facial artery & vein;
  Anastomotic branch of facial nerve;
  Infraorbital nerve.

Symptoms
  Epistaxis   Facial paralysis
  Nasal obstruction

Method of treatment
  Needle: 0.2 inch obliquely.
  Moxa: **Forbidden.**
  Feeling: Painful.
  Warning: Needle insertion readily causes tears and a runny nose.

LI 20; *Ying-Xiang*; 'Welcome Fragrance'

Location
  In nasolabial groove at midpoint of lateral border of ala nasi.

Regional anatomy
  Levator muscle of upper lip;
  Facial artery & vein;
  Branches of infraorbital artery & vein;
  Anastomotic branch of facial & infraorbital nerve.

Connecting point
  Meeting point of Hand & Foot Yang-*Ming* Meridians.

Functions
  Clears congestion in nose;
  Dispels wind & heat.

Symptoms
  Nasal obstruction   Epistaxis
  Facial paralysis   Itching & facial swelling

Clinical formula
  LI 20 + Bl 5 + GV 23 = Nasal obstruction

Method of treatment
  Needle: 0.3 inch obliquely.
  Moxa: **Forbidden.**
  Feeling: Painful.
  Warning: Needle insertion readily causes tears and a runny nose.

FOURTEEN MERIDIANS AND ACUPUNCTURE POINTS

3. Stomach Meridian of Foot Yang-Ming

This Meridian is characterized by high energy and high blood flows. The energy flow originates at St 1 under the eyeball, receives energy from the Large Intestine Meridian at LI 20 before ascending to Bl 1, then descends again to the lateral side of the nose to enter the upper gum, GV 26. Curving around the lip, it meets CV 24 at the mentolabial groove, crosses the lower part of the cheek to St 5 and across to St 6, then ascends to the front of the ear. It passes over GB 3, GB 4 and GB 6; after reaching the forehead at St 8, it connects with the Governor Vessel Meridian at GV 24.

From St 5 the Main Meridian continues up to St 9, where it gives off two branches. One branch proceeds along the throat, enters the supraclavicular fossa and descends through the diaphragm where, deep inside, it meets CV 12 and CV 13; it then connects with the Stomach and Spleen which are organs related to this Meridian. The other branch descends to St 30 on the lateral side of the lower abdomen where both the inner and superficial Meridians meet.

At St 30 the energy flows directly down to St 36 where it again divides into two branches; one descends to the second toe, St 45, while the other runs to the lateral side of the middle toe. The Stomach Meridian continues on from St 42 to terminate finally at the medial side of the tip of the great toe, where its energy flow links with the Spleen Meridian.

There are forty-five acupuncture points on each side of the Stomach Meridian.

Associated organs
- Belongs to Stomach;
- Related to Spleen;
- Directly connected to Heart, and Large and Small Intestines.

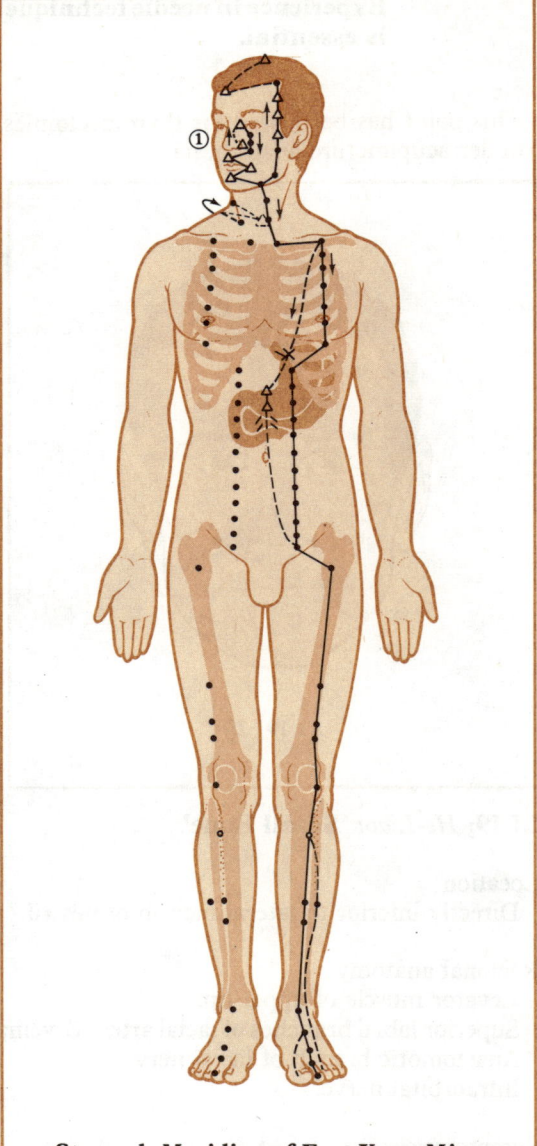

Stomach Meridian of Foot Yang-Ming

FOURTEEN MERIDIANS AND ACUPUNCTURE POINTS

Connecting points
　LI 20　Bl 1　GB 3　GB 4　GB 6　GV 14　GV 24
　GV 26　CV 12　CV 13　CV 24

Symptomatology
- Disorders along Meridian course
　　Fever　　　　　　Aphtha
　　Red complexion　Sore throat
　　Coma　　　　　　Swelling of neck
　　Mania　　　　　　Facial paralysis
　　Ophthalmalgia　　Pain in chest, legs
　　Dry nose　　　　　& feet
　　Epistaxis　　　　Cold feet

- Disorders in organ
　　Abdominal distention　Insomnia
　　Oedema　　　　　　　Indigestion

Acupuncture Points of Stomach Meridian

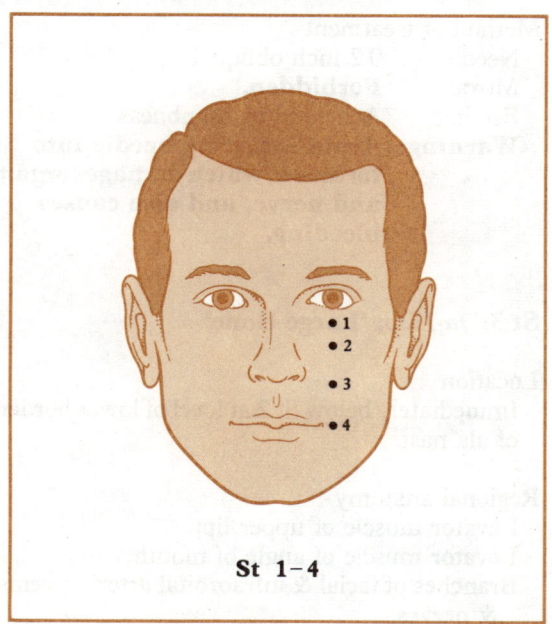

St 1-4

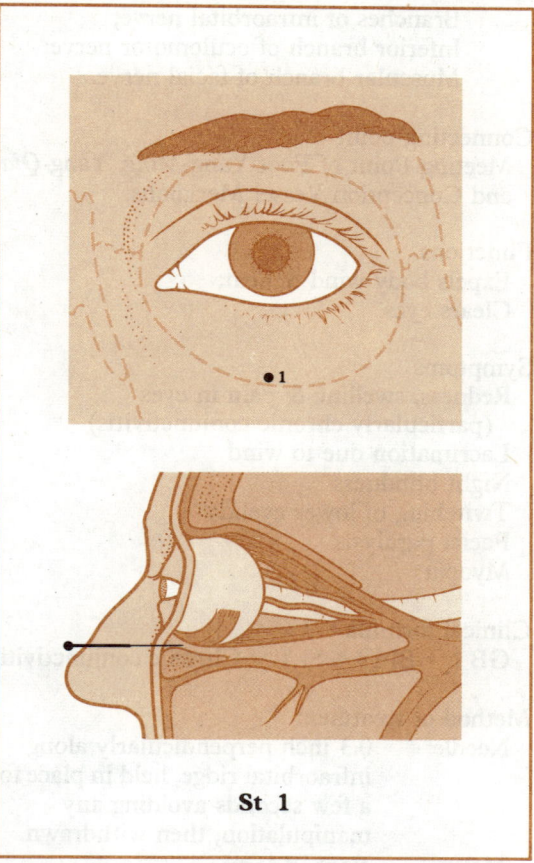

St 1

St 1; *Cheng-Qi*; **'Vase of Tears'**

Location
　Between eyeball and midpoint of infraorbital ridge.

Regional anatomy
　Orbicular muscle of eye (palpebral part);
　Inferior rectus muscle of eyeball;
　Inferior oblique muscle of eyeball;
　Branches of infraorbital & ophthalmic arteries
　　& veins;

Branches of infraorbital nerve;
Inferior branch of oculomotor nerve;
Muscular branch of facial nerve.

Connecting point
Meeting Point of Foot Yang-*Ming*, Yang-*Qiao* and Conception Vessel Meridians.

Functions
Expels body wind & heat;
Clears eyes.

Symptoms
Redness, swelling & pain in eyes (particularly chronic conjunctivitis)
Lacrimation due to wind
Night blindness
Twitching of lower eyelids
Facial paralysis
Myopia

Clinical formula
GB 1 + Bl 18 + St 1 = Chronic conjunctivitis

Method of treatment
Needle: 0.3 inch perpendicularly along infraorbital ridge, held in place for a few seconds avoiding any manipulation, then withdrawn.
Moxa: **Forbidden.**
Feeling: Ache/swelling/heaviness of eyes.
Warning: Experience and great care are essential for needling as bleeding is easily caused and the organ can be damaged. It is dangerous to retain the needle in this point for more than a few seconds.

St 2; *Si-Bai*; **'Four White Colours'**

Location
1 *cun* inferior to St 1 in depression of infraorbital foramen.

Regional anatomy
Orbicular muscle of eye (palpebral part);
Levator muscle of upper lip;
Branches of facial arteries, veins & nerves;
Infraorbital artery, vein & nerve.

Symptoms
Headache   Trigeminal neuralgia
Dizziness   Facial paralysis
Redness & pain in eyes

Clinical formula
St 2 + Bl 2 + GB 3 + St 7 + St 6 + St 36 = Trigeminal neuralgia

Method of treatment
Needle: 0.2 inch obliquely.
Moxa: **Forbidden.**
Feeling: Ache and/or numbness.
Warning: Avoid inserting needle into foramen, which damages organ and nerve, and also causes bleeding.

St 3; *Ju-Liao*; **'Large Bone'**

Location
Immediately below St 2 at level of lower border of ala nasi.

Regional anatomy
Levator muscle of upper lip;
Levator muscle of angle of mouth;
Branches of facial & infraorbital arteries, veins & nerves.

FOURTEEN MERIDIANS AND ACUPUNCTURE POINTS

Connecting point
  Meeting Point of Hand & Foot Yang-*Ming* Meridians & Yang-*Qiao* Meridian.

Symptoms
  Facial paralysis   Lip & cheek swelling
  Blurred vision   Trigeminal neuralgia

Clinical formula
  St 3 + SI 16 = Pain & swelling of cheek

Method of treatment
  Needle: 0.3 inch obliquely upwards.
  Moxa: Warm heating, 2 minutes.
  Feeling: Swelling and/or numbness.

St 4; *Di-Cang*; 'Earth Granary'

Location
  Immediately below St 3 lateral to corner of mouth.

Regional anatomy
  Orbicular muscle of mouth;
  Buccinator muscle;
  Facial artery & vein;
  Branches of facial & infraorbital nerves;
  Terminal branch of buccal nerve.

Connecting point
  Meeting Point of Hand & Foot Yang-*Ming* Meridians & Yang-*Qiao* Meridian.

Functions
  Expels pathogenic wind;
  Adjusts energy flow;
  Frees energy obstruction in joints.

Symptoms
  Facial paralysis   Aphasia
  Blurred vision   Trigeminal neuralgia

Clinical formula
  St 4 + St 5 + TH 17 + SI 19 + LI 4 + GV 26 = Facial paralysis

Method of treatment
  Needle: 0.3 inch obliquely with needle directed towards St 6.
  Moxa: Warm heating, 2 minutes.
  Feeling: Swelling and/or numbness.

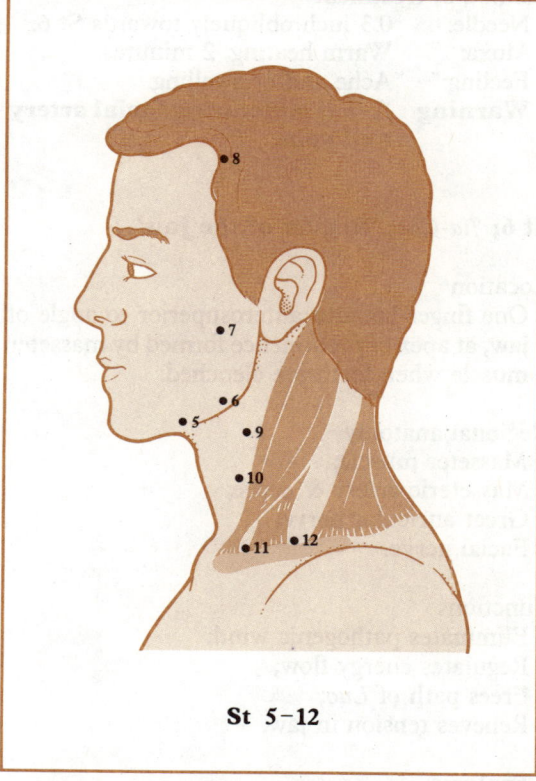

St 5–12

St 5; *Da-Ying*; 'Big Welcome'

Location
  0.5 *cun* in front of St 6, anterior to angle of mandible on anterior border of masseter muscle.

FOURTEEN MERIDIANS AND ACUPUNCTURE POINTS

Regional anatomy
 Anterior border of masseter muscle;
 Facial artery & vein;
 Facial & buccal nerves.

Symptoms
 Swollen cheek   Facial paralysis
 Trismus   Toothache

Method of treatment
 Needle: 0.3 inch obliquely towards St 6.
 Moxa: Warm heating, 2 minutes.
 Feeling: Ache and/or swelling.
 Warning: Avoid puncturing facial artery and vein.

St 6; *Jia-Che*; 'Region of the Jaw'

Location
 One finger-breadth anterosuperior to angle of jaw, at apex of prominence formed by masseter muscle when teeth are clenched.

Regional anatomy
 Masseter muscle;
 Masseteric artery & nerve;
 Great auricular nerve;
 Facial nerve.

Functions
 Eliminates pathogenic wind;
 Regulates energy flow;
 Frees path of *Luo*;
 Relieves tension in jaw.

Symptoms
 Trismus   Cheek swelling
 Facial paralysis   Stiff neck
 Toothache

Method of treatment
 Needle: 0.3 inch obliquely towards St 5.
 Moxa: Warm heating, 3 minutes.
 Feeling: Ache and/or swelling.
 Warning: Avoid puncturing facial artery and vein.

St 7; *Xia-Guan*; 'Lower Gate'

Location
 With mouth closed, point lies at lower border of zygomatic arch, anterior to condyloid process of mandible.

Regional anatomy
 Parotid gland;
 Masseter muscle;
 Transverse facial artery & vein;
 Maxillary artery & vein;
 Zygomatic branch of facial nerve;
 Branch of auriculotemporal nerve.

Connecting point
 Meeting Point of Foot Yang-*Ming* & Hand *Shao*-Yang Meridians.

Symptoms
 Facial paralysis   Trigeminal neuralgia
 Dislocation of jaw Tinnitus aurium

Method of treatment
 Needle: 0.3 inch perpendicularly.
 Moxa: **Forbidden.**
 Feeling: Ache and/or numbness.
 Warning: The mouth must be closed during needling.

St 8; *Tou-Wei*; 'Preservation of the Head'

FOURTEEN MERIDIANS AND ACUPUNCTURE POINTS

Location
  At superolateral corner of forehead, 0.5 *cun* within hairline.

Regional anatomy
  Temporal muscle;
  Frontal branches of superficial temporal artery & vein;
  Branch of auriculotemporal nerve;
  Temporal branch of facial nerve.

Connecting point
  Meeting Point of Foot Yang-*Ming* & Hand *Shao*-Yang Meridians, connected by a path to GV 24.

Functions
  Dispels wind & heat;
  Relieves pain in head;
  Clears eyes.

Symptoms
  Headache   Blurred vision
  Ophthalmalgia   Lacrimation caused by wind

Clinical formulae
  St 8 + *Tai*-Yang + LI 4 + GV 20 + GV 24 = Headache; St 8 + Pc 7 = Ophthalmalgia

Method of treatment
  Needle: 0.3 inch horizontally.
  Moxa: **Forbidden.**
  Feeling: Pain and/or swelling.

St 9; *Ren-Ying*; **'Man Welcome'**

Location
  At medial border of sternocleidomastoid muscle, level with tip of thyroid cartilage (Adam's apple), just on course of common carotid artery.

Regional anatomy
  Platysma muscle;
  Sternocleidomastoid muscle;
  Superior thyroid artery;
  External & internal jugular veins;
  Bifurcation of internal & external carotid arteries;
  Cutaneous cervical nerve;
  Cervical branch of facial nerve;
  Sympathetic trunk;
  Descending branch of hypoglossal nerve;
  Vagus nerve.

Connecting point
  Meeting Point of Foot Yang-*Ming* & Hand *Shao*-Yang Meridians.

Symptoms
  Dyspnoea   Throat swelling
  Fullness in chest

Method of treatment
  Needle: 0.3 inch perpendicularly.
  Moxa: **Forbidden.**
  Feeling: Ache and/or swelling.
  Warning: Experience is essential for needle insertion at this point.

Note
This point gives the pulse of the internal organs and is always used for comparison with the pulse of the radial artery.

This energy point is often used for strengthening energy flow and balancing energy of the face and head. Massage is better than the needle at this point.

The ancient Chinese philosophers always forbade use of the needle at this point because, if punctured too deeply, the patient can die. However, with experience and an understanding of anatomy, needling can be quite safe.

FOURTEEN MERIDIANS AND ACUPUNCTURE POINTS

St 10; *Shui-Men (Shui-Tu)*; 'Water Gate'

Location
Midway between St 9 and St 11 at anterior border of sternocleidomastoid muscle.

Regional anatomy
Platysma muscle;
Sternocleidomastoid muscle;
Omohyoid muscle;
Common carotid artery;
Cutaneous cervical nerve;
Superior cardiac nerve issuing from sympathetic nerve & trunk.

Symptoms
Dyspnoea
Throat swelling
Shortness of breath

Method of treatment
Needle: 0.3 inch perpendicularly.
Moxa: Warm heating, 2 minutes.
Feeling: Ache and/or swelling.
Warning: Avoid puncturing the common carotid artery.

St 11; *Qi-She*; 'Place of Energy'

Location
At superior border of sternal end of clavicle between the two heads of sternocleidomastoid muscle.

Regional anatomy
Platysma muscle;
Sternocleidomastoid muscle;
External jugular vein;
Common carotid artery;
Medial supraclavicular nerve;
Muscular branch of ansa hypoglossi.

Symptoms
Stiff neck
Throat swelling
Shortness of breath
Coughing

Method of treatment
Needle: 0.3 inch perpendicularly.
Moxa: Warm heating, 2 minutes.
Feeling: Ache and/or swelling.
Warning: Avoid inserting needle too deeply.

St 12; *Que-Pen*; 'Small Bowl'

Location
Midpoint of supraclavicular fossa.

Regional anatomy
Platysma muscle;
Omohyoid muscle;
Transverse cervical artery;
Intermediate supraclavicular nerve;
Supraclavicular portion of brachial network;
Pleural cupola;
Apex of lung.

Symptoms
Fullness in chest
Shortness of breath
Pain in supraclavicular fossa

Method of treatment
Needle: 0.2 inch perpendicularly.
Moxa: Warm heating, 2 minutes.
Feeling: Ache and/or swelling.
Warning: Puncturing too deeply at this point damages the lung and leads to difficulty in breathing. Correct needling comes with experience. Needling in pregnancy is forbidden.

FOURTEEN MERIDIANS AND ACUPUNCTURE POINTS

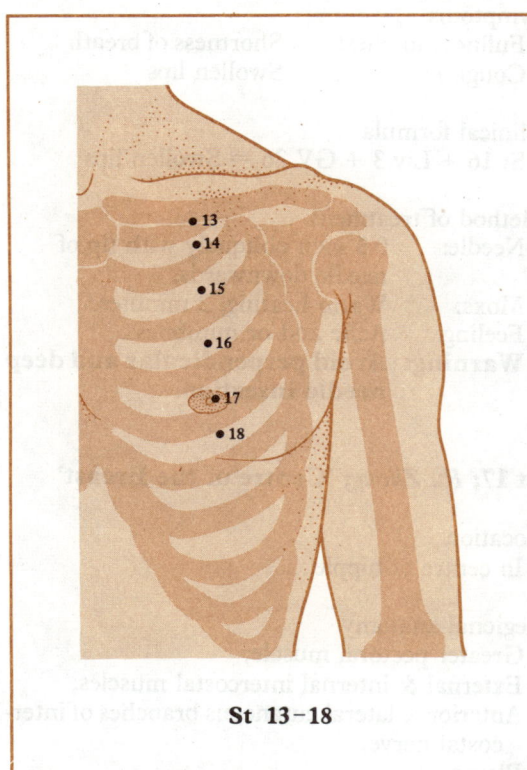

St 13-18

St 13; *Qi-Hu*; 'Home of Energy'

Location
  Below clavicle on mammillary line.

Regional anatomy
  Greater pectoral muscle;
  Subclavius muscle;
  Branches of thoracoacromial artery & vein;
  Subclavicular vein;
  Branches of supraclavicular nerve;
  Anterior thoracic nerve;
  Pleural cupola;
  Apex of lung.

Symptoms
  Coughing   Fullness in chest
  Shortness of breath   Pain in chest & back

Method of treatment
  Needle: 0.3 inch obliquely.
  Moxa: Warm heating, 2 minutes.
  Feeling: Ache and/or swelling.
  Warning: When inserting needles in intercostal spaces, particularly between true ribs, care must be taken with needle direction and depth to avoid penetration of vital viscera.

St 14; *Ku-Fang*; 'Store Room'

Location
  In first intercostal space on mammillary line.

Regional anatomy
  Greater & smaller pectoral muscles;
  External & internal intercostal muscles;
  Thoracoacromial artery & vein;
  Branches of lateral thoracic artery & vein;
  Branch of anterior thoracic nerve;
  Pleura;
  Lungs.

Symptoms
  Fullness in chest   Coughing
  Shortness of breath

Method of treatment
  Needle: 0.3 inch obliquely with tip of needle downwards.
  Moxa: Warm heating, 2 minutes.
  Feeling: Ache and/or numbness.
  Warning: Avoid perpendicular and deep needle insertion.

FOURTEEN MERIDIANS AND ACUPUNCTURE POINTS

St 15; *Wu-yi*; 'House of the Nebula'

Location
  In second intercostal space on mammillary line.

Regional anatomy
  Greater & smaller pectoral muscles;
  External & internal intercostal muscles;
  Thoracoacromial artery & vein;
  Branches of lateral thoracic artery & vein;
  Branch of anterior thoracic nerve;
  Pleura;
  Lungs.

Symptoms
  Coughing
  Dyspnoea
  General body swelling (oedema)

Method of treatment
  Needle: 0.3 inch obliquely with tip of needle downwards.
  Moxa: Warm heating, 2 minutes.
  Feeling: Ache and/or numbness.
  Warning: Avoid perpendicular and deep needle insertion.

St 16; *Ying-Chuang*; 'Breast Window'

Location
  In third intercostal space on mammillary line.

Regional anatomy
  Greater pectoral muscle;
  External & internal intercostal muscles;
  Lateral thoracic artery & vein;
  Branch of anterior thoracic nerve;
  Pleura;
  Lungs.

Symptoms
  Fullness in chest   Shortness of breath
  Coughing   Swollen lips

Clinical formula
  St 16 + Liv 3 + GV 26 = Swollen lips

Method of treatment
  Needle: 0.3 inch obliquely with tip of needle downwards.
  Moxa: Warm heating, 2 minutes.
  Feeling: Ache and/or numbness.
  Warning: Avoid perpendicular and deep needle insertion.

St 17; *Ru-Zhong*; 'Centre of the Breast'

Location
  In centre of nipple.

Regional anatomy
  Greater pectoral muscle;
  External & internal intercostal muscles;
  Anterior & lateral cutaneous branches of intercostal nerve;
  Pleura;
  Lungs.

• **Acupuncture and moxibustion are both forbidden at this point.**

St 18; *Ru-Gen*; 'Breast Root'

Location
  In fifth intercostal space on mammillary line.

Regional anatomy
  Greater pectoral muscle;
  External & internal intercostal muscles;
  Branches of intercostal artery & vein;

FOURTEEN MERIDIANS AND ACUPUNCTURE POINTS

Branch of intercostal nerve;
Pleura;
Lungs.

Symptoms
Fullness & pain in chest   Shortness of breath
Coughing   Lactation deficiency

Clinical formula
St 18 + CV 17 + SI 1 = Lactation deficiency

Method of treatment
Needle: 0.3 inch obliquely with tip of needle upwards.
Moxa: Warm heating, 2 minutes.
Feeling: Ache and/or swelling.
Warning: Do not puncture perpendicularly or too deeply. Do not overheat with moxa.

St 19; *Bu-Rong*; 'No Admittance'

Location
2 *cun* lateral to CV 14 and 6 *cun* above umbilicus.

Regional anatomy
Anterior layer of rectus sheath;
Rectus muscle of abdomen;
Transverse muscle of abdomen;
Peritoneum;
Branches of intercostal artery, vein & nerve;
Branches of superior epigastric artery & vein;
Stomach;
Liver.

Symptoms
Abdominal distention   Loss of appetite
Vomiting   Pain in chest & back
Gastric pain

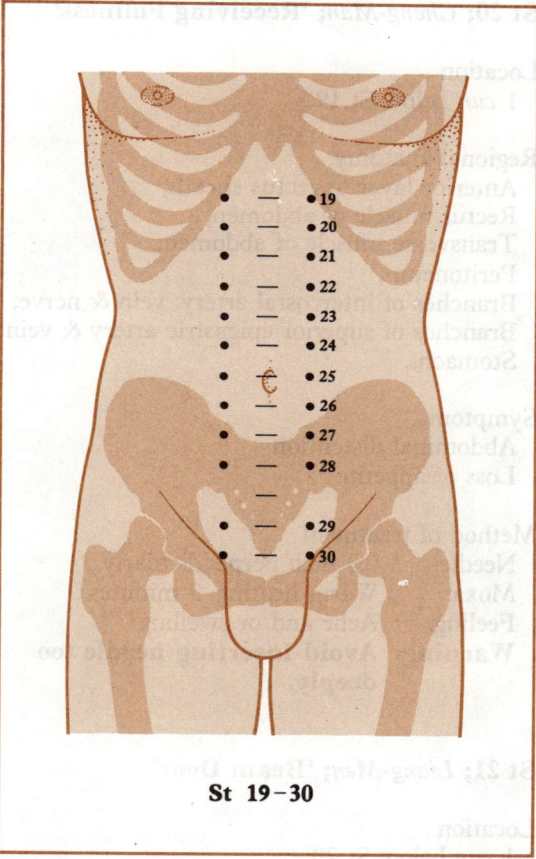

St 19–30

Clinical formula
St 19 + CV 12 + Pc 6 = Vomiting

Method of treatment
Needle: 0.4 inch perpendicularly.
Moxa: Warm heating, 2 minutes.
Feeling: Ache and/or swelling.
Warning: Avoid inserting needle too deeply.

FOURTEEN MERIDIANS AND ACUPUNCTURE POINTS

St 20; *Cheng-Man*; 'Receiving Fullness'

Location
  1 *cun* below St 19.

Regional anatomy
  Anterior layer of rectus sheath;
  Rectus muscle of abdomen;
  Transverse muscle of abdomen;
  Peritoneum;
  Branches of intercostal artery, vein & nerve;
  Branches of superior epigastric artery & vein;
  Stomach.

Symptoms
  Abdominal distention
  Loss of appetite

Method of treatment
  Needle: 0.3 inch perpendicularly.
  Moxa: Warm heating, 2 minutes.
  Feeling: Ache and/or swelling.
  Warning: Avoid inserting needle too deeply.

St 21; *Liang-Men*; 'Beam Door'

Location
  1 *cun* below St 20.

Regional anatomy
  Anterior layer of rectus sheath;
  Rectus muscle of abdomen;
  Transverse muscle of abdomen;
  Peritoneum;
  Branches of intercostal & superior epigastric arteries & veins;
  Branch of intercostal nerve;
  Duodenum;
  Stomach.

Functions
  Regulates energy flow;
  Balances Stomach & Intestine functions;
  Increases digestion.

Symptoms
  Indigestion   Abdominal distention
  Loss of appetite   Loose stools

Method of treatment
  Needle: 0.3 inch perpendicularly.
  Moxa: Warm heating, 2 minutes.
  Feeling: Ache and/or swelling.
  Warning: Pregnant women must not be treated with moxibustion/moxa cones.

St 22; *Guan-Men*; 'Closed Door'

Location
  1 *cun* below St 21.

Regional anatomy
  Rectus sheath;
  Rectus muscle of abdomen;
  Peritoneum;
  Branches of intercostal & superior epigastric arteries & veins;
  Branch of intercostal nerve;
  Transverse colon.

Symptoms
  Abdominal pain   Oedema
  Indigestion   Enuresis
  Diarrhoea

Clinical formula
  St 22 + Lu 1 + H 7 = Enuresis

Method of treatment
  Needle: 0.5 inch perpendicularly.

Moxa: Warm heating, 2 minutes.
Feeling: Ache and/or swelling.

St 23; *Tai-Yi*; 'Celestial Stem'

Location
  1 *cun* below St 22.

Regional anatomy
  Rectus sheath;
  Rectus muscle of abdomen;
  Peritoneum;
  Branches of intercostal arteries, veins & nerves;
  Inferior epigastric artery & vein;
  Transverse colon.

Symptoms
  Mania
  Restlessness

Method of treatment
  Needle: 0.5 inch perpendicularly.
  Moxa: Warm heating, 2 minutes.
  Feeling: Ache and/or swelling.

St 24; *Hua-Rou-Men*; 'Door to Fresh Meat'

Location
  1 *cun* below St 23.

Regional anatomy
  Rectus sheath;
  Rectus muscle of abdomen;
  Peritoneum;
  Branches of intercostal artery, vein & nerve;
  Inferior epigastric artery & vein;
  Small intestine.

Symptoms
  Stiff tongue   Vomiting
  Mania

Clinical formula
  St 24 + H 3 + LI 7 = Stiff tongue

Method of treatment
  Needle: 0.5 inch perpendicularly.
  Moxa: Warm heating, 2 minutes.
  Feeling: Ache and/or swelling.

St 25; *Tian-Shu*; 'Celestial Pivot'

Location
  2 *cun* lateral to CV 8 at level of umbilicus.

Regional anatomy
  Rectus sheath;
  Rectus muscle of abdomen;
  Peritoneum;
  Branches of intercostal artery & vein;
  Inferior epigastric artery & vein;
  Intercostal nerve;
  Small intestine.

Connecting point
  Front-*Mu* Point of Large Intestine.

Functions
  Harmonizes function of Large Intestine;
  Strengthens 'Earth' function;
  Expels damp in body;
  Harmonizes *Jing* blood & Meridian energy flow;
  Clears energy obstruction in Large Intestine.

Symptoms
  Diarrhoea   Oedema
  Indigestion   Pain around umbilicus
  Abdominal distention Irregular menstruation

FOURTEEN MERIDIANS AND ACUPUNCTURE POINTS

Clinical formulae
  St 25 + CV 8 + CV 4 = Diarrhoea
  St 25 + Sp 6 + CV 4 = Menstrual tension

Method of treatment
  Needle: 0.5 inch perpendicularly.
  Moxa: Warm heating, 3 minutes.
  Feeling: Ache and/or swelling.
  Warning: Avoid strong manipulation of needle. Moxa cones must not be used on pregnant women.

St 26; *Wai-Ling*; 'Beside the Hill'

Location
  1 *cun* below St 25.

Regional anatomy
  Rectus sheath;
  Rectus muscle of abdomen;
  Branches of intercostal & inferior epigastric arteries & veins;
  Branch of intercostal nerve;
  Peritoneum;
  Small intestine.

Symptoms
  Abdominal pain
  Lower abdominal pain during menstruation

Method of treatment
  Needle: 0.5 inch perpendicularly.
  Moxa: Warm heating, 2 minutes.
  Feeling: Ache and/or swelling.

St 27; *Da-Ju*; 'The Greatest'

Location
  1 *cun* below St 26.

Regional anatomy
  Rectus sheath;
  Rectus muscle of abdomen;
  Branches of intercostal artery, vein & nerve;
  Inferior epigastric artery & vein;
  Peritoneum;
  Small intestine.

Symptoms
  Abdominal distention
  Dysuria
  Insomnia due to fear
  Weakness in extremities

Method of treatment
  Needle: 0.5 inch perpendicularly.
  Moxa: Warm heating, 2 minutes.
  Feeling: Ache and/or swelling.

St 28; *Shui-Dao*; 'Water Path'

Location
  1 *cun* below St 27.

Regional anatomy
  Rectus sheath;
  Rectus muscle of abdomen;
  Branches of intercostal artery, vein & nerve;
  Inferior epigastric artery & vein;
  Peritoneum;
  Small intestine.

Symptoms
  Stiff spine & lumbar region
  Lower abdominal pain
  Urine retention
  Menstrual tension

Method of treatment
  Needle: 0.5 inch perpendicularly.
  Moxa: Warm heating, 2 minutes.

FOURTEEN MERIDIANS AND ACUPUNCTURE POINTS

Feeling: Ache and/or swelling.

St 29; *Gui-Lai*; 'The Return'

Location
1 *cun* below St 28.

Regional anatomy
Anterior layer of rectus sheath;
Rectus muscle of abdomen;
Internal oblique muscle of abdomen;
Tendon of transverse muscle of abdomen;
Inferior epigastric artery & vein;
Iliohypogastric nerve.

Symptoms
Abdominal distention
Amenorrhoea

Method of treatment
Needle: 0.5 inch perpendicularly.
Moxa: Warm heating, 2 minutes.
Feeling: Ache and/or swelling.

St 30; *Qi-Chong*; 'Thoroughfare of Energy'

Location
1 *cun* below St 29.

Regional anatomy
Tendon of external oblique muscle of abdomen;
Internal oblique muscle of abdomen;
Transverse muscle of abdomen;
Branches of superficial epigastric artery & vein;
Inferior epigastric artery & vein;
Pathway of ilioinguinal nerve.

Functions
Relieves tension in tendon;
Expels damp & pathogenic energy;
Regulates Bladder energy flow;
Harmonizes *Jing* blood & Meridian energy flow.

Symptoms
Pain in genitalia   Dysmenorrhoea
Lumbar pain   Sterility
Abdominal pain &   Weakness of Stomach
  distention   & Spleen

Method of treatment
Needle: 0.3 inch perpendicularly or prick with three-edged needle to cause bleeding.
Moxa: Warm heating, 2 minutes.
Feeling: Ache/heaviness/swelling.
Warning: Avoid needle penetration into blood vessel. Experienced needle technique is essential to avoid accidents. Do not overheat with moxa.

Note
This point is on an important energy flow path relating to blood and energy circulations of the internal organs and lower extremities.

St 31; *Bi-Guan*; 'Thigh Gate'

Location
With thigh flexed, point lies directly below anterior superior iliac spine in lateral depression of sartorius muscle.

Regional anatomy
Tensor muscle of fascia lata;
Sartorius muscle;
Branches of lateral circumflex femoral artery & vein;
Lateral femoral cutaneous nerve.

FOURTEEN MERIDIANS AND ACUPUNCTURE POINTS

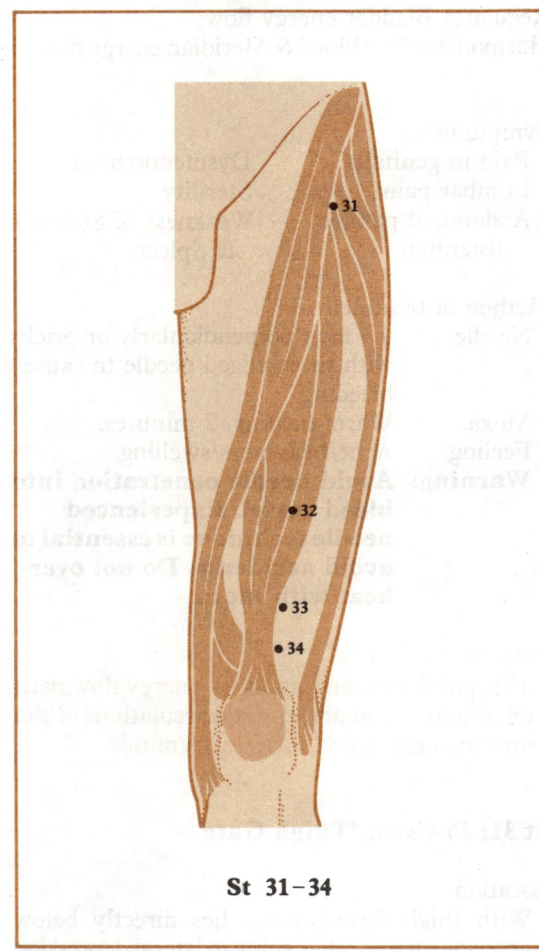

St 31–34

Symptoms
- Lumbar pain
- Pain in thigh
- Pain in knee
- Muscular atrophy
- Numbness in lower extremities

Method of treatment
- Needle: 0.6 inch perpendicularly.
- Moxa: Warm heating, 3 minutes.
- Feeling: Ache and/or swelling.

St 32; *Fu-Tu*; 'Prostrate Hare'

Location
6 *cun* above laterosuperior border of patella, on line connecting anterior superior iliac spine and lateral border of patella.

Regional anatomy
- Rectus muscle of thigh;
- Branches of lateral circumflex femoral artery & vein;
- Anterior & lateral femoral cutaneous nerves.

Symptoms
- Pain & cold in knee
- Abdominal distention

Method of treatment
- Needle: 0.5 inch perpendicularly.
- Moxa: **Forbidden.**
- Feeling: Ache and/or swelling.

St 33; *Yin-Shi*; 'Yin Market'

Location
3 *cun* above laterosuperior border of patella.

Regional anatomy
- Rectus muscle of thigh;
- Lateral vastus muscle of thigh;
- Descending branch of lateral circumflex femoral artery;
- Anterior & lateral femoral cutaneous nerves.

Symptoms
- Pain & cold in thigh & knee
- Abdominal pain & distention

Method of treatment
- Needle: 0.3 inch perpendicularly.

| Moxa: | Warm heating, 2 minutes; no moxa cone. |
| Feeling: | Ache and/or swelling. |

ST 34; *Liang-Qiu*; 'Ridge on Hill'

Location
2 *cun* above laterosuperior border of patella.

Regional anatomy
Rectus muscle of thigh;
Lateral vastus muscle of thigh;
Descending branch of lateral circumflex femoral artery;
Anterior & lateral femoral cutaneous nerves.

Connecting point
Xi-Cleft Point.

Functions
Regulates Stomach energy flow;
Harmonizes Middle Heater energy flow & sends Stomach energy downwards;
Expels wind & damp from Middle Heater.

Symptoms
Pain & swelling in knee   Cold feet
Pain in lower extremities   Fear

Method of treatment
Needle:	0.3 inch perpendicularly.
Moxa:	Warm heating, 2 minutes.
Feeling:	Ache and/or numbness.

St 35; *Du-Bi*; 'Nose of Calf'

Location
With knee bent, point (also known as external 'knee-eye' point) lies in depression below patella

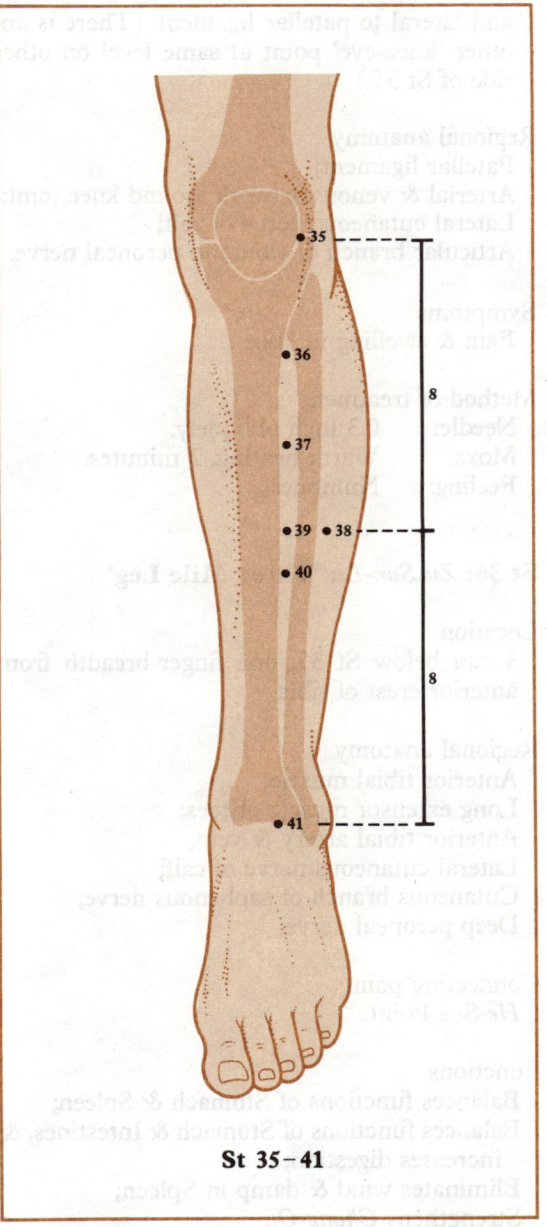

St 35–41

FOURTEEN MERIDIANS AND ACUPUNCTURE POINTS

and lateral to patellar ligament. (There is another 'knee-eye' point at same level on other side of St 35.)

Regional anatomy
    Patellar ligament;
    Arterial & venous network around knee joint;
    Lateral cutaneous nerve of calf;
    Articular branch of common peroneal nerve.

Symptoms
    Pain & swelling in knee

Method of treatment
    Needle: 0.3 inch obliquely.
    Moxa: Warm heating, 2 minutes.
    Feeling: Numbness.

St 36; *Zu-San-Li*; 'Three Mile Leg'

Location
    3 *cun* below St 35, one finger-breadth from anterior crest of tibia.

Regional anatomy
    Anterior tibial muscle;
    Long extensor muscle of toes;
    Anterior tibial artery & vein;
    Lateral cutaneous nerve of calf;
    Cutaneous branch of saphenous nerve;
    Deep peroneal nerve.

Connecting point
    He-Sea Point.

Functions
    Balances functions of Stomach & Spleen;
    Balances functions of Stomach & Intestines, & increases digestion;
    Eliminates wind & damp in Spleen;
    Strengthens *Chong-Qi*;
    Regulates Meridian blood & energy flows.

Symptoms
    Fatigue   Indigestion
    Body weakness   Loss of appetite
    Dizziness   Weakness of knee & leg
    Abdominal pain & distention   Hemiplegia

Clinical formulae
    St 36 + St 25 + LI 4 + CV 4 = Indigestion
    St 36 + LI 11 + CV 4 + GV 20 = Body weakness

Method of treatment
    Needle: 0.5 inch perpendicularly.
    Moxa: Warm heating, 3 minutes.
    Feeling: Ache and/or swelling. The sensation travels towards back of foot or to toe.
    Warning: **As application of moxibustion at this point increases Yang energy flow, it is only suitable for patients with chronic disease causing body weakness or for old people who have a deficiency of Yang energy. Treating the young or physically strong with moxibustion causes headaches.**

St 37; *Shang-Ju-Xu*; 'Upper Great Void'

Location
    3 *cun* below St 36.

FOURTEEN MERIDIANS AND ACUPUNCTURE POINTS

Regional anatomy
  Anterior tibial muscle;
  Anterior tibial artery & vein;
  Lateral cutaneous nerve of calf;
  Cutaneous branch of saphenous nerve;
  Deep peroneal nerve.

Connecting point
  He-Sea Point of Large Intestine.

Functions
  Balances functions of Stomach & Spleen;
  Increases movement & digestion of Intestines;
  Balances blood circulation.

Symptoms
  Weakness in Spleen &   Diarrhoea
    Stomach   Indigestion
  Fatigue   Pain in knee & leg

Clinical formula
  St 37 + St 39 = Diarrhoea

Method of treatment
  Needle: 0.3 inch perpendicularly.
  Moxa: Warm heating, 2 minutes.
  Feeling: Ache and/or swelling.

St 38; *Tiao-Kou*; 'A Narrow Region'

Location
  2 *cun* below St 37 lateral to tibia.

Regional anatomy
  Anterior tibial muscle;
  Anterior tibial artery & vein;
  Lateral cutaneous nerve of calf;
  Cutaneous branch of saphenous nerve;
  Deep peroneal nerve.

Symptoms
  Numbness in leg   Muscle spasm in leg
  Pain in leg   Shoulder pain

Method of treatment
  Needle: 0.5 inch perpendicularly.
  Moxa: Warm heating, 2 minutes.
  Feeling: Ache and/or swelling.

St 39; *Xia-Ju-Xu*; 'Lower Great Void'

Location
  3 *cun* below St 37.

Regional anatomy
  Anterior tibial muscle;
  Long extensor muscle of toes;
  Long extensor muscle of great toe;
  Anterior tibial artery & vein;
  Branches of superficial peroneal nerve;
  Deep peroneal nerve.

Connecting point
  He-Sea Point of Small Intestine.

Symptoms
  Deficient Small   Pain in lower abdomen
    Intestine energy   Pain & paralysis of leg
  Loss of appetite   Pain in heel
  Dry lips

Method of treatment
  Needle: 0.3 inch perpendicularly.
  Moxa: Warm heating, 2 minutes.
  Feeling: Ache and/or swelling.

St 40; *Feng-Long*; 'Rich and Prosperous'

Location
  8 *cun* below St 35 lateral to fibula, between long

FOURTEEN MERIDIANS AND ACUPUNCTURE POINTS

extensor muscle of toes and short peroneal muscle.

Regional anatomy
  Long extensor muscle of toes;
  Short peroneal muscle;
  Branches of anterior tibial artery & vein;
  Superficial peroneal nerve.

Connecting point
  Luo-Connecting Point.

Functions
  Harmonizes Stomach energy;
  Eliminates damp & phlegm from Lungs;
  Clears mind & *Shen*.

Symptoms
  Shortness of breath   Pain in abdomen
  Chest pain   Restlessness
  Fatigue   Pain & paralysis of leg

Clinical formula
  St 40 + GB 40 = Chest pain

Method of treatment
  Needle: 0.3 inch perpendicularly.
  Moxa: Warm heating, 2 minutes.
  Feeling: Ache and/or swelling.

St 41; *Jie-Xi*; 'Divided Brook'

Location
  At junction of dorsum of foot and leg, between tendons of long extensor muscles of toes and great toe, approximately at tip of external malleolus.

Regional anatomy
  Tendons of long extensor muscles of toes & great toe;

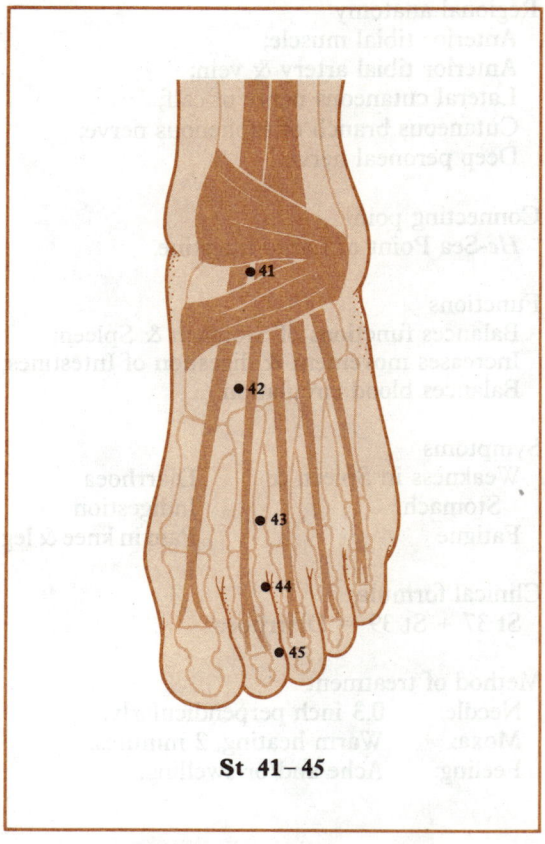

St 41–45

Anterior tibial artery & vein;
Superficial & deep peroneal nerves.

Connecting point
  Jing-River Point.

Functions
  Strengthens Spleen energy;
  Dispels damp in Spleen;
  Eliminates heat from Stomach;
  Clears mind & *Shen*.

FOURTEEN MERIDIANS AND ACUPUNCTURE POINTS

Symptoms
   Facial oedema   Dizziness
   Abdominal distention   Pain in eyebrows
   Headache   Pain in ankle & foot

Clinical formula
   St 41 + GB 40 + Sp 5 = Pain in ankle

Method of treatment
   Needle: 0.3 inch obliquely.
   Moxa: Warm heating, 2 minutes.
   Feeling: Ache and/or numbness.

St 42; *Chong-Yang*; 'Thoroughfare of Yang'

Location
   Distal to St 41 at highest point of dorsum of foot, in depression between second and third metatarsals and cuneiform bones.

Regional anatomy
   Tendon of long extensor muscle of toes;
   Dorsal artery & vein of foot;
   Dorsal venous network of foot;
   Medial dorsal cutaneous nerve of foot;
   Deep peroneal nerve.

Connecting point
   Yuan-Source Point.

Functions
   Strengthens 'Earth' & dispels damp in Spleen;
   Harmonizes Stomach energy & clears Shen.

Symptoms
   Facial paralysis   Headache
   Loss of appetite   Mania
   Pain & swellng in   Restlessness
     dorsum of foot

Clinical formula
   St 42 + H 7 + SI 3 = Mania & Restlessness

Method of treatment
   Needle: 0.2 inch obliquely.
   Moxa: Warm heating, 2 minutes.
   Feeling: Ache and/or numbness.
   Warning: **Avoid puncturing dorsal artery of foot.**

St 43; *Xian-Gu*; 'Depth of the Valley'

Location
   In depression between second and third metatarsal bones distal to joint.

Regional anatomy
   Plantar interosseous muscles;
   Dorsal venous network of foot;
   Medial dorsal cutaneous nerve of foot.

Connecting point
   Shu-Stream Point.

Symptoms
   Facial oedema   Pain in dorsum of foot
   Abdominal distention

Method of treatment
   Needle: 0.2 inch obliquely.
   Moxa: Warm heating, 2 minutes.
   Feeling: Ache.

St 44; *Nei-Ting*; 'Inner Court'

Location
   Proximal to web margin between second and third toes, in depression distal and lateral to second metatarsophalangeal joint.

Regional anatomy
　Dorsal venous network of foot where lateral branch of medial dorsal cutaneous nerve divides into dorsal digital nerve.

Connecting point
　Ying-Spring Point.

Functions
　Draws Stomach energy downwards;
　Balances functions of Intestines;
　Dispels damp in Intestines.

Symptoms
　Abdominal distention　　Toothache
　Sore throat　　　　　　Epistaxis
　Facial paralysis

Clinical formulae
　St 44 + LI 4 = Toothache
　St 44 + Sp 6 = Abdominal distention

Method of treatment
　Needle:　　0.2 inch perpendicularly.
　Moxa:　　　Warm heating, 2 minutes.
　Feeling:　　Ache and/or swelling.

St 45; *Li-Dui*; 'Exchange of Wildness'

Location
　On lateral side of second toe about 0.1 *cun* posterior to corner of nail.

Regional anatomy
　Arterial & venous network formed by dorsal digital artery & vein of foot;
　Dorsal digital nerve derived from superficial peroneal nerve.

Connecting point
　Jing-Well Point.

Functions
　Frees energy obstruction in Meridian;
　Revives from unconsciousness;
　Clears mind;
　Eliminates heat in Yang-*Ming* Meridians.

Symptoms
　Coma　　　　　　　　Pain & cold in leg
　Abdominal distention　　& foot
　Facial oedema　　　　　Epistaxis
　Facial paralysis　　　　Dream-disturbed sleep
　Toothache　　　　　　Fear

Clinical formula
　St 45 + Sp 1 = Dream-disturbed sleep

Method of treatment
　Needle:　　0.1 inch obliquely or bleed with three-edged needle.
　Moxa:　　　Warm heating, 1 minute.
　Feeling:　　Soreness.

4. Spleen Meridian of Foot Tai-Yin

This Meridian is characterized by high energy flow and low blood flow. The energy flow originates in the big toe at Sp 1 and travels along the medial aspect of the foot to the frontal region of the medial malleolus. From there, it travels up the anterior and outer surface of the leg and thigh to the groin, Sp 13, and connects with CV 3 and CV 4. At Sp 15 it links with CV 10. A branch from CV 10 goes to Sp 16, passes over GB 14 and Liv 14 up to Sp 17, and thence to Sp 21. From there it joins Lu 1 and ascends to the throat, terminating under the tongue.

　The Main Meridian from CV 10 enters the abdomen, continues into the Spleen and connects with the Stomach. From here it passes through the diaphragm and flows to the Heart to link with the Heart Meridian.

　There are twenty-one acupuncture points on

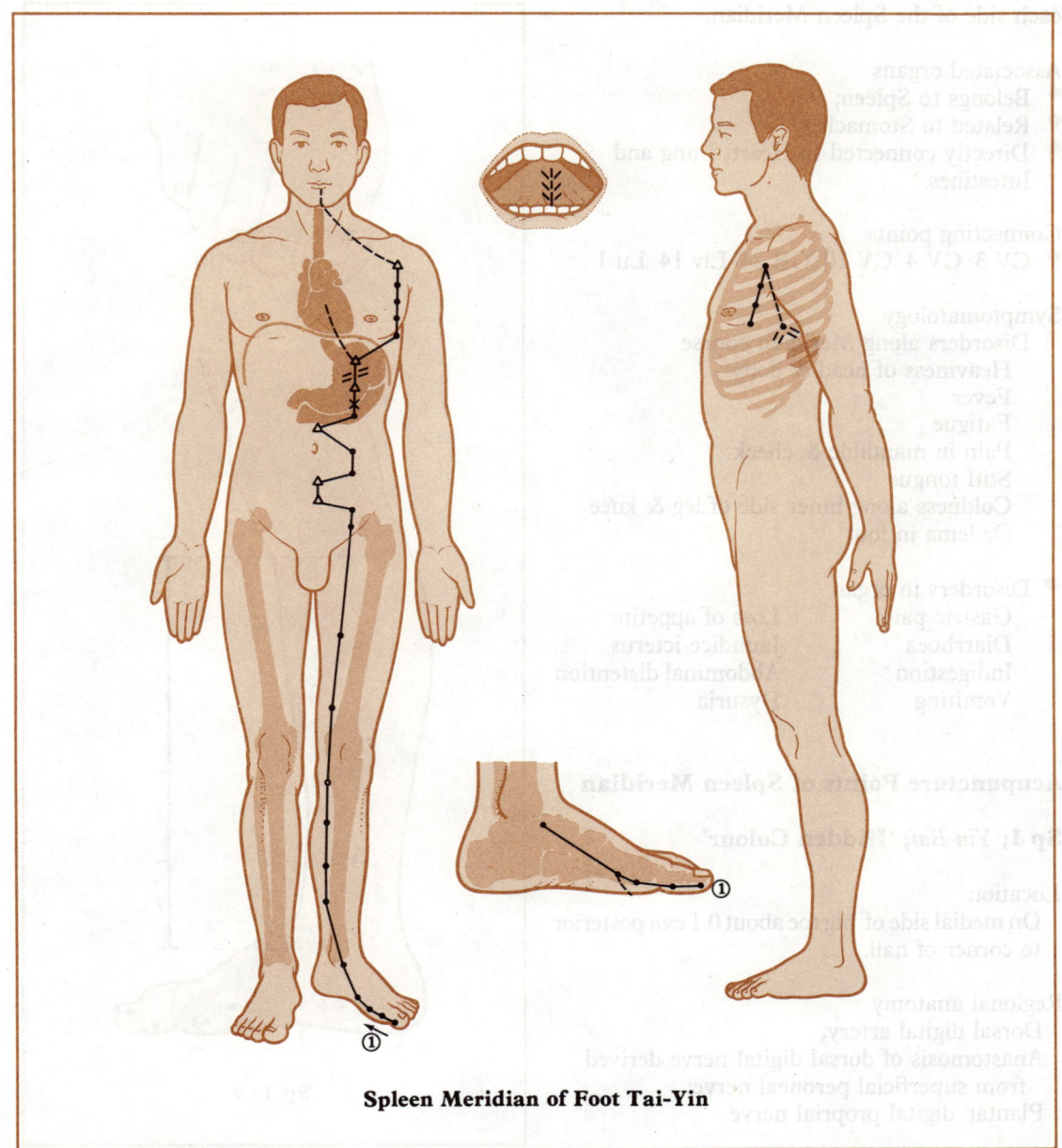

Spleen Meridian of Foot Tai-Yin

FOURTEEN MERIDIANS AND ACUPUNCTURE POINTS

each side of the Spleen Meridian.

Associated organs
- Belongs to Spleen;
- Related to Stomach;
- Directly connected to Heart, Lung and Intestines.

Connecting points
- CV 3 CV 4 CV 10 GB 24 Liv 14 Lu 1

Symptomatology
- Disorders along Meridian course
    Heaviness of head & body
    Fever
    Fatigue
    Pain in mandible & cheek
    Stiff tongue
    Coldness along inner side of leg & knee
    Oedema in foot

- Disorders in organ
    Gastric pain   Loss of appetite
    Diarrhoea   Jaundice icterus
    Indigestion   Abdominal distention
    Vomiting   Dysuria

Acupuncture Points of Spleen Meridian

Sp 1; *Yin-Bai*; **'Hidden Colour'**

Location
   On medial side of big toe about 0.1 *cun* posterior to corner of nail.

Regional anatomy
   Dorsal digital artery;
   Anastomosis of dorsal digital nerve derived from superficial peroneal nerve;
   Plantar digital proprial nerve.

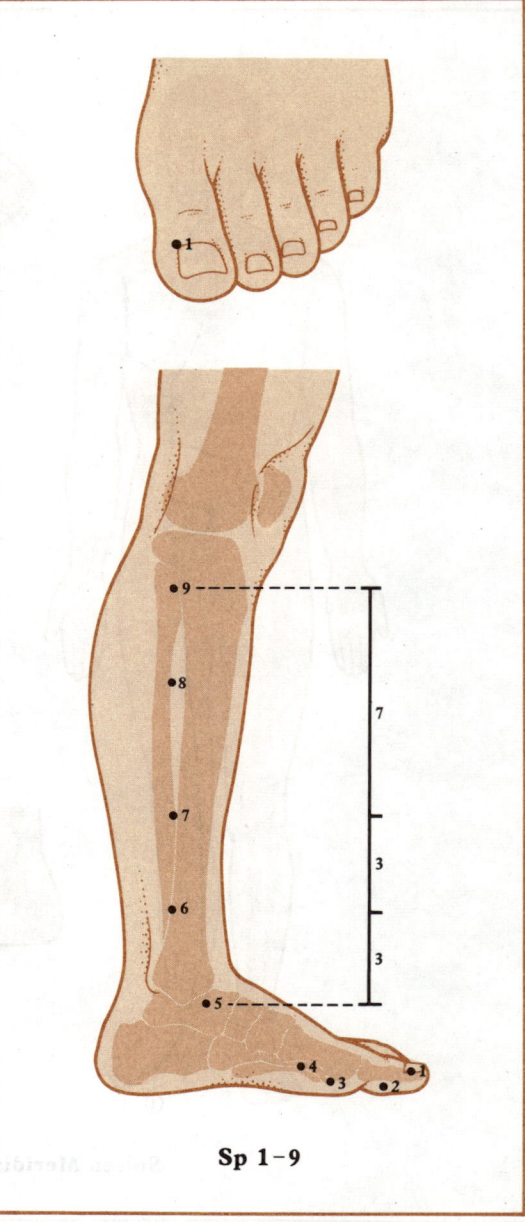

Sp 1–9

FOURTEEN MERIDIANS AND ACUPUNCTURE POINTS

Connecting point
  Jing-Well Point.

Functions
  Regulates blood circulation;
  Tones Spleen;
  Clears mind and *Shen*;
  Strengthens Yang energy flow;
  Revives from unconsciousness.

Symptoms
  Abdominal distension   Shortness of breath
  Vomiting   Uterine bleeding
  Diarrhoea   Cold feet

Clinical formula
  Sp 1 + Sp 10 + H 7 = Uterine bleeding

Method of treatment
  Needle: 0.1 inch obliquely or bleed with
            three-edged needle.
  Moxa: Warm heating, 1 minute.
  Feeling: Soreness.

Sp 2; *Da-Du*; 'Big Capital'

Location
  On medial side of big toe, distal and inferior
  to the first metatarsophalangeal joint.

Regional anatomy
  Abductor muscle of great toe;
  Branches of medial plantar artery & vein;
  Plantar digital proprial nerve derived from
    medial plantar nerve.

Connecting point
  Ying-Spring Point.

Symptoms
  General body ache   Lumbar pain
    & pain   Abdominal distention
  Fever   Gastric pain

Method of treatment
  Needle: 0.2 inch obliquely.
  Moxa: Warm heating, 2 minutes.
  Feeling: Ache and/or swelling.
  Warning: Moxa should not be used at this point during pregnancy or for three months after childbirth.

Sp 3; *Tai-Bai*; 'Supreme Whiteness'

Location
  On medial side of foot, inferior to head of first
  metatarsal bone.

Regional anatomy
  Abductor muscle of great toe;
  Dorsal venous network of foot;
  Medial plantar artery;
  Branches of medial tarsal artery;
  Branches of saphenous & superficial peroneal
    nerves.

Connecting points
  Shu-Stream Point; *Yuan*-Source Point.

Functions
  Strengthens Spleen function;
  Harmonizes Middle Heater function;
  Regulates Meridian energy flow;
  Increases functions of digestion, absorption &
    transportation.

Symptoms
  Abdominal distension   Gastric pain
  Indigestion   Sluggishness

115

FOURTEEN MERIDIANS AND ACUPUNCTURE POINTS

Vomiting
Diarrhoea
Muscular spasm in leg

Method of treatment
- Needle: 0.3 inch obliquely.
- Moxa: Warm heating, 2 minutes.
- Feeling: Ache and/or swelling.

Sp 4; *Gong-Sun*; 'Surname'

Location
In depression distal and inferior to base of first metatarsal bone.

Regional anatomy
Abductor muscle of great toe;
Medial artery & dorsal venous plexus of foot;
Saphenous nerve;
Branch of superficial peroneal nerve.

Connecting points
Luo-Connecting Point;
One of Eight Confluent Points connecting with *Chong-Mai*.

Functions
Strengthens functions of Spleen and Stomach;
Regulates blood circulation in Uterus;
Regulates *Chong-Mai* energy flow.

Symptoms
Loss of appetite   Facial swelling
Vomiting   Abdominal distention
Restlessness

Method of treatment
- Needle: 0.4 inch obliquely.
- Moxa: Warm heating, 2 minutes.
- Feeling: Ache and/or swelling.

Sp 5; *Shang-Qiu*; 'Merchant Hill'

Location
In depression distal and inferior to medial malleolus, midway between tuberosity of navicular bone and tip of medial malleolus.

Regional anatomy
Medial tarsal artery;
Great saphenous vein;
Medial cutaneous nerve of leg;
Branch of superficial peroneal nerve.

Connecting point
Jing-River Point.

Symptoms
Abdominal distention   Drowsiness
Lower abdominal pain   Body heaviness
Weak Spleen   Sterility
Stiff tongue   Pain in foot & ankle
Gloom

Clinical formula
Sp 5 + St 41 + GB 40 = Pain in ankle

Method of treatment
- Needle: 0.3 inch obliquely.
- Moxa: Warm heating, 2 minutes.
- Feeling: Ache.

Sp 6; *San-Yin-Jiao*; 'Reunion of Three Yin'

Location
3 *cun* above tip of medial malleolus on posterior border of tibia.

Regional anatomy
Soleus muscle;
Long flexor muscle of toes;
Great saphenous vein;

FOURTEEN MERIDIANS AND ACUPUNCTURE POINTS

Posterior tibial artery & vein;
Medial cutaneous nerve of leg;
Tibial nerve.

Connecting point
  Meeting Point of Spleen, Liver and Kidney Meridians.

Functions
  Strengthens Spleen function;
  Increases functions of digestion, absorption and transportation;
  Frees energy obstruction in Three Yin Meridians;
  Regulates Lower Heater function;
  Harmonizes blood and energy flows of reproductive system;
  Eliminates wind and damp in *Jing-Luo*.

Symptoms
  Weakness of Spleen & Stomach
  Abdominal distention
  Loss of appetite
  Oedema
  Irregular menstruation
  Amenorrhoea
  Sterility
  Difficult labour
  Pain in external genitalia
  Enuresis
  Seminal emission

Clinical formulae
  Sp 6 + Sp 10 + CV 6 + CV 4 = Irregular menstruation
  Sp 6 + CV 4 = Enuresis

Method of treatment
  Needle: 0.3 inch perpendicularly.
  Moxa: Warm heating, 3 minutes.
  Feeling: Ache and/or numbness.
  Warning: No needle is used during pregnancy and moxa should be done with care. Only an experienced practitioner should use needle technique for difficult labour.

Note
This is one of the most important acupuncture points for the reproductive system.

Sp 7; *Lou-Gu*; 'Leaking Valley'

Location
  3 *cun* above Sp 6.

Regional anatomy
  Soleus muscle;
  Long flexor muscle of toes;
  Great saphenous vein;
  Posterior tibial artery & vein;
  Medial cutaneous nerve of leg;
  Tibial nerve.

Symptoms
  Abdominal distention
  Pain in leg & knee

Method of treatment
  Needle: 0.3 inch perpendicularly.
  Moxa: **Forbidden.**
  Feeling: Ache and/or swelling.

Sp 8; *Pi-She (Di-Ji)*; 'Earth Home'

Location
  4 *cun* above Sp 7.

Regional anatomy
  Soleus muscle;
  Great saphenous vein;
  Branch of genu suprema artery;
  Posterior tibial artery & vein;
  Medial cutaneous nerve of leg;
  Tibial nerve.

FOURTEEN MERIDIANS AND ACUPUNCTURE POINTS

Connecting point
  Xi-Cleft Point.

Functions
  Harmonizes function of Spleen and Uterus.

Symptoms
  Lower back pain
  Diarrhoea
  Abdominal distention
  Oedema
  Dysuria
  Irregular menstruation

Method of treatment
  Needle: 0.3 inch perpendicularly.
  Moxa: Warm heating, 2 minutes.
  Feeling: Ache and/or numbness.

Sp 9; *Yin-Ling-Quan*; 'Yin Hill Rivulet'

Location
  On lower border of medial condyle of tibia, in depression between posterior border of tibia and gastrocnemius muscle.

Regional anatomy
  Gastrocnemius muscle;
  Soleus muscle;
  Great saphenous vein;
  Genu suprema artery;
  Posterior tibial artery & vein;
  Medial cutaneous nerve of leg;
  Tibial nerve.

Connecting point
  He-Sea Point.

Functions
  Strengthens Middle Heater function;
  Dispels damp;
  Strengthens Bladder function;
  Expels wind and cold.

Symptoms
  Oedema
  Dysuria
  Seminal emission
  Dyspnoea
  Pain in chest & lower back
  Diarrhoea

Clinical formulae
  Sp 9 + CV 6 + Sp 6 = Dysuria
  Sp 9 + CV 9 = Oedema

Method of treatment
  Needle: 0.5 inch perpendicularly.
  Moxa: Warm heating, 2 minutes.
  Feeling: Ache.

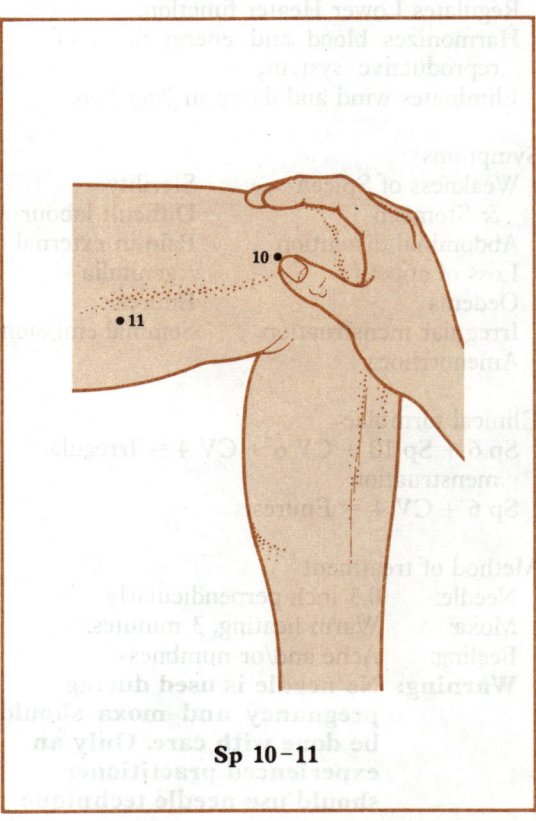

Sp 10–11

FOURTEEN MERIDIANS AND ACUPUNCTURE POINTS

Sp 10; *Xue-Hai*; 'Sea of Blood'

Location
2 *cun* above mediosuperior border of patella on bulge of medial portion of quadriceps muscle of thigh, with knee flexed. (To locate, right-hand palm is placed over left patella; tip of thumb rests on point.)

Regional anatomy
Quadriceps muscle of thigh;
Muscular branch of femoral artery & vein;
Anterior femoral cutaneous nerve;
Muscular branch of femoral nerve.

Functions
Regulates blood circulation;
Regulates Lower Heater function;
Clears blood.

Symptoms
Irregular menstruation	Uterine bleeding
Amenorrhoea	Eczema
Dysmenorrhoea	Urticaria

Method of treatment
Needle: 0.5 inch perpendicularly.
Moxa: Warm heating, 3 minutes.
Feeling: Ache.

Sp 11; *Ji-Men*; 'Screen Door'

Location
6 *cun* above Sp 10.

Regional anatomy
Sartorius muscle;
Great adductor muscle;
Great saphenous vein;
Femoral artery & vein;
Anterior femoral cutaneous nerve;
Saphenous nerve.

Symptoms
Urine retention
Enuresis
Pain & swelling in inguinal region

Method of treatment
Needle: 0.3 inch perpendicularly.
Moxa: Warm heating, 2 minutes.
Feeling: Ache and/or swelling.
Warning: Avoid inserting needle too deeply to avoid the femoral artery and vein lying just below.

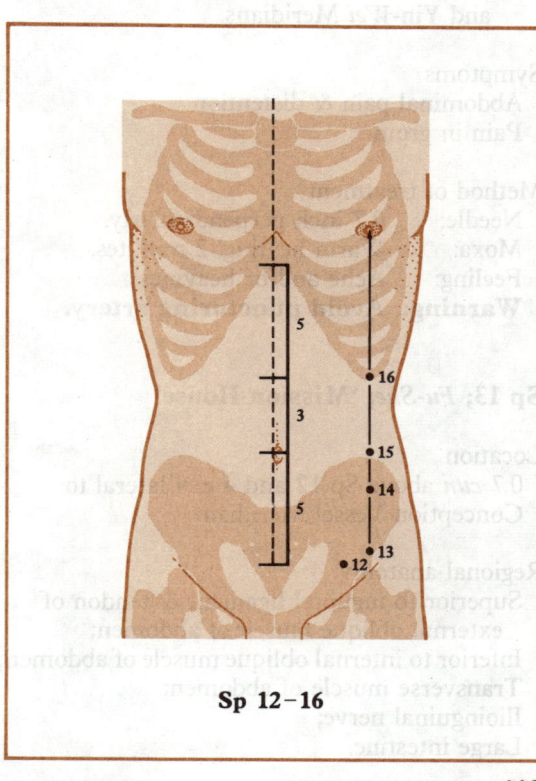

Sp 12–16

FOURTEEN MERIDIANS AND ACUPUNCTURE POINTS

Sp 12; *Chong-Men*; 'Door to Thoroughfare'

Location
  Superior to lateral end of inguinal groove on lateral side of femoral artery, at level of upper border of pubic symphysis, 3.5 *cun* lateral to CV 2.

Regional anatomy
  Superior to inguinal ligament & tendon of external oblique muscle of abdomen;
  Inferior to internal oblique muscle of abdomen;
  Femoral artery & nerve.

Connecting point
  Meeting Point of Foot *Tai*-Yin, Foot *Jue*-Yin and Yin-*Wei* Meridians.

Symptoms
  Abdominal pain & distention
  Pain in groin

Method of treatment
  Needle: 0.7 inch perpendicularly.
  Moxa: Warm heating, 2 minutes.
  Feeling: Ache and/or heaviness.
  Warning: Avoid puncturing artery.

Sp 13; *Fu-She*; 'Mission House'

Location
  0.7 *cun* above Sp 12 and 4 *cun* lateral to Conception Vessel Meridian.

Regional anatomy
  Superior to inguinal ligament & tendon of external oblique muscle of abdomen;
  Inferior to internal oblique muscle of abdomen;
  Transverse muscle of abdomen;
  Ilioinguinal nerve;
  Large intestine.

Connecting points
  Meeting Point of Foot *Tai*-Yin, Foot *Jue*-Yin and Yin-*Wei* Meridians;
  Meeting Point of *Tai*-Yin-*Xi*, three Yin Meridians and Yang-*Ming* Divergent Meridian.

Symptoms
  Abdominal pain & distention
  Pain in groin

Method of treatment
  Needle: 0.7 inch perpendicularly.
  Moxa: Warm heating, 2 minutes.
  Feeling: Ache and/or swelling.

Sp 14; *Fu-Jie*; 'Abdominal Knot'

Location
  3 *cun* above Sp 13.

Regional anatomy
  External & internal oblique muscles of abdomen;
  Transverse muscle of abdomen;
  Intercostal artery, vein & nerve.

Symptoms
  Coughing   Pain around umbilicus
  Diarrhoea

Method of treatment
  Needle: 0.7 inch perpendicularly.
  Moxa: Warm heating, 3 minutes.
  Feeling: Ache and/or swelling.

Sp 15; *Da-Heng*; 'Big Transversal'

Location
  Lateral to centre of umbilicus on same level as mammillary line.

FOURTEEN MERIDIANS AND ACUPUNCTURE POINTS

Regional anatomy
    External & internal oblique muscles of abdomen;
    Transverse muscle of abdomen;
    Intercostal artery, vein & nerve.

Connecting point
    Meeting Point of Foot *Tai*-Yin and Yin-*Wei* Meridians.

Symptoms
    Diarrhoea
    Gloom

Method of treatment
    Needle: 0.7 inch perpendicularly.
    Moxa: Warm heating, 3 minutes.
    Feeling: Ache and/or swelling.

Sp 16; *Fu-Ai*; 'Sorrow of the Abdomen'

Location
    3 *cun* above Sp 15.

Regional anatomy
    External & internal oblique muscles of abdomen;
    Transverse muscle of abdomen;
    Intercostal artery, vein & nerve;
    Liver (right side);
    Large intestine.

Connecting point
    Meeting Point of Foot *Tai*-Yin and Yin-*Wei* Meridians.

Symptoms
    Indigestion
    Abdominal pain

Method of treatment
    Needle: 0.3 inch perpendicularly.
    Moxa: Warm heating, 2 minutes.
    Feeling: Ache and/or swelling.

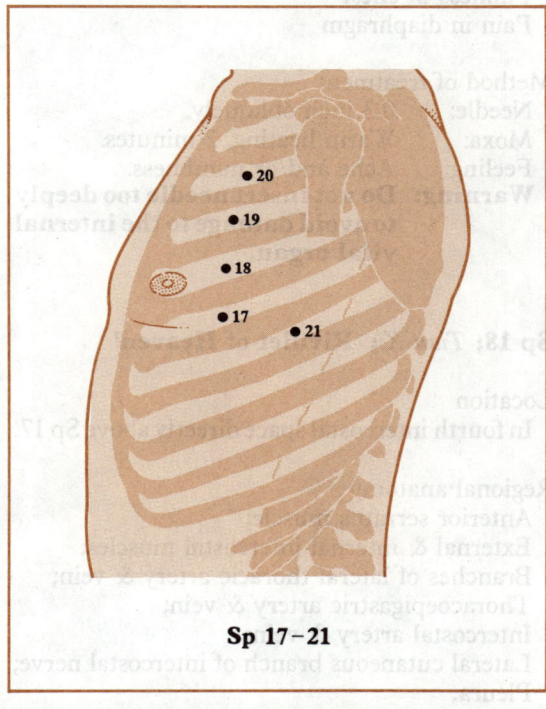

Sp 17–21

Sp 17; *Shi-Dou*; 'Food Recipient'

Location
    2 *cun* lateral to mammillary line in fifth intercostal space.

Regional anatomy
    Anterior serratus muscle;
    External & internal intercostal muscles;
    Thoracoepigastric vein;
    Lateral cutaneous branch of intercostal nerve;
    Pleura;
    Lung;

FOURTEEN MERIDIANS AND ACUPUNCTURE POINTS

Pericardium;
Heart.

Symptoms
Fullness in chest
Pain in diaphragm

Method of treatment
Needle: 0.3 inch obliquely.
Moxa: Warm heating, 2 minutes.
Feeling: Ache and/or numbness.
Warning: Do not insert needle too deeply to avoid damage to the internal vital organ.

Sp 18; *Tian-Xi*; 'Rivulet of Heaven'

Location
In fourth intercostal space directly above Sp 17.

Regional anatomy
Anterior serratus muscle;
External & internal intercostal muscles;
Branches of lateral thoracic artery & vein;
Thoracoepigastric artery & vein;
Intercostal artery & vein;
Lateral cutaneous branch of intercostal nerve;
Pleura;
Lung;
Pericardium;
Heart.

Symptoms
Fullness & pain in chest
Coughing

Method of treatment
Needle: 0.3 inch obliquely.
Moxa: Warm heating, 2 minutes.
Feeling: Ache and/or swelling.
Warning: Do not insert needle too deeply to avoid damage to the internal vital organ.

Sp 19; *Xiong-Xiang*; 'Chest Village'

Location
In third intercostal space directly above Sp 18.

Regional anatomy
Greater & smaller pectoral muscles;
Anterior serratus muscle;
External & internal intercostal muscles;
Lateral thoracic artery & vein;
Intercostal artery, vein & nerve;
Pleura;
Lung;
Pericardium;
Heart.

Symptoms
Fullness in chest
Pain in back & chest

Method of treatment
Needle: 0.3 inch obliquely.
Moxa: Warm heating, 2 minutes.
Feeling: Ache and/or numbness.
Warning: Avoid inserting needle too deeply.

Sp 20; *Zhou-Rong*; 'Encircling Glory'

Location
In second intercostal space directly below Lu 1.

Regional anatomy
Greater & smaller pectoral muscles;
External & internal intercostal muscles;
Lateral thoracic artery & vein;
Intercostal branch of anterior thoracic nerve;

Pleura;
Lung.

Symptoms
Fullness & pain in chest
Coughing

Method of treatment
Needle: 0.3 inch obliquely.
Moxa: Warm heating, 2 minutes.
Feeling: Ache and/or swelling.
Warning: Avoid puncturing too deeply.

Sp 21; *Da-Bao*; 'Big Package'

Location
On midaxillary line in sixth intercostal space.

Regional anatomy
Anterior serratus muscle;
Latissimus dorsi muscle;
Thoracodorsal artery & vein;
Intercostal artery, vein & nerve;
Terminal branch of long thoracic nerve;
Pleura;
Lung.

Connecting point
Major *Luo*-Connecting Point of Spleen.

Functions
Regulates *Luo* Meridian energy flow;
Strengthens functions of tendons and muscles.

Symptoms
Pain in chest
Shortness of breath
General weakness & body ache

Method of treatment
Needle: 0.3 inch obliquely.
Moxa: Warm heating, 2 minutes.
Feeling: Ache and/or swelling.
Warning: Avoid puncturing too deeply.

5. Heart Meridian of Hand Shao-Yin

This Meridian is characterized by high energy flow and low blood flow. The energy flow originates in the Heart and connects with the great vessels entering and leaving the Heart, and descends through the diaphragm to link with the Small Intestine, its related organ.

A branch from the Heart ascends the oesophagus and pharynx to connect with the eye. The main Meridian leaves the Heart, traverses the Lung and emerges at the axilla at H 1. From here it continues along the posterior border of the medial aspect of the arm, behind the Lung and Pericardium Meridians, to terminate at the little finger, H 9, where it links with the Small Intestine Meridian.

There are nine acupuncture points on each side of the Heart Meridian.

Associated organs
- Belongs to Heart;
- Related to Small Intestine;
- Directly connected to Lung and Kidney.

Symptomatology
- Disorders along Meridian course
  Fever   Dry throat
  Headache   Pain in shoulder
  Ophthalmalgia   & inner arm
  Chest & back pain

- Disorders in organ
  Cardiac pain   Shortness of breath
  Fullness & pain   Insomnia
  in chest   Vertigo
  Palpitations   Fear & anxiety
  Restlessness   Sadness & dejection

FOURTEEN MERIDIANS AND ACUPUNCTURE POINTS

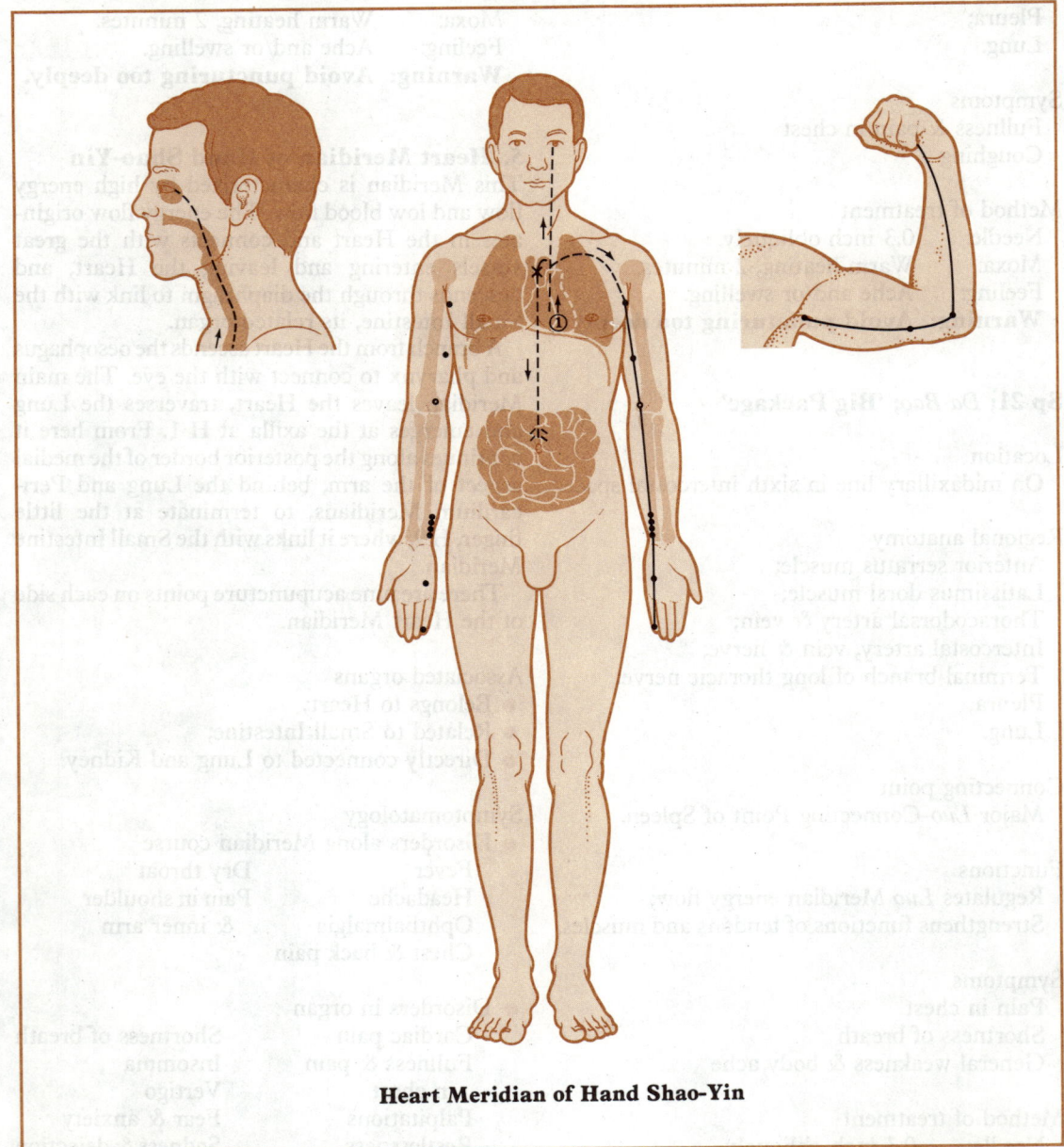

Heart Meridian of Hand Shao-Yin

FOURTEEN MERIDIANS AND ACUPUNCTURE POINTS

Acupuncture Points of Heart Meridian

H 1; *Ji-Quan*; 'Deep Stream'

Location
Centre of axilla on medial side of axillary artery.

Regional anatomy
Greater pectoral muscle;
Coracobrachial muscle;
Lateral axillary artery;
Ulnar & median nerves, & medial branch of cutaneous nerve.

Symptoms
Pain in arm
Pain in costal & cardiac regions
Fullness in chest
Thirst

Method of treatment
Needle: 0.3 inch perpendicularly.
Moxa: Warm heating, 2 minutes.
Feeling: Ache and/or numbness.
Warning: Avoid puncturing artery or vein. After insertion, the patient's arm must not be moved until the needle has been withdrawn.

H 2; *Qing-Ling*; 'Green Spirit'

Location
3 *cun* above H 3.

Regional anatomy
Biceps & triceps muscles of arm;
Basilic vein;
Superior ulnar collateral artery;
Medial cutaneous nerves of forearm & of arm;
Ulnar nerve.

Symptoms
Pain in hypochondriac region
Pain in shoulder & arm

Method of treatment
Needle: 0.3 inch perpendicularly.
Moxa: Warm heating, 2 minutes.
Feeling: Ache and/or swelling.

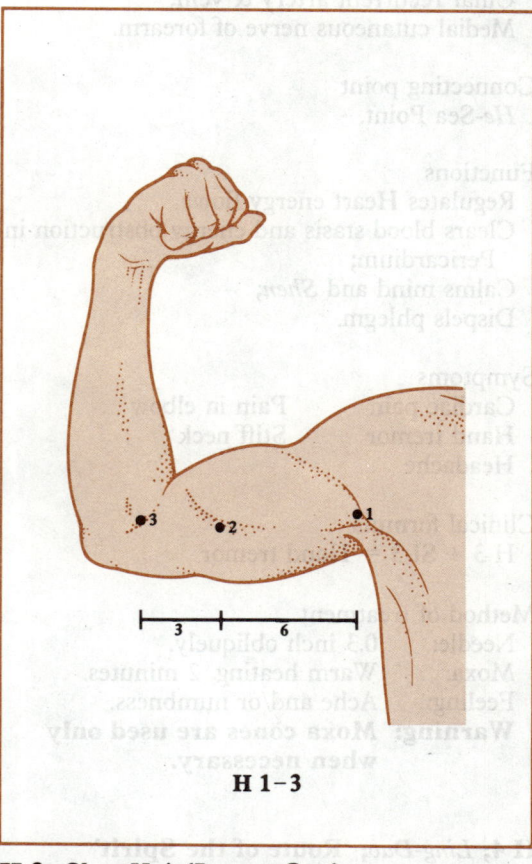

H 1–3

H 3; *Shao-Hai*; 'Lesser Sea'

Location
In depression between medial end of transverse

cubital crease and medial epicondyle of humerus, with arm bent.

Regional anatomy
Round pronator muscle;
Brachial muscle;
Basilic vein;
Inferior ulnar collateral artery;
Ulnar recurrent artery & vein;
Medial cutaneous nerve of forearm.

Connecting point
He-Sea Point.

Functions
Regulates Heart energy flow;
Clears blood stasis and energy obstruction in Pericardium;
Calms mind and *Shen*;
Dispels phlegm.

Symptoms
Cardiac pain   Pain in elbow
Hand tremor   Stiff neck
Headache

Clinical formula
H 3 + SI 3 = Hand tremor

Method of treatment
Needle: 0.3 inch obliquely.
Moxa: Warm heating, 2 minutes.
Feeling: Ache and/or numbness.
Warning: Moxa cones are used only when necessary.

H 4; *Ling-Dao*; 'Route of the Spirit'

Location
1.5 *cun* above H 7.

Regional anatomy
Tendon of ulnar flexor muscle of wrist;
Superficial & deep flexor muscles of fingers;
Ulnar artery & nerve;
Medial cutaneous nerve of forearm.

Connecting point
Jing-River Point.

Symptoms
Cardiac pain   Pain in forearm
Sadness & fear   Sudden hoarseness of voice

Clinical formula
H 4 + CV 20 + SI 16 = Sudden loss of voice

Method of treatment
Needle: 0.3 inch perpendicularly.
Moxa: Warm heating, 2 minutes.
Feeling: Ache and/or numbness.
Warning: Avoid puncturing tendon or artery.

H 5; *Tong-Li*; 'Communication with the Interior'

Location
1 *cun* above H 7.

Regional anatomy
Tendon of ulnar flexor muscle of wrist;
Superficial & deep flexor muscles of fingers;
Ulnar artery & nerve;
Medial cutaneous nerve of forearm.

Connecting point
Luo-Connecting Point.

Functions
Creates quiet in Heart and *Shen*;

FOURTEEN MERIDIANS AND ACUPUNCTURE POINTS

Dispels wind;
Regulates *Jing* blood.

Symptoms
Headache   Excessive menstruation
Dizziness   (heavy bleeding)
Palpitations   Pain in wrist

Clinical formula
H 5 + LI 2 + Sp 6 = Excessive menstruation (heavy bleeding)

Method of treatment
Needle: 0.3 inch perpendicularly.
Moxa: Warm heating, 2 minutes.
Feeling: Ache and/or numbness.
Warning: Avoid puncturing tendon and artery.

H 6; *Yin-Xi*; 'Yin Cleft'

Location
0.5 *cun* above H 7.

Regional anatomy
Tendon of ulnar flexor muscle of wrist;
Superficial & deep flexor muscles of fingers;
Ulnar artery & nerve;
Medial cutaneous nerve of forearm.

Connecting point
Xi-Cleft Point.

Functions
Eases Heart Fire;
Balances Yin and Yang energies in Heart;
Creates quiet in mind and *Shen*;
Protects *Wei* energy.

Symptoms
Epistaxis
Fullness in chest
Cardiac pain & palpitations

Method of treatment
Needle: 0.3 inch perpendicularly.
Moxa: Warm heating, 2 minutes.
Feeling: Ache and/or numbness.
Warning: Avoid puncturing tendon and artery.

H 7; *Shen-Men*; 'Door of the Spirit'

Location
On transverse crease of wrist, in articular region between pisiform and ulna bones, in depression on radial side of tendon of ulnar flexor muscle of wrist.

Regional anatomy
Tendon of ulnar flexor muscle of wrist;
Superficial & deep flexor muscles of fingers;
Ulnar artery & nerve;
Medial cutaneous nerve of forearm.

Connecting points
Shu-Stream and *Yuan*-Source Points.

Functions
Creates quiet in Heart and *Shen*;
Eases Heart Fire;
Balances *Jing* blood;
Expels excess heat from Heart;
Regulates Heart energy flow.

Symptoms
Restlessness   Cardiac pain
Dry mouth   Fear & palpitations
Insomnia   Loss of memory
Loss of appetite

FOURTEEN MERIDIANS AND ACUPUNCTURE POINTS

Clinical formulae
H 7 + Pc 6 + Sp 6 = Insomnia
H 7 + Lu 10 + Pc 7 = Fear and palpitations

Method of treatment
Needle: 0.3 inch perpendicularly.
Moxa: Warm heating, 2 minutes.
Feeling: Ache and/or numbness.
Warning: Avoid puncturing tendon or artery.

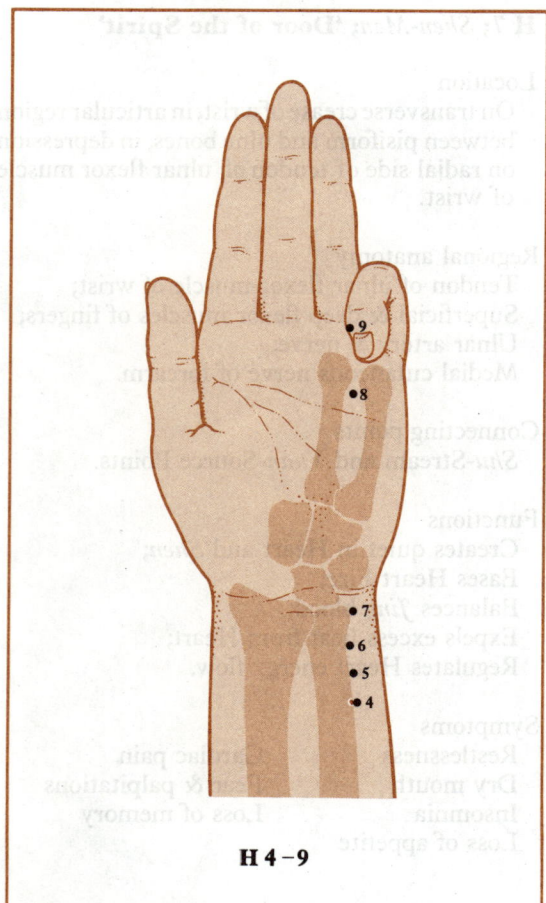

H 4–9

H 8; *Shao-Fu*; 'Little House'

Location
On palmar surface between fourth and fifth metacarpal bones. When forming a fist, tip of little finger rests on this point.

Regional anatomy
Lumbrical muscles of hand;
Tendons of superficial & deep flexor muscles of fingers;
Palmar interosseous muscles;
Common palmar digital artery, vein & nerve.

Connecting point
Ying-Spring Point.

Symptoms
Fullness in chest   Enuresis
Dysuria   Pain in little finger
Sadness & fear

Clinical formula
H 8 + St 36 = Dysuria

Method of treatment
Needle: 0.2 inch perpendicularly.
Moxa: Warm heating, 2 minutes.
Feeling: Soreness and/or swelling.

H 9; *Shao-Chong*; 'Small Thoroughfare'

Location
On radial side of little finger, about 0.1 *cun* posterior to corner of nail.

Regional anatomy
Arterial & venous network formed by palmar digital proprial artery & vein;

Palmar digital proprial nerve.

Connecting point
Jing-Well Point.

Functions
Opens 'Heart Gate';
Clears mind and *Shen*;
Revives from unconsciousness;
Expels excess heat from body.

Symptoms
Cardiac pain   Fever
Pain in chest   Pain in forearm

Method of treatment
Needle: 0.1 inch obliquely or bleed with three-edged needle.
Moxa: Warm heating, 1 minute.
Feeling: Painful.

6. Small Intestine Meridian of Hand Tai-Yang

This Meridian is characterized by high blood flow and low energy flow. The energy flow originates in the little finger at SI 1, flows up the ulnar side of the dorsum of hand and along the posterior aspect of the forearm and upper arm to the shoulder joint. It circles around the scapular region from SI 13 to Bl 41, turns back to SI 14 and continues on to Bl 11. It then runs back to SI 15, emerges at GV 14 and proceeds to the supraclavicular fossa. From here, a branch enters the oesophagus and Heart, then descends through the diaphragm to reach the Stomach where it connects (deeply) with CV 12 and CV 13. The branch then terminates at the Small Intestine from where a further branch descends to connect with St 39, the Inferior *He*-Sea Point of the Small Intestine.

The main Meridian ascends from the supraclavicular fossa to the neck, SI 17, and onto the cheek at SI 18, from where a branch ascends to the outer canthus to connect with GB 1, then turns back to TH 22 and descends to SI 19 to enter the ear. The main Meridian continues on from SI 18 to the inner canthus to Bl 1, where it links with the Bladder Meridian.

There are nineteen acupuncture points on each side of the Small Intestine Meridian.

Associated organs
- Belongs to Small Intestine;
- Related to Heart;
- Directly connected to Stomach.

Connecting points
GV 14 CV 12 CV 13 Bl 1 Bl 11 Bl 41 TH 22 GB 1

Symptomatology
- Disorders along Meridian course
  Ulcers in mouth & on tongue
  Pain in cheek area
  Sore throat
  Lacrimation
  Stiff neck
  Pain in shoulder & arm

- Disorders in organ
  Pain & distention of abdomen
  Pain in lower back & lower abdomen
  Diarrhoea or constipation

Acupuncture Points of Small Intestine

SI 1; *Shao-Ze;* **'Lesser Marsh'**

Location
On ulnar side of little finger, about 0.1 *cun* posterior to corner of nail.

FOURTEEN MERIDIANS AND ACUPUNCTURE POINTS

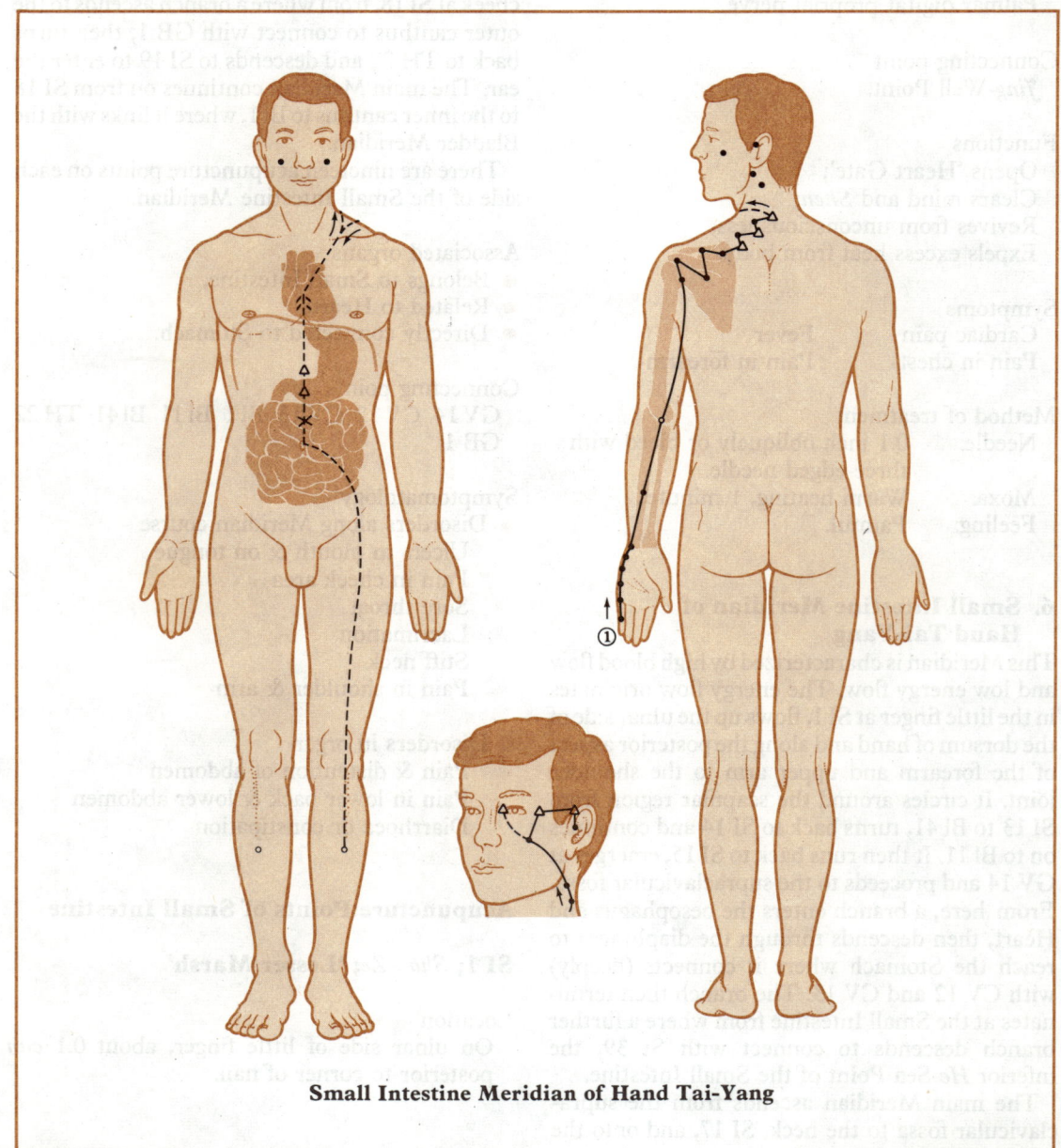

Small Intestine Meridian of Hand Tai-Yang

FOURTEEN MERIDIANS AND ACUPUNCTURE POINTS

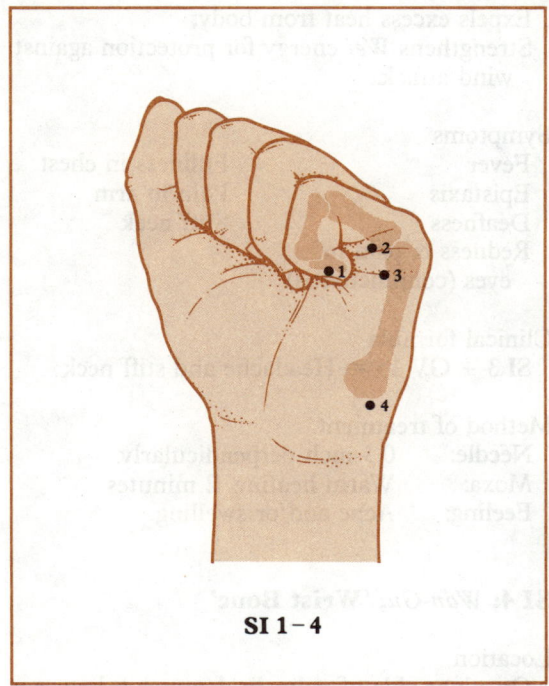

SI 1-4

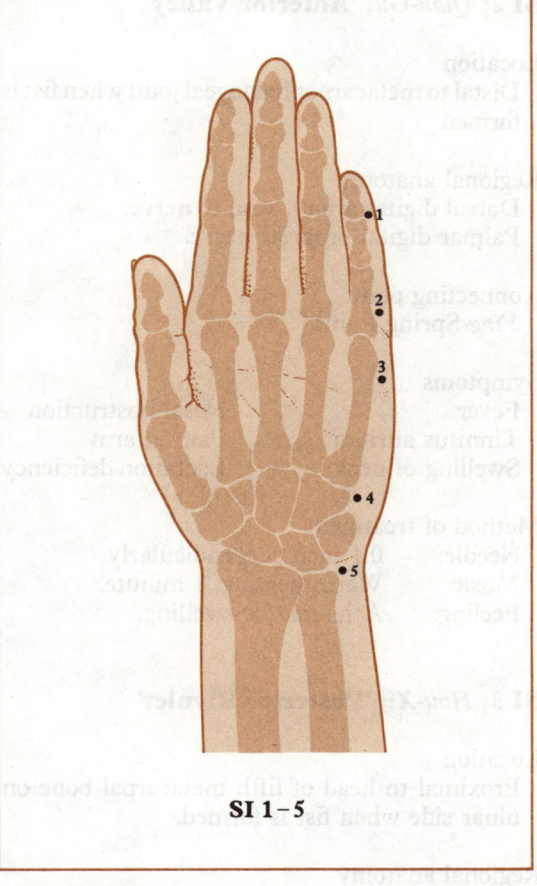

SI 1-5

Regional anatomy
    Arterial & venous network formed by palmar & dorsal digital proprial arteries & veins;
    Palmar & dorsal digital nerves.

Connecting point
    Jing-Well Point.

Functions
    Eases tension & Heart Fire;
    Expels excess heat from body.

Symptoms
Fever	Headache
Restlessness	Stiff neck
Dry mouth	Lactation deficiency
Stiff tongue	

Clinical formula
    SI 1 + LI 4 + CV 17 = Lactation deficiency

Method of treatment
    Needle: 0.1 inch obliquely or bleed with three-edged needle.
    Moxa: Warm heating, 1 minute.
    Feeling: Painful.
    Warning: Do not bleed this point when treating lactation deficiency.

FOURTEEN MERIDIANS AND ACUPUNCTURE POINTS

SI 2; *Qian-Gu*; 'Anterior Valley'

Location
  Distal to metacarpophalangeal joint when fist is formed.

Regional anatomy
  Dorsal digital artery, vein & nerve;
  Palmar digital proprial nerve.

Connecting point
  Ying-Spring Point.

Symptoms
  Fever   Nasal obstruction
  Tinnitus aurium   Pain in arm
  Swelling of neck   Lactation deficiency

Method of treatment
  Needle: 0.1 inch perpendicularly.
  Moxa: Warm heating, 1 minute.
  Feeling: Ache and/or swelling.

SI 3; *Hou-Xi*; 'Posterior Rivulet'

Location
  Proximal to head of fifth metacarpal bone on ulnar side when fist is formed.

Regional anatomy
  Origin of abductor muscle of little finger;
  Dorsal digital artery & vein;
  Dorsal venous network of hand;
  Dorsal branch of ulnar nerve.

Connecting points
  Shu-Stream Point; one of Eight Confluent Points connected to Governor Vessel Meridian.

Functions
  Creates quiet in mind and *Shen*;
  Expels excess heat from body;
  Strengthens *Wei* energy for protection against wind attack.

Symptoms
  Fever   Fullness in chest
  Epistaxis   Pain in arm
  Deafness   Stiff neck
  Redness & pain in
    eyes (conjunctivitis)

Clinical formula
  SI 3 + GV 15 = Headache and stiff neck

Method of treatment
  Needle: 0.3 inch perpendicularly.
  Moxa: Warm heating, 2 minutes.
  Feeling: Ache and/or swelling.

SI 4; *Wan-Gu*; 'Wrist Bone'

Location
  On ulnar side of palm in depression between base of fith metacarpal bone and triquetral bone.

Regional anatomy
  Abductor muscle of little finger;
  Posterior artery of wrist;
  Dorsal venous network of hand;
  Dorsal branch of ulnar nerve.

Connecting point
  Yuan-Source Point.

Functions
  Frees energy obstruction in *Tai*-Yang Meridian;
  Expels excess heat and damp from Small Intestine.

Symptoms
  Fever   Tinnitus aurium

FOURTEEN MERIDIANS AND ACUPUNCTURE POINTS

Pain in chest
Headache
Swelling of neck
Pain in wrist
Restlessness

Clinical formula
SI 4 + Pc 7 + Pc 5 + LI 3 = Pain in wrist and fingers

Method of treatment
Needle: 0.2 inch perpendicularly.
Moxa: Warm heating, 2 minutes.
Feeling: Ache and/or swelling.

SI 5; *Yang-Gu*; 'Valley of Yang'

Location
On ulnar side of wrist in depression between styloid process of ulna and triquetral bone.

Regional anatomy
Tendon of ulnar extensor muscle of wrist;
Posterior artery of wrist;
Dorsal branch of ulnar nerve.

Connecting point
Jing-River Point.

Symptoms
Fever
Pain in chest
Swelling of neck
Deafness
Tinnitus aurium

Clinical formula
SI 5 + LI 1 + GV 20 = Tinnitus aurium

Method of treatment
Needle: 0.2 inch obliquely.
Moxa: Warm heating, 2 minutes.
Feeling: Ache and/or heaviness.

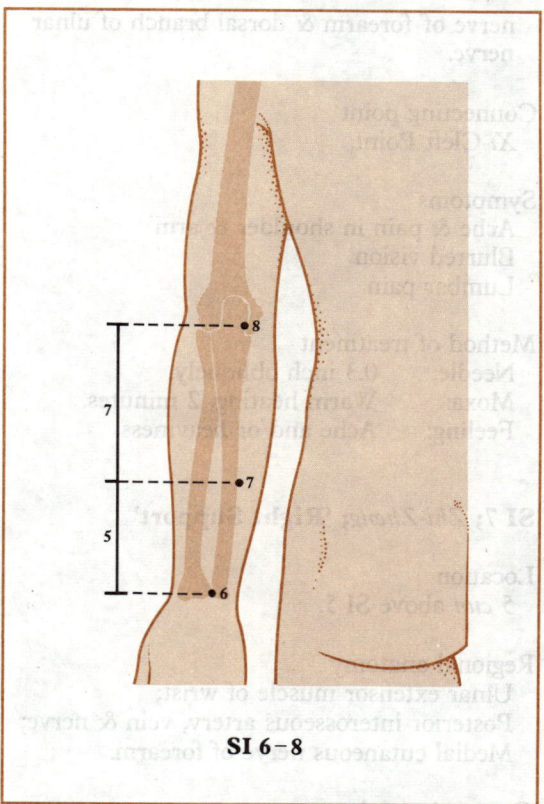

SI 6–8

SI 6; *Yang-Lao*; 'Provision for the Aged'

Location
Dorsal to head of ulna. When palm is facing chest, in bony cleft on radial side of styloid process of ulna.

Regional anatomy
Tendon of ulnar extensor muscle of wrist;
Tendon of extensor muscle of little finger;
Terminal branches of posterior interosseous artery & vein;
Dorsal venous network of wrist;
Anastomotic branches of posterior cutaneous

FOURTEEN MERIDIANS AND ACUPUNCTURE POINTS

nerve of forearm & dorsal branch of ulnar nerve.

Connecting point
Xi-Cleft Point.

Symptoms
Ache & pain in shoulder & arm
Blurred vision
Lumbar pain

Method of treatment
Needle: 0.3 inch obliquely.
Moxa: Warm heating, 2 minutes.
Feeling: Ache and/or heaviness.

SI 7; *Zhi-Zheng*; 'Right Support'

Location
5 *cun* above SI 5.

Regional anatomy
Ulnar extensor muscle of wrist;
Posterior interosseous artery, vein & nerve;
Medial cutaneous nerve of forearm.

Connecting point
Luo-Connecting Point.

Functions
Clears mind and *Shen*;
Dispels superficial heat;
Frees energy obstruction in Meridian.

Symptoms
Sadness & fear
Body weakness
Pain & spasm in arm & forearm
Pain in fingers
Pain in neck & lower back

Method of treatment
Needle: 0.3 inch perpendicularly.
Moxa: Warm heating, 2 minutes.
Feeling: Ache and/or heaviness.

SI 8; *Xiao-Hai*; 'Small Sea'

Location
Between olecranon of ulna and medial epicondyle of humerus when elbow is flexed.

Regional anatomy
Origin of ulnar flexor muscle of wrist;
Superior & inferior ulnar collateral arteries & veins;
Ulnar recurrent artery & vein;
Medial cutaneous nerve of forearm;
Ulnar nerve.

Connecting point
He-Sea Point.

Functions
Frees energy obstruction in *Tai*-Yang Meridian;
Expels excess heat from Small Intestine;
Dispels wind;
Clears mind and *Shen*.

Symptoms
Stiff neck
Pain in arm & forearm
Swelling of cheek & gum
Lower abdominal pain

Method of treatment
Needle: 0.3 inch obliquely.
Moxa: Warm heating, 2 minutes.
Feeling: Ache and/or numbness.

Note
St 39 is the main *He*-Sea Point of the Small

FOURTEEN MERIDIANS AND ACUPUNCTURE POINTS

Intestine and is used mainly for treating disorders of this organ.

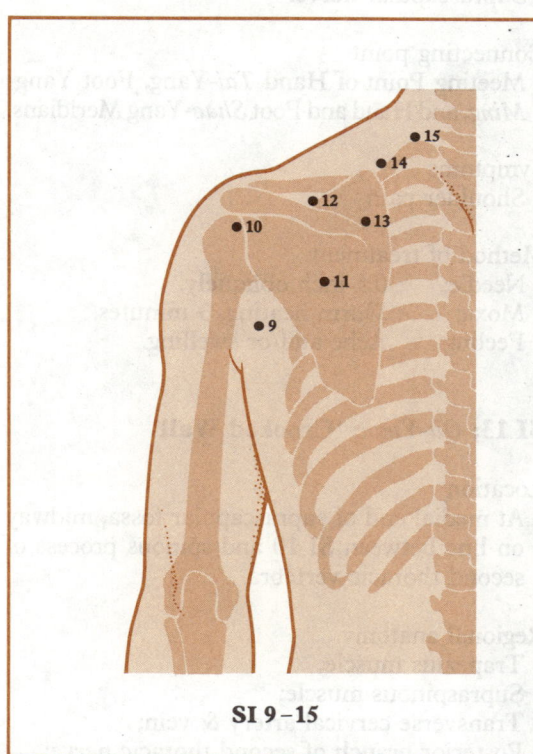

SI 9–15

SI 9; *Jian-Zhen*; 'Shoulder Strength'

Location
  1 *cun* above posterior end of axillary fold when arm is adducted.

Regional anatomy
  Deltoid muscle;
  Teres major muscle;
  Circumflex scapular artery & vein;
  Branch of axillary nerve;
  Radial nerve.

Symptoms
  Fever
  Deafness
  Tinnitus aurium
  Pain in supraclavicular fossa
  Numbing of fingers

Clinical formula
  SI 9 + SI 11 + SI 14 = Shoulder pain

Method of treatment
  Needle: 0.5 inch perpendicularly.
  Moxa: Warm heating, 3 minutes.
  Feeling: Ache and/or swelling.

SI 10; *Nao-Shu*; 'Shu Point of Shoulder Blade'

Location
  Directly above SI 9 in depression inferolateral to scapular spine.

Regional anatomy
  Deltoid muscle;
  Infraspinous muscle;
  Posterior circumflex humeral artery & vein;
  Suprascapular artery & vein;
  Posterior cutaneous nerve of arm;
  Axillary nerve;
  Suprascapular nerve.

Connecting point
  Meeting Point of Hand *Tai*-Yang, Yang-*Wei* and Yang-*Qiao* Meridians.

Symptoms
  Ache & pain in shoulder & arm

Method of treatment
  Needle: 0.8 inch perpendicularly.
  Moxa: Warm heating, 3 minutes.
  Feeling: Ache and/or swelling.

FOURTEEN MERIDIANS AND ACUPUNCTURE POINTS

SI 11; *Tian-Zong*; 'Celestial Principle'

Location
In infrascapular fossa, forming a triangle with SI 10 and SI 9.

Regional anatomy
Middle of dorsum of scapula
Infraspinous muscle;
Muscular branches of circumflex scapular artery & vein;
Suprascapular nerve.

Functions
Eases energy obstruction in *Tai*-Yang Meridian;
Frees energy obstruction in chest and ribs.

Symptoms
Ache & pain in shoulder & arm
Swelling of cheek & neck

Clinical formula
SI 11 + CV 17 = Pain in chest

Method of treatment
Needle: 0.5 inch perpendicularly.
Moxa: Warm heating, 3 minutes.
Feeling: Very sensitive to the touch; the needle sensation moves down the arm to the little finger.

SI 12; *Bing-Feng*; 'Wind Receiver'

Location
Directly above SI 11 in centre of suprascapular fossa in depression formed when arm is raised.

Regional anatomy
Trapezius muscle;
Supraspinous muscle;
Suprascapular artery & vein;
Lateral suprascapular nerve;
Accessory nerve;
Suprascapular nerve.

Connecting point
Meeting Point of Hand *Tai*-Yang, Foot Yang-*Ming*, and Hand and Foot *Shao*-Yang Meridians.

Symptoms
Shoulder pain

Method of treatment
Needle: 0.5 inch obliquely.
Moxa: Warm heating, 3 minutes.
Feeling: Ache and/or swelling.

SI 13; *Qu-Yuan*; 'Crooked Wall'

Location
At medial end of suprascapular fossa, midway on line between SI 10 and spinous process of second thoracic vertebra.

Regional anatomy
Trapezius muscle;
Supraspinous muscle;
Transverse cervical artery & vein;
Posterior branch of second thoracic nerve;
Accessory nerve;
Muscular branch of suprascapular artery, vein & nerve.

Symptoms
Pain in scapular region

Method of treatment
Needle: 0.5 inch obliquely.
Moxa: Warm heating, 2 minutes.
Feeling: Ache.

SI 14; Jian-Wai-Shu; 'Shu Point of External Shoulder'

Location
3 cun lateral to GV 13 on a vertical line from vertebral border of scapula.

Regional anatomy
Trapezius muscle;
Levator muscle of scapula;
Lesser rhomboid muscle;
Transverse cervical artery & vein;
Medial cutaneous branches of posterior branches of first & second thoracic nerves;
Accessory nerve;
Dorsal scapular nerve.

Symptoms
Ache & pain in back & shoulder
Stiff neck

Method of treatment
Needle: 0.6 inch perpendicularly.
Moxa: Warm heating, 3 minutes.
Feeling: Ache and/or numbness.

SI 15; Jian-Zhong-Shu; 'Shu Point of Middle Shoulder'

Location
2 cun lateral to GV 14.

Regional anatomy
Trapezius muscle;
Levator muscle of scapula;
Lesser rhomboid muscle;
Transverse cervical artery & vein;
Medial cutaneous branches of posterior branches of first & second thoracic nerves;
Accessory nerve;
Dorsal scapular nerve.

Symptoms
Coughing   Pain in back & shoulder
Shortness of breath   Blurred vision

Method of treatment
Needle: 0.3 inch perpendicularly.
Moxa: Warm heating, 3 minutes.
Feeling: Ache and/or numbness.

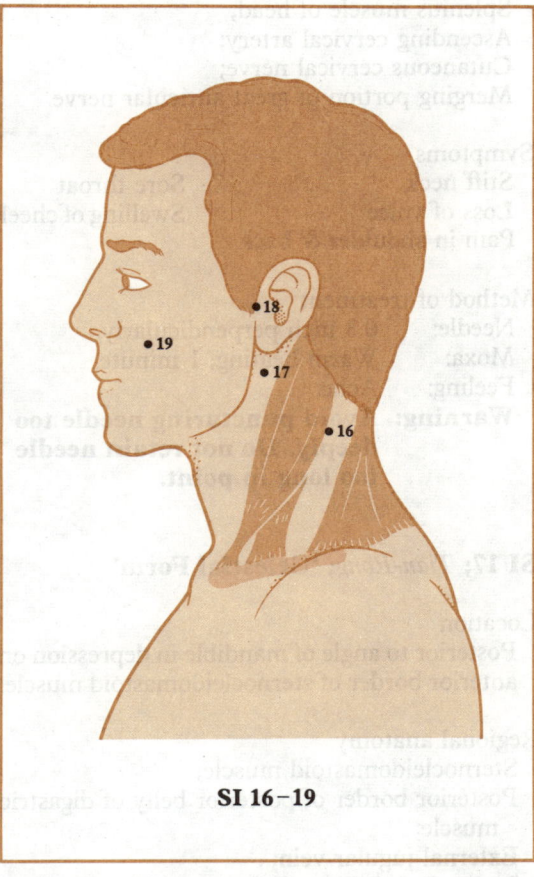

SI 16–19

FOURTEEN MERIDIANS AND ACUPUNCTURE POINTS

SI 16; *Tian-Chuang*; 'Heavenly Window'

Location
At posterior border of sternocleidomastoid muscle, posterosuperior to LI 18.

Regional anatomy
Anterior border of trapezius muscle;
Posterior border of levator muscle of scapula;
Splenius muscle of head;
Ascending cervical artery;
Cutaneous cervical nerve;
Merging portion of great auricular nerve.

Symptoms

Stiff neck	Sore throat
Loss of voice	Swelling of cheek
Pain in shoulder & back	

Method of treatment
Needle: 0.3 inch perpendicularly.
Moxa: Warm heating, 1 minute.
Feeling: Ache.
Warning: Avoid puncturing needle too deeply. Do not retain needle too long in point.

SI 17; *Tian-Rong*; 'Celestial Form'

Location
Posterior to angle of mandible in depression on anterior border of sternocleidomastoid muscle.

Regional anatomy
Sternocleidomastoid muscle;
Posterior border of posterior belly of digastric muscle;
External jugular vein;
Internal carotid artery & internal jugular vein;
Anterior branch of great auricular nerve;
Cervical branch of facial nerve;
Superior cervical ganglion of sympathetic trunk.

Symptoms

Sore throat	Shortness of breath
Stiff neck	Deafness
Chest pain	Tinnitus aurium

Method of treatment
Needle: 0.2 inch perpendicularly.
Moxa: Warm heating, 1 minute.
Feeling: Ache and/or numbness.
Warning: Avoid inserting needle too deeply. Experience in needle technique is required.

SI 18; *Quan-Liao*; 'Zygomatic Bone'

Location
Directly below outer canthus in depression on lower border of zygomatic bone.

Regional anatomy
Origin of masseter muscle;
Zygomatic muscle;
Branches of transverse facial artery & vein;
Facial & infraorbital nerves.

Connecting point
Meeting Point of Hand *Shao*-Yang and Hand *Tai*-Yang Meridians.

Symptoms

Facial paralysis	Toothache
Twitching of eyelids	Trigeminal neuralgia

Method of treatment
Needle: 0.3 inch perpendicularly.
Moxa: **Forbidden.**
Feeling: Ache and/or swelling.

FOURTEEN MERIDIANS AND ACUPUNCTURE POINTS

Note
This point has been used for forehead region operations under acupuncture anaesthesia.

SI 19; *Ting-Gong*; 'Listening Palace'

Location
Between tragus and mandibular joint where depression is formed when mouth is slightly open.

Regional anatomy
Auricular branches of superficial temporal artery & vein;
Branch of facial nerve;
Auriculotemporal nerve.

Connecting point
Meeting Point of Hand and Foot *Shao*-Yang and Hand *Tai*-Yang Meridians.

Functions
Frees and opens 'Gate of the Ear';
Creates quiet in mind and *Shen*.

Symptoms
Loss of voice   Tinnitus aurium
Deafness

Method of treatment
Needle: 0.3 inch perpendicularly.
Moxa: Warm heating, 1 minute.
Feeling: Swelling.
Warning: When treating deafness, it is necessary to insert needle about 1 inch. The practitioner must be experienced.

7. Bladder Meridian of Foot Tai-Yang

This Meridian is characterized by high blood flow and low energy flow. The energy flow originates at the inner canthus, Bl 1, ascends to the forehead to meet GV 24 and GB 15, and runs up to Bl 7 to join GV 20 at the vertex, where a branch runs down to the temple, then carries on to connect with GB 7, GB 8, GB 10, GB 11 and GB 12.

The main Meridian runs from the vertex to Bl 9, enters the Brain, meets GV 17 and comes out again at Bl 10. Here it again divides. One branch proceeds to GV 14, GV 13 and then to Bl 11, running alongside the spinal column to arrive at Bl 23. This branch first enters the Kidney and then the Bladder. The other branch goes to Bl 41, running parallel with the vertebral column and 3 *cun* from the Governor Vessel Meridian. Proceeding downwards, it passes over the gluteal region, GB 30, and meets the other branch (from Bl 23) at Bl 40.

The main Meridian continues down through the gluteal region to the popliteal fossa, Bl 40, then travels down the leg, past the external malleolus, to end at the little toe, Bl 67. From this point it runs to K 1 where it links with the Kidney Meridian.

There are sixty-seven acupuncture points on each side of the Bladder Meridian.

Associated organs
- Belongs to Bladder;
- Related to Kidneys;
- Directly connected to Brain and Heart.

Connecting points
- GB 7 GB 8 GB 10 GB 11 GB 12 GB 15
GB 30 GV 13 GV 14 GV 17 GV 20

Symptomatology
- Disorders along Meridian course
Fever   Ophthalmalgia
Headache   Lacrimation

FOURTEEN MERIDIANS AND ACUPUNCTURE POINTS

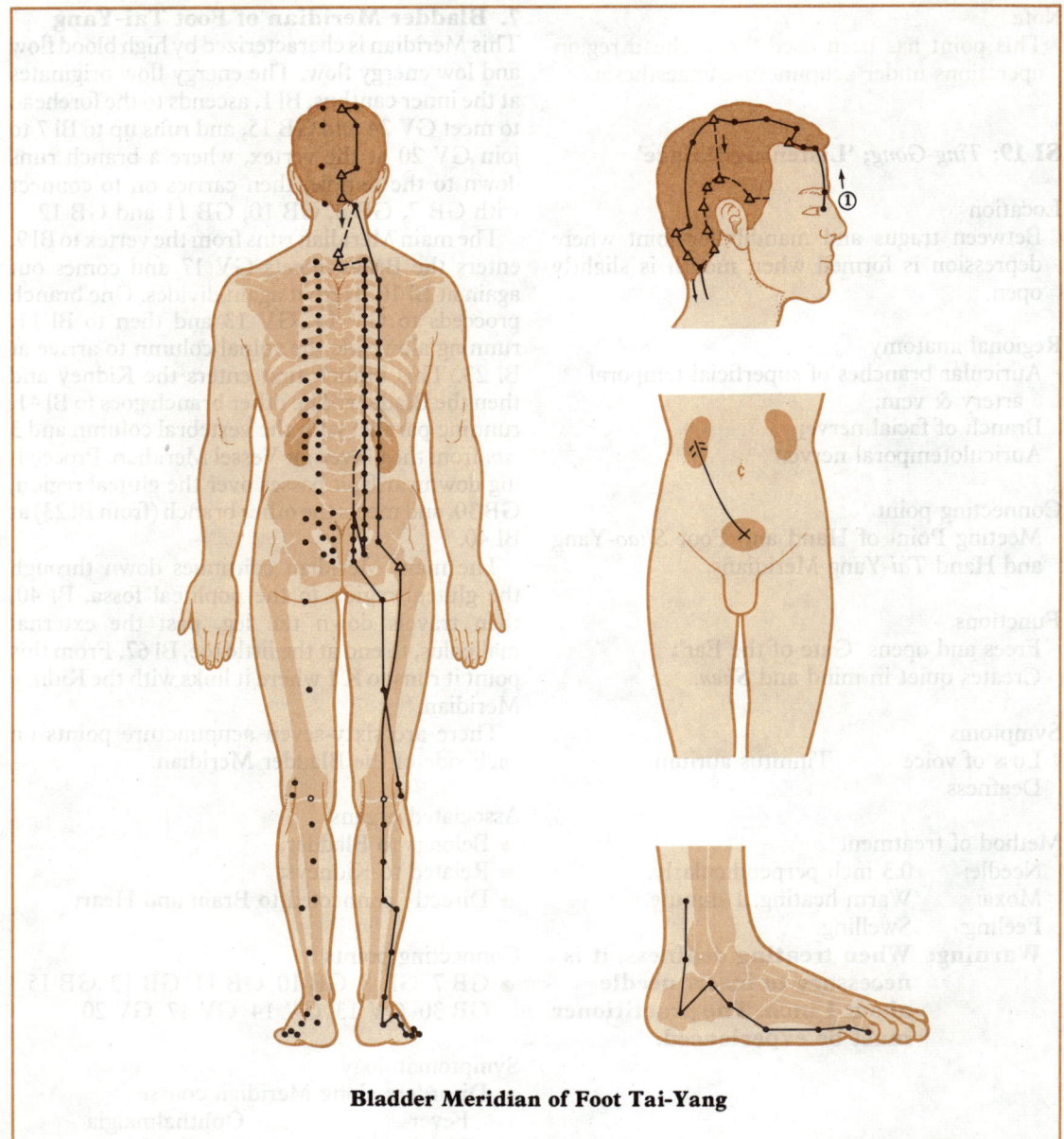

Bladder Meridian of Foot Tai-Yang

FOURTEEN MERIDIANS AND ACUPUNCTURE POINTS

Stiff neck
Pain in spine & lower back
Nasal obstruction
Pain along thigh, knee, popliteal fossa, leg & foot

• Disorders in organ
Lower abdominal distention & pain
Dysuria
Enuresis
Mental disorders

Acupuncture Points of Bladder Meridian

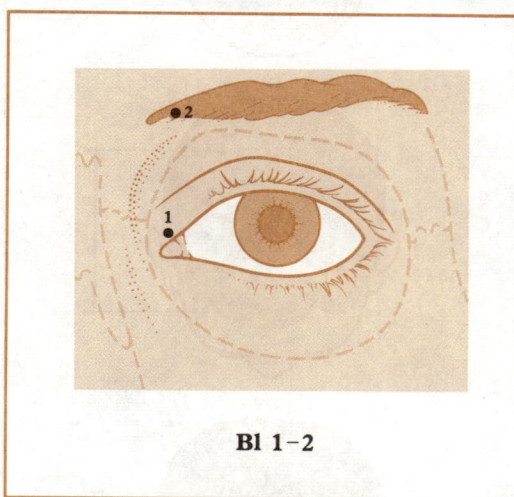

Bl 1–2

Bl 1; *Jing-Ming*; 'Bright Eyes'

Location
0.1 *cun* superior to inner canthus.

Regional anatomy
Medial rectus muscle of eyeball;
Angular artery & vein;
Ophthalmic artery & vein;
Supra- & infratrochlear nerves;
Branches of oculomotor nerve;
Ophthalmic nerve;
Lacrimal canaliculi;
Lacrimal sac;
Nasolacrimal duct.

Connecting point
Meeting Point of five Meridians: Hand and Foot *Tai*-Yang, Foot Yang-*Ming*, Yang- and Yin-*Qiao* Meridians.

Functions
Dispels wind and eliminates heat;
Nourishes water which clears eyes.

Symptoms
Myopia
Lacrimation
Headache
Redness, swelling & pain in eyes
Itching of inner canthus

Clinical formula
Bl 1 + Bl 2 + St 36 + St 44 = Redness, swelling and pain in eyes

Method of treatment
Needle: 0.2 inch perpendicularly.
Moxa: **Forbidden.**
Feeling: Ache/swelling/great pain around eyeballs or behind the eyes.
Warning: Skilled needle technique is very important. Without experience, puncturing may be dangerous.

Bl 2; *Zan-Zhu*; 'Holding the Bamboo'

Location
Directly above Bl 1 in depression on medial extremity of eyebrow at edge of orbit.

Regional anatomy
Frontal muscle;
Superciliary corrugator muscle;

141

FOURTEEN MERIDIANS AND ACUPUNCTURE POINTS

Frontal artery & vein;
Medial branch of frontal nerve.

Functions
Eliminates wind;
Clears eyes.

Symptoms
Blurred vision   Palpebral spasm
Lacrimation   Headache
Itching of eyes   Trigeminal neuralgia
Ophthalmalgia

Clinical formula
Bl 2 + St 8 = Ophthalmalgia

Method of treatment
Needle: 0.2 inch horizontally with needle tip inferiorly or laterally, or prick with three-edged needle to cause bleeding.
Moxa: **Forbidden.**
Feeling: Ache and/or swelling.
Warning: This point bleeds easily.

Bl 3; *Mei-Chong*; 'Thoroughfare of Eyebrow'

Location
On a line above Bl 2, 0.5 *cun* inside hairline, level with GV 24.

Regional anatomy
Frontal muscle;
Frontal artery & vein;
Medial branch of frontal nerve.

Symptoms
Headache
Nasal obstruction
(Epilepsy)

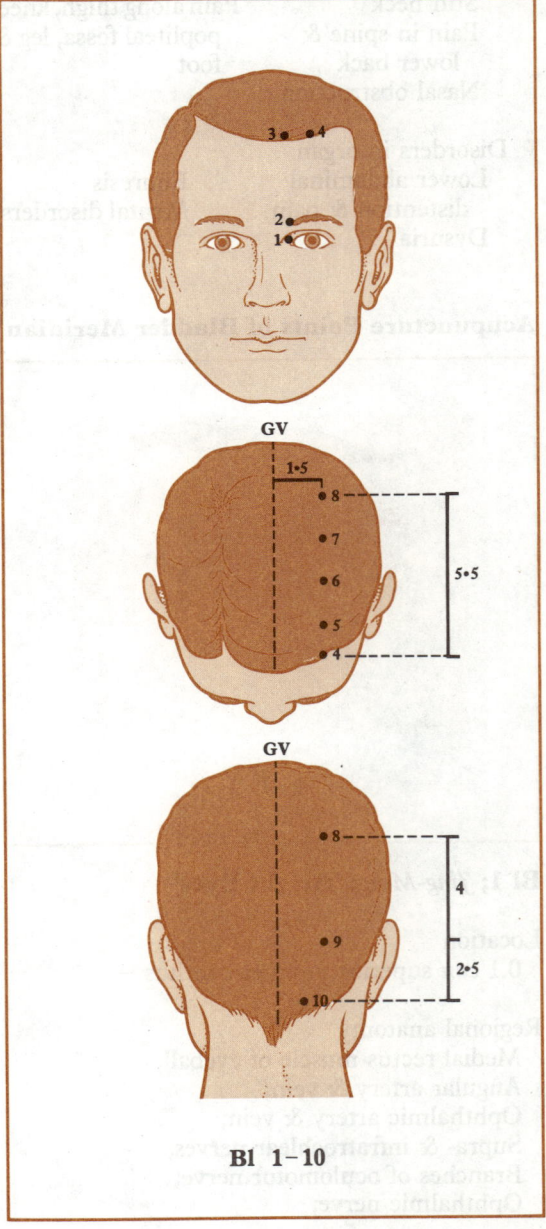

Bl 1–10

FOURTEEN MERIDIANS AND ACUPUNCTURE POINTS

Method of treatment
  Needle: 0.3 inch horizontally, directed upwards.
  Moxa: **Forbidden.**
  Feeling: Swelling and/or heaviness.

Bl 4; *Qu-Chai*; 'Crooked Curve'

Location
  Same level as Bl 3, 1.5 *cun* lateral to GV 24.

Regional anatomy
  Frontal muscle;
  Frontal artery, vein & nerve.

Symptoms
  Blurred vision   Restlessness
  Epistaxis   Headache
  Nasal obstruction

Method of treatment
  Needle: 0.2 inch horizontally, directed upwards.
  Moxa: Warm heating, 1 minute.
  Feeling: Swelling and/or heaviness.

Bl 5; *Wu-Chu*; 'Five Regions'

Location
  Directly above Bl 4, 1 *cun* inside anterior hairline.

Regional anatomy
  Frontal muscle;
  Frontal artery, vein & nerve.

Symptoms
  Headache
  Blurred vision
  (Epilepsy)

Method of treatment
  Needle: 0.3 inch horizontally, directed upwards.
  Moxa: Warm heating, 1 minute.
  Feeling: Swelling and/or heaviness.

Bl 6; *Cheng-Guang*; 'Receive Light'

Location
  1.5 *cun* posterior to Bl 5.

Regional anatomy
  Galea aponeurotica;
  Occipitofrontal muscle aponeurosis;
  Frontal artery, vein & nerve;
  Superficial temporal artery & vein;
  Occipital artery & vein;
  Branch of greater occipital nerve.

Symptoms
  Headache & giddiness   Facial paralysis
  Restlessness   Blurred vision
  Nasal obstruction

Method of treatment
  Needle: 0.3 inch horizontally, directed upwards.
  Moxa: **Forbidden.**
  Feeling: Swelling and/or heaviness.

Bl 7; *Tong-Tian*; 'Penetrating Heaven'

Location
  1.5 *cun* posterior to Bl 6.

Regional anatomy
  Galea aponeurotica;
  Occipitofrontal muscle aponeurosis;
  Anastomotic network of superficial temporal artery & vein;

FOURTEEN MERIDIANS AND ACUPUNCTURE POINTS

Occipital artery & vein;
Branch of greater occipital nerve.

Symptoms
Stiff neck   Rhinorrhoea
Epistaxis   Dyspnoea
Nasal obstruction   Headache

Method of treatment
Needle: 0.3 inch horizontally, directed upwards;
Moxa: Warm heating, 1 minute.
Feeling: Swelling and/or heaviness.

Bl 8; *Luo-Que*; 'Luo-Cleft'

Location
1.5 *cun* posterior to Bl 7.

Regional anatomy
Insertion of occipital muscle;
Branches of occipital artery & vein;
Branch of greater occipital nerve.

Symptoms
Dizziness   Mental confusion
Tinnitus aurium   Blurred vision

Method of treatment
Needle: 0.3 inch horizontally, directed upwards.
Moxa: Warm heating, 1 minute.
Feeling: Swelling and/or heaviness.

Bl 9; *Yu-Zhen*; 'Jade Pillow'

Location
1.5 *cun* posterior to Bl 8 and 1.3 *cun* lateral to GV 17, on lateral side of superior border of external occipital protuberance.

Regional anatomy
Occipital muscle;
Occipital artery & vein;
Branch of greater occipital nerve.

Symptoms
Ophthalmalgia   Headache
Myopia   Nasal obstruction

Method of treatment
Needle: 0.3 inch horizontally, directed downwards.
Moxa: Warm heating, 1 minute.
Feeling: Ache and/or heaviness.

Bl 10; *Tian-Zhu*; 'Celestial Column'

Location
1.3 *cun* lateral to GV 15 inside posterior hairline on lateral side of trapezius muscle.

Regional anatomy
Origin of trapezius muscle;
Splenius muscle of neck;
Occipital artery & vein;
Greater occipital nerve.

Symptoms
Pain in shoulder & back   Nasal obstruction
Blurred vision   Stiff neck
Headache

Clinical formula
Bl 10 + SI 6 = Pain in shoulder and back

Method of treatment
Needle: 0.3 inch perpendicularly.
Moxa: **Forbidden.**
Feeling: Ache and/or swelling.

FOURTEEN MERIDIANS AND ACUPUNCTURE POINTS

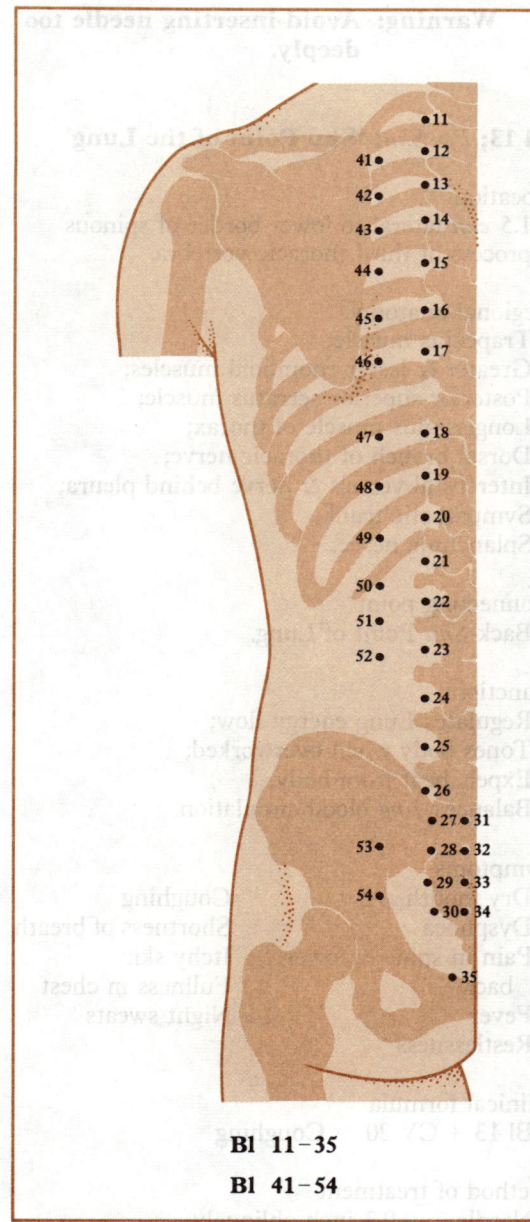

Bl 11–35
Bl 41–54

Bl 11; *Da-Shu*; 'Big Shuttle'

Location
1.5 *cun* lateral to lower border of spinous process of first thoracic vertebra.

Regional anatomy
Trapezius muscle;
Greater & lesser rhomboid muscles;
Posterior superior serratus muscle;
Longissimus muscle of thorax;
Dorsal branch of thoracic nerve;
Intercostal vessels & nerve behind pleura;
Sympathetic trunk;
Splanchnic nerve.

Connecting points
Meeting Point of Hand and Foot *Tai*-Yang and *Shao*-Yang Meridians; Divergent Meridian of Governor Vessel Meridian; one of 'Eight Influential Points' dominating bone.

Functions
Dispels wind;
Expels excess heat from body;
Frees movement of tendons;
Regulates function of bones & joints.

Symptoms
Pain in spine & lower back   Coughing
Fever   Abdominal pain
Stiff neck   Pain in knee
Dizziness   (Epilepsy)

Method of treatment
Needle: 0.3 inch obliquely.
Moxa: Not used unless absolutely necessary; needle is preferable.
Feeling: Ache and/or swelling.
Warning: Inserting the needle too deeply in the region of the first to tenth thoracic vertebrae will

145

FOURTEEN MERIDIANS AND ACUPUNCTURE POINTS

will damage the vital internal organ.

Warning: Avoid inserting needle too deeply.

Bl 12; *Feng-Men*; 'Wind Gate'

Location
  1.5 *cun* lateral to lower border of spinous process of second thoracic vertebra.

Regional anatomy
  Trapezius muscle;
  Greater & lesser rhomboid muscles;
  Posterior superior serratus muscle;
  Longissimus muscle of thorax;
  Dorsal branch of thoracic nerve;
  Intercostal vessels & nerve behind pleura;
  Sympathetic trunk;
  Splanchnic nerve.

Connecting point
  Meeting Point of Governor Vessel Meridian and Foot *Tai*-Yang Meridian.

Functions
  Dispels wind;
  Strengthens function of Lungs;
  Frees energy flow;
  Eases cold and heat in body.

Symptoms
  Fever   Pain in chest & back
  Shortness of breath Acute rhinitis
  Coughing   Stiff neck

Clinical formula
  Bl 12 + Lu 5 + GV 13 = Common cold

Method of treatment
  Needle: 0.3 inch obliquely.
  Moxa: Warm heating, 2 minutes.
  Feeling: Ache and/or swelling.

Bl 13; *Fei-Shu*; 'Shu Point of the Lung'

Location
  1.5 *cun* lateral to lower border of spinous process of third thoracic vertebra.

Regional anatomy
  Trapezius muscle;
  Greater & lesser rhomboid muscles;
  Posterior superior serratus muscle;
  Longissimus muscle of thorax;
  Dorsal branch of thoracic nerve;
  Intercostal vessels & nerve behind pleura;
  Sympathetic trunk;
  Splanchnic nerve.

Connecting point
  Back-*Shu* Point of Lung.

Functions
  Regulates Lung energy flow;
  Tones body when overworked;
  Expels heat from body;
  Balances *Jing* blood circulation.

Symptoms
  Dry mouth   Coughing
  Dyspnoea   Shortness of breath
  Pain in spine & lower Itchy skin
    back   Fullness in chest
  Fever   Night sweats
  Restlessness

Clinical formula
  Bl 13 + CV 20 = Coughing

Method of treatment
  Needle: 0.3 inch obliquely.

Bl 14; *Jue-Yin-Shu*; 'Shu Point of the Pericardium'

Location
1.5 *cun* lateral to inferior border of spinous process of fourth thoracic vertebra.

Regional anatomy
  Trapezius muscle;
  Greater & lesser rhomboid muscles;
  Posterior superior serratus muscle;
  Longissimus muscle of thorax;
  Dorsal branch of thoracic nerve;
  Intercostal vessels & nerve behind pleura;
  Sympathetic trunk;
  Splanchnic nerve.

Connecting point
  Back-*Shu* Point of Pericardium.

Symptoms
  Coughing   Restlessness
  Shortness of breath   Fullness in chest
  Cardiac pain

Method of treatment
  Needle: 0.3 inch obliquely.
  Moxa: Warm heating, 2 minutes.
  Feeling: Ache and/or swelling.
  Warning: Avoid inserting needle too deeply.

Bl 15; *Xin-Shu*; 'Shu Point of the Heart'

Location
1.5 *cun* lateral to lower border of spinous process of fifth thoracic vertebra.

Regional anatomy
  Trapezius muscle;
  Greater & lesser rhomboid muscles;
  Posterior superior serratus muscle;
  Longissimus muscle of thorax;
  Dorsal branch of thoracic nerve;
  Intercostal vessels & nerve behind pleura;
  Sympathetic trunk;
  Splanchnic nerve.

Connecting point
  Back-*Shu* Point of Heart.

Functions
  Creates quiet in mind and *Shen*;
  Strengthens & harmonizes Heart function.

Symptoms
  Hemiplegia   Sadness
  Palpitations   Loss of memory
  Cardiac pain   Coughing
  Restlessness   Hemoptysis

Clinical formula
  Bl 15 + H 7 + H 3 + Lu 7 = Loss of memory

Method of treatment
  Needle: 0.3 inch obliquely.
  Moxa: Warm heating, 2 minutes.
  Feeling: Ache and/or swelling.
  Warning: Avoid puncturing needle too deeply.

FOURTEEN MERIDIANS AND ACUPUNCTURE POINTS

Bl 16; *Du-Shu*; 'Shu Point of Governor Vessel'

Location
1.5 *cun* lateral to inferior border of spinous process of sixth thoracic vertebra.

Regional anatomy
Trapezius muscle;
Latissimus dorsi muscle;
Longissimus muscle of thorax;
Intercostal artery & vein;
Descending branch of transverse cervical artery;
Dorsal scapular nerve;
Dorsal branch of thoracic nerve;
Intercostal nerve;
Sympathetic trunk;
Splanchnic nerve.

Connecting point
Shu Point of Governor Vessel Meridian.

Functions
Harmonizes Stomach function;
Stops vomiting.

Symptoms
Fever   Abdominal pain
Cardiac pain   Vomiting

Method of treatment
Needle: 0.3 inch obliquely.
Moxa: Warm heating, 2 minutes.
Feeling: Ache and/or swelling.
Warning: Avoid inserting needle too deeply.

Bl 17; *Ge-Shu*; 'Shu Point of the Diaphragm'

Location
1.5 *cun* lateral to lower border of spinous process of seventh thoracic vertebra.

Regional anatomy
Trapezius muscle;
Latissimus dorsi muscle;
Longissimus muscle of thorax;
Intercostal artery & vein;
Dorsal branch of thoracic nerve;
Intercostal nerve;
Sympathetic trunk;
Splanchnic nerve.

Connecting points
Shu Point of Diaphragm; one of 'Eight Influential Points' which controls blood.

Functions
Expels excess heat from blood;
Tones body when overworked;
Harmonizes function of Stomach;
Improves movement of diaphragm.

Symptoms
Cardiac pain   Sweating
Vomiting   Fever
Hiccups   Body heaviness
Fatigue   Fullness & pain in chest
Drowsiness

Method of treatment
Needle: 0.3 inch obliquely.
Moxa: Warm heating, 2 minutes.
Feeling: Ache and/or swelling.
Warning: Avoid inserting needle too deeply.

Bl 18; *Gan-Shu*; 'Shu Point of the Liver'

Location
1.5 *cun* lateral to inferior border of spinous process of ninth thoracic vertebra.

Regional anatomy
  Latissimus dorsi muscle;
  Longissimus muscle of thorax;
  Iliocostal muscle;
  Intercostal artery & vein;
  Dorsal branch of thoracic nerve;
  Intercostal nerve;
  Sympathetic trunk;
  Splanchnic nerve.

Connecting point
  Back-*Shu* Point of Liver.

Functions
  Tones *Jing* blood;
  Disperses blood stasis in Liver;
  Expels excess heat and damp from Liver and Gall Bladder;
  Creates quiet in mind and *Shen*;
  Clears vision.

Symptoms
Anger	Cough
Dry mouth	Shortness of breath
Dizziness	Muscular spasm
Blurred vision	

Clinical formula
  Bl 18 + St 36 = Eye disorder

Method of treatment
  Needle: 0.3 inch obliquely.
  Moxa: Warm heating, 2 minutes.
  Feeling: Ache and/or swelling.
  Warning: Avoid inserting needle too deeply.

Bl 19; *Dan-Shu*; 'Shu Point of the Gall Bladder'

Location
1.5 *cun* lateral to lower border of spinous process of tenth thoracic vertebra.

Regional anatomy
  Latissimus dorsi muscle;
  Longissimus muscle of thorax;
  Iliocostal muscle;
  Intercostal artery & vein;
  Dorsal branch of thoracic nerve;
  Intercostal nerve;
  Sympathetic trunk;
  Splanchnic nerve.

Connecting point
  Back-*Shu* Point of Gall Bladder.

Functions
  Expels excess heat and damp from Gall Bladder;
  Harmonizes function of Stomach;
  Improves movement of diaphragm;
  Clears vision.

Symptoms
Headache	Dry mouth
Sore throat	Bitter taste in mouth
Swelling in hypochondriac region	

Method of treatment
  Needle: 0.3 inch obliquely.
  Moxa: Warm heating, 2 minutes.
  Feeling: Ache and/or swelling.
  Warning: Avoid inserting needle too deeply.

FOURTEEN MERIDIANS AND ACUPUNCTURE POINTS

Bl 20; *Pi-Shu*; 'Shu Point of the Spleen'

Location
1.5 *cun* lateral to lower border of spinous process of eleventh thoracic vertebra.

Regional anatomy
Latissimus dorsi muscle;
Longissimus muscle of thorax;
Iliocostal muscle;
Intercostal artery & vein;
Dorsal branch of thoracic nerve;
Intercostal nerve;
Sympathetic trunk;
Splanchnic nerve.

Connecting point
Back-*Shu* Point of Spleen.

Functions
Strengthens 'Earth' function;
Dispels damp in Spleen;
Balances functions of Spleen and Stomach;
Increases digestive, absorptive and transport functions of Spleen and Stomach.

Symptoms
Abdominal distention	Diarrhoea
Pain in chest & back	Oedema
Indigestion	Anorexia

Clinical formula
Bl 20 + Bl 21 = Indigestion

Method of treatment
Needle: 0.3 inch obliquely.
Moxa: Warm heating, 2 minutes.
Feeling: Ache and/or swelling.
Warning: Avoid inserting needle too deeply.

Bl 21; *Wei-Shu*; 'Shu Point of the Stomach'

Location
1.5 *cun* lateral to inferior border of spinous process of twelfth thoracic vertebra.

Regional anatomy
Lumbodorsal fascia;
Longissimus muscle of thorax;
Iliocostal muscle;
Intercostal artery & vein;
Dorsal branch of thoracic nerve;
Intercostal nerve;
Sympathetic trunk;
Splanchnic nerve.

Connecting point
Back-*Shu* Point of Stomach.

Functions
Balances functions of Middle Heater and Stomach;
Dispels damp;
Improves digestion;
Strengthens body energy flow.

Symptoms
Abdominal distention	Loss of appetite
Gastric pain	Fullness in chest
Vomiting	

Clinical formula
Bl 21 + Bl 23 = Abdominal distention

Method of treatment
Needle: 0.3 inch obliquely.
Moxa: Warm heating, 2 minutes.
Feeling: Ache and/or swelling.
Warning: Avoid inserting needle too deeply.

Bl 22; *San-Jiao-Shu*; 'Shu Point of the Three Heater'

Location
1.5 *cun* lateral to inferior border of spinous process of first lumbar vertebra.

Regional anatomy
Lumbodorsal fascia;
Longissimus muscle of thorax;
Iliocostal muscle;
Posterior branch of lumbar artery & vein;
Dorsal branch of thoracic nerve;
Iliohypogastric nerve;
Sympathetic trunk.

Connecting point
Back-*Shu* Point of Three Heater.

Functions
Harmonizes Stomach function;
Regulates Three Heater function;
Regulates water metabolism.

Symptoms
Pain in shoulder, back & lower back	Diarrhoea
Abdominal distention	Headache
Indigestion	Dizziness

Method of treatment
Needle: 0.5 inch obliquely.
Moxa: Warm heating, 2 minutes.
Feeling: Ache and/or numbness.

Bl 23; *Shen-Shu*; 'Shu Point of the Kidney'

Location
1.5 *cun* lateral to inferior border of spinous process of second lumbar vertebra.

Regional anatomy
Lumbodorsal fascia;
Longissimus muscle of thorax;
Iliocostal muscle;
Posterior branch of lumbar artery & vein;
Ilioinguinal nerve;
Sympathetic trunk.

Connecting point
Back-*Shu* Point of Kidney.

Functions
Tones Kidneys;
Increases function of *Ming-Men-Huo*;
Eliminates damp and water;
Strengthens function of lumbar spine;
Balances function between Water (Kidney) and Fire (Heart);
Clears vision;
Improves hearing.

Symptoms
General weakness	Seminal emission
Deafness	Weakness of leg
Oedema	Irregular menstruation
Abdominal distention	Impotence
Lower back pain	Enuresis
Pain in lower abdomen	Leucorrhoea

Clinical formula
Bl 23 + CV 4 = Impotence

Method of treatment
Needle: 0.3 inch perpendicularly.
Moxa: Warm heating, 3 minutes.
Feeling: Ache and/or numbness.

Bl 24; *Qi-Hai-Shu*; 'Shu Point of the Centre Energy'

Location
1.5 *cun* lateral to inferior border of spinous process of third lumbar vertebra.

Regional anatomy
Lumbodorsal fascia;
Longissimus muscle of thorax;
Iliocostal muscle;
Lumbar artery & vein;
Lateral cutaneous nerve of thigh;
Sympathetic trunk.

Connecting point
Shu Point of Centre Energy.

Symptoms
Lower back pain
(Haemorrhoids)

Method of treatment
Needle: 0.3 inch perpendicularly.
Moxa: Warm heating, 3 minutes.
Feeling: Ache and/or numbness.

Bl 25; *Da-Chang-Shu*; 'Shu Point of the Large Intestine'

Location
1.5 *cun* lateral to inferior border of spinous process of fourth lumbar vertebra.

Regional anatomy
Lumbodorsal fascia;
Longissimus muscle of thorax;
Iliocostal muscle;
Lumbar artery & vein;
Femoral nerve;
Sympathetic trunk.

Connecting point
Back-*Shu* Point of Large Intestine.

Functions
Regulates and balances functions of Large and Small Intestines;
Frees movement of Large Intestine.

Symptoms
Lumbar pain
Lower abdominal pain
Abdominal pain & distention
Indigestion
Difficulty in bladder & bowel movements (especially after general anaesthesia in lumbar region)

Method of treatment
Needle: 0.3 inch perpendicularly.
Moxa: Warm heating, 3 minutes.
Feeling: Ache and/or swelling.

Bl 26; *Guan-Yuan-Shu*; 'Shu Point of the Door of Vital Essence'

Location
1.5 *cun* lateral to inferior border of spinous process of fifth lumbar vertebra.

Regional anatomy
Erector muscle of spine;
Lumbar artery & vein;
Lumbosacral trunk nerve;
Sympathetic nerve.

Connecting point
Back-*Shu* Point of 'Door of Vital Essence'.

Symptoms
Lumbar pain   Dysuria
Diarrhoea   Enuresis

FOURTEEN MERIDIANS AND ACUPUNCTURE POINTS

Method of treatment
- Needle: 0.3 inch perpendicularly.
- Moxa: Warm heating, 3 minutes.
- Feeling: Ache and/or numbness.

Bl 27; *Xiao-Chang-Shu*; 'Shu Point of the Small Intestine'

Location
1.5 *cun* lateral to midline of back at level of first posterior sacral foramen.

Regional anatomy
Origin of erector muscle of spine;
Greatest gluteal muscle;
Posterior branches of lateral sacral artery & vein;
Lateral branches of posterior branch of first sacral nerve.

Connecting point
Back-*Shu* Point of Small Intestine.

Functions
Harmonizes and strengthens function of Small Intestine;
Harmonizes function of Bladder;
Regulates movements of Small Intestine and Bladder.

Symptoms
Dysuria	Swelling of legs
Diarrhoea	Leucorrhoea
Dry mouth	(Haemorrhoids)
Lower abdominal distention	

Method of treatment
- Needle: 0.3 inch perpendicularly.
- Moxa: Warm heating, 3 minutes.
- Feeling: Ache and/or numbness.

Bl 28; *Pang-Guang-Shu*; 'Shu Point of the Bladder'

Location
1.5 *cun* lateral to midline of back at level of second posterior sacral foramen.

Regional anatomy
Origin of erector muscle of spine;
Greatest gluteal muscle;
Posterior branches of lateral sacral artery & vein;
Lateral branches of posterior branch of first & second sacral nerves.

Connecting point
Back-*Shu* Point of Bladder.

Functions
Harmonizes function of Bladder;
Regulates function of Lower Heater;
Frees movement of lumbar spine;
Dispels wind and damp in Bladder.

Symptoms
Lumbar pain	Abdominal distention
Urine retention	Constipation
Enuresis	Weakness in knee & leg

Method of treatment
- Needle: 0.3 inch perpendicularly.
- Moxa: Warm heating, 3 minutes.
- Feeling: Ache and/or numbness.

Bl 29; *Zhong-Lu-Shu*; 'Shu Point of Middle of Back Bone'

Location
1.5 *cun* lateral to Governor Vessel Meridian at level of third posterior sacral foramen.

FOURTEEN MERIDIANS AND ACUPUNCTURE POINTS

Regional anatomy
   Greatest gluteal muscle;
   Origin of sacrotuberous ligament;
   Posterior branches of lateral sacral artery & vein;
   Branches of inferior gluteal artery & vein;
   Lateral branches of posterior branch of third & fourth sacral nerves.

Symptoms
   Lower back pain
   Diarrhoea
   Abdominal distention

Method of treatment
   Needle: 0.3 inch perpendicularly.
   Moxa: Warm heating, 3 minutes.
   Feeling: Ache.

Bl 30; *Bai-Huan-Shu*; 'Shu Point of the White Circle'

Location
   1.5 *cun* lateral to Governor Vessel Meridian at level of fourth posterior sacral foramen.

Regional anatomy
   Greatest gluteal muscle;
   Inferior to sacrotuberous ligament;
   Inferior gluteal artery & vein;
   Internal pudendal artery & vein;
   Lateral branches of posterior branches of third & fourth sacral nerves;
   Inferior gluteal nerve.

Symptoms
   Pain in lower back & spine
   Dysuria
   Pain in hip & leg

Method of treatment
   Needle: 0.5 inch perpendicularly.

Moxa: Warm heating, 3 minutes; No moxa cone.
Feeling: Ache.

Bl 31; *Shang-Liao*; 'Upper Hole'

Location
   In first posterior sacral foramen, midway between posterior superior iliac spine and Governor Vessel Meridian.

Regional anatomy
   Origin of erector muscle of spine;
   Origin of greatest gluteal muscle;
   Posterior branches of lateral sacral artery & vein;
   Posterior branch of first sacral nerve.

Symptoms
   Urine retention   Pain in lower back & knee
   Leucorrhoea   Sterility

Method of treatment
   Needle: 0.3 inch perpendicularly.
   Moxa: Warm heating, 3 minutes.
   Feeling: Ache and/or numbness.

Note
There are eight acupuncture points in the eight sacral foramina. The principal treatment at this point is for lower back pain, including external problems with muscles and tendons, and for internal problems such as menstrual pain and disorder in the uterus or bladder.

Bl 32; *Ci-Liao*; 'Second Hole'

Location
   In second posterior sacral foramen.

FOURTEEN MERIDIANS AND ACUPUNCTURE POINTS

Regional anatomy
  Origin of greatest gluteal muscle;
  Posterior branches of lateral sacral artery & vein;
  Posterior branch of second sacral nerve.

Symptoms
  Frequent micturition   Leucorrhoea
  Lower back pain   Lower abdominal pain
  Diarrhoea

Method of treatment
  Needle: 0.3 inch perpendicularly.
  Moxa: Warm heating, 3 minutes.
  Feeling: Ache and/or numbness.

Bl 33; *Zhong-Liao*; 'Third Hole'

Location
  In third posterior sacral foramen.

Regional anatomy
  Origin of greatest gluteal muscle;
  Posterior branches of lateral sacral artery & vein;
  Posterior branch of third sacral nerve.

Connecting point
  Meeting Point of Foot *Jue*-Yin and Foot *Shao*-Yang Meridians.

Symptoms
  Urine retention   Irregular
  Abdominal distention   menstruation
  Diarrhoea   Sterility

Method of treatment
  Needle: 0.3 inch perpendicularly.
  Moxa: Warm heating, 3 minutes.
  Feeling: Ache and/or numbness.

Bl 34; *Xia-Liao*; 'Lower Hole'

Location
  In fourth posterior sacral foramen.

Regional anatomy
  Origin of greatest gluteal muscle;
  Branches of inferior gluteal artery & vein;
  Posterior branch of fourth sacral nerve.

Symptoms
  Urine retention   Lower abdominal pain
  Diarrhoea   Leucorrhoea
  Lumbar pain

Method of treatment
  Needle: 0.3 inch perpendicularly.
  Moxa: Warm heating, 3 minutes.
  Feeling: Ache and/or numbness.

Bl 35; *Hui-Yang*; 'Reunion of Yang'

Location
  On either side of tip of coccyx, 0.5 *cun* lateral to Governor Vessel Meridian.

Regional anatomy
  Greatest gluteal muscle;
  Branches of inferior gluteal artery & vein;
  Coccygeal nerve.

Symptoms
  Abdominal pain   Lower back pain
  Diarrhoea   Impotence
  Deficiency of Yang energy (Haemorrhoids)

Method of treatment
  Needle: 0.3 inch perpendicularly.
  Moxa: Warm heating, 3 minutes.
  Feeling: Ache and/or numbness.

FOURTEEN MERIDIANS AND ACUPUNCTURE POINTS

Bl 36; *Chen-Fu*; 'Receive and Support'

Location
In middle of transverse gluteal fold when lying in prone position.

Regional anatomy
Greatest gluteal muscle;
Biceps muscle of thigh;
Sciatic artery & vein;
Posterior femoral cutaneous nerve;
Sciatic nerve.

Symptoms
Haemorrhoids (relieves symptoms)
Pain in lower back, sacral, gluteal & femoral areas
Dysuria
Lower abdominal pain

Method of treatment
Needle: 0.7 inch perpendicularly.
Moxa: Warm heating, 3 minutes.
Feeling: Ache and/or numbness.

Bl 37; *Yin-Men*; 'Prosperous Gate'

Location
6 *cun* below Bl 36.

Regional anatomy
Biceps muscle of thigh;
Semitendinous muscle;
Third perforating branches of deep femoral artery & vein;
Posterior femoral cutaneous nerve;
Sciatic nerve.

Symptoms
Pain in lower back & thigh
Diarrhoea

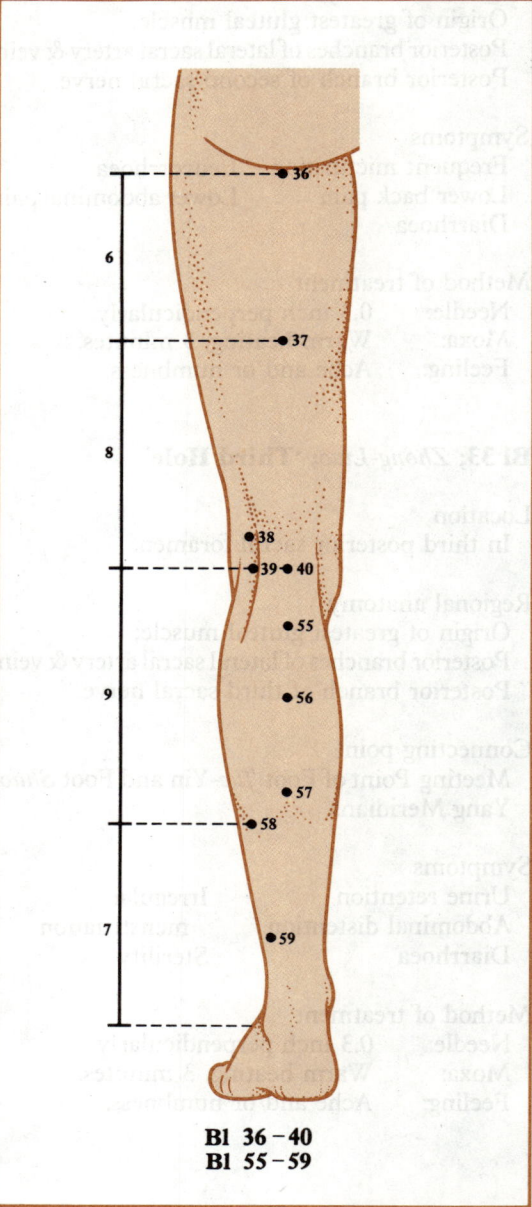

Bl 36–40
Bl 55–59

FOURTEEN MERIDIANS AND ACUPUNCTURE POINTS

Connecting points
   Inferior *He*-Sea Point of Three Heater Meridian;
   Divergent Meridian of Foot *Tai*-Yang Meridian.

Functions
   Frees function of Three Heater;
   Regulates water metabolism;
   Strengthens Bladder function.

Method of treatment
   Needle: 0.7 inch perpendicularly.
   Moxa: Warm heating, 3 minutes;
            No moxa cone.
   Feeling: Ache and/or numbness.

Bl 38; *Fu-Xi*; 'Surface Cleft'

Location
   1 *cun* above Bl 39, on medial side of tendon of biceps muscle of thigh.

Regional anatomy
   Biceps muscle of thigh;
   Superolateral genicular artery & vein;
   Posterior femoral cutaneous nerve;
   Common peroneal nerve.

Symptoms
   Muscle & tendon spasms
   Pain in gluteal & femoral areas
   Constipation

Method of treatment
   Needle: 0.5 inch obliquely.
   Moxa: Warm heating, 2 minutes.
   Feeling: Ache and/or numbness.

Bl 39; *Wei-Yang*; 'Entrust Yang'

Location
   Lateral to Bl 40, on medial border of tendon of biceps muscle of thigh.

Regional anatomy
   Biceps muscle of thigh;
   Superolateral genicular artery & vein;
   Posterior femoral cutaneous nerve;
   Common peroneal nerve.

Symptoms
   Pain & swelling in axillary region
   Fullness in chest
   Muscle & tendon spasms
   Dysuria

Clinical formula
   Bl 39 + Pc 1 = Pain and swelling in axillary region

Method of treatment
   Needle: 0.7 inch perpendicularly.
   Moxa: Warm heating, 3 minutes.
   Feeling: Ache and/or swelling.

Bl 40; *Wei-Zhong*; 'Entrust the Centre'

Location
   Midpoint of transverse crease of popliteal fossa, between tendons of biceps muscle of thigh and semitendinous muscle.

Regional anatomy
   Tendons of biceps muscle of thigh;
   Semitendinous muscle;
   Femoropopliteal vein;
   Popliteal vein & artery;
   Posterior femoral cutaneous nerve;
   Tibial nerve.

FOURTEEN MERIDIANS AND ACUPUNCTURE POINTS

Connecting point
  He-Sea Point of Bladder; Cleft of blood.

Functions
  Clears blood;
  Expels excess heat;
  Frees function of tendons;
  Frees *Luo*-Meridian energy flow;
  Dispels wind & damp;
  Strengthens lumbar & knee movements.

Symptoms
  Pain in knee, thigh & lower back
  Enuresis
  Abdominal distention & pain
  Fever

Clinical formula
  Bl 40 + Bl 23 + Bl 60 = Lower back pain

Method of treatment
  Needle: 0.5 inch perpendicularly.
  Moxa: Warm heating, 2 minutes;
            No moxa cone.
  Feeling: Ache and/or numbness.
  Warning: This point can be bled with a three-edged needle, but take care not to puncture the large blood vessel to avoid internal bleeding.

Bl 41; *Fu-Fen*; 'Supplementary Segment'

Location
  3 *cun* lateral to inferior border of spinous process of second thoracic vertebra (at level of Bl 12 and 3 *cun* lateral to Governor Vessel Meridian at superior point on Bladder Meridian).

Regional anatomy
  Trapezius muscle;
  Greater & lesser rhomboid muscles;
  Iliocostal muscle;
  Transverse cervical artery;
  Intercostal artery & vein;
  Dorsal branch of thoracic nerve;
  Dorsal scapular nerve;
  Intercostal nerve;
  Lung.

Connecting point
  Meeting Point of Foot and Hand *Tai*-Yang Meridians.

Symptoms
  Pain in shoulder, back, arm & elbow
  Stiff neck

Method of treatment
  Needle: 0.3 inch obliquely.
  Moxa: Warm heating, 2 minutes.
  Feeling: Ache and/or swelling.
  Warning: Avoid inserting needle too deeply.

Bl 42; *Po-Hu*; 'Home of the Animal Spirit'

Location
  3 *cun* lateral to inferior border of spinous process of third thoracic vertebra (at level of Bl 13).

Regional anatomy
  Trapezius muscle;
  Greater & lesser rhomboid muscles;
  Iliocostal muscle;
  Transverse cervical artery;
  Intercostal artery & vein;
  Dorsal branch of thoracic nerve;
  Dorsal scapular nerve;
  Intercostal nerve;
  Lung.

Symptoms
  Pain in back & arm
  Dyspnoea
  Stiff neck
  Fullness in chest
  Weak Lungs
  Coughing

Method of treatment
  Needle: 0.5 inch obliquely.
  Moxa: Warm heating, 3 minutes.
  Feeling: Ache and/or swelling.
  Warning: Avoid inserting needle too deeply.

Bl 43; *Gao-Huang-Shu*; 'Shu Point of Centre of Vital Energy'

Location
3 *cun* lateral to inferior border of spinous process of fourth thoracic vertebra (at level of Bl 14).

Regional anatomy
  Trapezius muscle;
  Greater & lesser rhomboid muscles;
  Iliocostal muscle;
  Transverse cervical artery;
  Intercostal artery & vein;
  Dorsal branch of thoracic nerve;
  Dorsal scapular nerve;
  Intercostal nerve;
  Lung.

Functions
  Strengthens functions of Lungs and Spleen;
  Tones body following overwork and fatigue;
  Balances functions of Heart and Kidneys;
  Strengthens *Yuan* energy.

Symptoms
  General weakness of body
  Fatigue
  Dyspnoea
  Poor memory
  Seminal emission
  Coughing
  Night sweats

Clinical formula
  Bl 43 + CV 6 + St 36 = Body weakness after chronic weakness

Method of treatment
  Needle: 0.3 inch obliquely.
  Moxa: Warm heating, 5 minutes.
  Feeling: Ache and/or swelling.
  Warning: Avoid inserting needle too deeply.

Note
This is an important point for strengthening the physical body after chronic illness. In this instance, moxa is better than needling.

Bl 44; *Shen-Tang*; 'Palace of Spirit'

Location
3 *cun* lateral to inferior border of spinous process of fifth thoracic vertebra (at level of Bl 15).

Regional anatomy
  Trapezius muscle;
  Greater & lesser rhomboid muscles;
  Iliocostal muscle;
  Transverse cervical artery;
  Intercostal artery & vein;
  Dorsal branch of thoracic nerve;
  Dorsal scapular nerve;
  Intercostal nerve;
  Lung.

Symptoms
  Pain in back, lower back & spine
  Fullness in chest

FOURTEEN MERIDIANS AND ACUPUNCTURE POINTS

Method of treatment
    Needle: 0.3 inch obliquely.
    Moxa: Warm heating, 3 minutes.
    Feeling: Ache and/or swelling.
    Warning: Avoid inserting needle too deeply.

Bl 45; *Yi-Xi*; 'Sighing/Giggling'

Location
3 *cun* lateral to inferior border of spinous process of sixth thoracic vertebra (at level of Bl 16).

Regional anatomy
    Trapezius muscle;
    Iliocostal muscle;
    Intercostal artery & vein;
    Dorsal branch of thoracic nerve;
    Intercostal nerve;
    Lung.

Symptoms
Pain in chest, back & lower back	Blurred vision
Fullness in chest	Ophthalmalgia
Abdominal distention	Epistaxis
	Dyspnoea

Method of treatment
    Needle: 0.6 inch obliquely.
    Moxa: Warm heating, 3 minutes.
    Feeling: Ache and/or swelling.
    Warning: Avoid inserting needle too deeply.

Bl 46; *Ge-Guan*; 'Gate of Diaphragm'

Location
3 *cun* lateral to inferior border of spinous process of seventh thoracic vertebra (at level of Bl 17).

Regional anatomy
    Latissimus dorsi muscle;
    Iliocostal muscle;
    Intercostal artery & vein;
    Dorsal branch of thoracic nerve;
    Intercostal nerve;
    Lung.

Symptoms
Pain in back	Fullness in chest
Stiff spine	Difficulty in swallowing

Method of treatment
    Needle: 0.5 inch obliquely.
    Moxa: Warm heating, 2 minutes.
    Feeling: Ache and/or swelling.
    Warning: Avoid inserting needle too deeply.

Bl 47; *Hun-Men*; 'Door of the Soul'

Location
3 *cun* lateral to inferior border of spinous process of ninth thoracic vertebra (at level of Bl 18).

Regional anatomy
    Latissimus dorsi muscle;
    Iliocostal muscle;
    Intercostal artery & vein;
    Dorsal branch of thoracic nerve;
    Intercostal nerve.

Symptoms
    Pain in chest & back
    Difficulty in swallowing
    Abdominal distention

FOURTEEN MERIDIANS AND ACUPUNCTURE POINTS

Method of treatment
  Needle: 0.5 inch perpendicularly.
  Moxa: Warm heating, 2 minutes.
  Feeling: Ache and/or swelling.

Bl 48; *Yang-Gang*; 'Essential of Yang'

Location
  3 *cun* lateral to inferior border of spinous process of tenth thoracic vertebra (at level of Bl 19).

Regional anatomy
  Latissimus dorsi muscle;
  Iliocostal muscle;
  Intercostal artery & vein;
  Dorsal branch of thoracic nerve;
  Intercostal nerve.

Functions
  Balances functions of Gall Bladder and Stomach;
  Dispels damp and heat.

Symptoms
  Abdominal pain & distention   Loss of appetite
  Diarrhoea   Fatigue

Method of treatment
  Needle: 0.5 inch perpendicularly.
  Moxa: Warm heating, 2 minutes.
  Feeling: Ache and/or numbness.

Bl 49; *Yi-She*; 'Lodge of Ideas'

Location
  3 *cun* lateral to inferior border of spinous process of eleventh thoracic vertebra (at level of Bl 20).

Regional anatomy
  Latissimus dorsi muscle;
  Iliocostal muscle;
  Intercostal artery & vein;
  Dorsal branch of thoracic nerve;
  Intercostal nerve.

Symptoms
  Abdominal distention   Pain in back
  Diarrhoea   Vomiting

Method of treatment
  Needle: 0.5 inch obliquely.
  Moxa: Warm heating, 2 minutes.
  Feeling: Ache.

Bl 50; *Wei-Cang*; 'Granary of the Stomach'

Location
  3 *cun* lateral to inferior border of spinous process of twelfth thoracic vertebra (at level of Bl 21).

Regional anatomy
  Latissimus dorsi muscle;
  Iliocostal muscle;
  Subcostal artery & vein;
  Dorsal branch of thoracic nerve;
  Intercostal nerve.

Functions
  Harmonizes Stomach function;
  Dispels damp in Spleen;
  Balances energy flow;
  Frees Middle Heater function.

Symptoms
  Abdominal distention
  Oedema
  Pain in spine & back

Method of treatment
- Needle: 0.5 inch obliquely.
- Moxa: Warm heating, 2 minutes.
- Feeling: Ache.

Bl 51; *Huang-Men*; 'Door of Vital Centre'

Location
3 *cun* lateral to inferior border of spinous process of first lumbar vertebra (at level of Bl 22).

Regional anatomy
- Latissimus dorsi muscle;
- Iliocostal muscle;
- Posterior branches of lumbar artery & vein;
- Dorsal branch of thoracic nerve;
- Iliohypogastric nerve.

Symptoms
- Gastric pain
- Constipation

Method of treatment
- Needle: 0.5 inch obliquely.
- Moxa: Warm heating, 2 minutes.
- Feeling: Ache.

Bl 52; *Zhi-Shi*; 'Lodge of the Will'

Location
3 *cun* lateral to inferior border of spinous process of second lumbar vertebra (at level of Bl 23).

Regional anatomy
- Latissimus dorsi muscle;
- Iliocostal muscle;
- Lumbar artery & vein;
- Dorsal branch of thoracic nerve;
- Lateral cutaneous nerve of thigh (L2-L3).

Functions
- Tones Kidney organ;
- Strengthens Kidney *Ching*;
- Harmonizes Bladder function.

Symptoms
Pain & swelling of genital region	Stiff lower back & spine
Pain in back	Stiff abdomen
Seminal emission	Pain in rib

Method of treatment
- Needle: 0.5 inch obliquely.
- Moxa: Warm heating, 3 minutes.
- Feeling: Ache and/or numbness.
- **Warning: Avoid inserting needle too deeply.**

Bl 53; *Bao-Huang*; 'Womb and Vitals'

Location
3 *cun* lateral to inferior border of spinous process of second sacral vertebra (at level of Bl 32).

Regional anatomy
- Greatest, middle & least gluteal muscles;
- Superior gluteal artery & vein;
- Superior clunial nerves;
- Superior gluteal nerve.

Symptoms
Pain in spine & lumbar region	Constipation
Abdominal distention	Dysuria

Method of treatment
- Needle: 0.5 inch perpendicularly.
- Moxa: Warm heating, 3 minutes.

Feeling: Ache and/or numbness.

Bl 54; *Zhi-Bian*; 'Side of the Sacral'

Location
3 *cun* lateral to Governor Vessel Meridian directly below Bl 53 at level of Bl 30.

Regional anatomy
Greatest gluteal muscle;
Piriform muscle;
Inferior gluteal artery, vein & nerve;
Posterior femoral cutaneous nerve;
Sciatic nerve.

Symptoms
Haemorrhoids (relieves symptoms)
Pain in lumbosacral region & lower extremities

Method of treatment
Needle: 0.5 inch perpendicularly.
Moxa: Warm heating, 3 minutes.
Feeling: Ache and/or numbness.

Bl 55; *He-Yang*; 'Union of Yang'

Location
2 *cun* directly below Bl 40.

Regional anatomy
Gastrocnemius muscle;
Small saphenous vein;
Popliteal artery & vein;
Medial cutaneous nerve of calf;
Tibial nerve.

Symptoms
Abdominal pain due to stiff lower back muscle & spine
Pain & ache in genital area
Leucorrhoea

Method of treatment
Needle: 0.6 inch perpendicularly.
Moxa: Warm heating, 2 minutes.
Feeling: Ache and/or numbness.

Bl 56; *Cheng-Jin*; 'Support for the Tendons'

Location
In centre of belly of gastrocnemius muscle midway between Bl 55 and Bl 57.

Regional anatomy
Gastrocnemius muscle;
Small saphenous vein;
Posterior tibial artery & vein;
Medial cutaneous nerve of calf;
Tibial nerve.

Symptoms
Stiff back & lower back
Constipation
Relieves symptoms of haemorrhoids
Numb leg
Pain in heel
Ache & spasm of gastrocnemius muscle

Method of treatment
Needle: **Forbidden.**
Moxa: Warm heating, 3 minutes.
Feeling:

Bl 57; *Cheng-Shan*; 'Support for the Mountain'

Location
8 *cun* below Bl 40.

FOURTEEN MERIDIANS AND ACUPUNCTURE POINTS

Regional anatomy
  Gastrocnemius muscle;
  Small saphenous vein;
  Posterior tibial artery & vein;
  Medial cutaneous nerve of calf;
  Tibial nerve.

Functions
  Strengthens tendons;
  Cools blood;
  Harmonizes function of Intestines;
  Relieves symptoms of haemorrhoids.

Symptoms
  Constipation
  Swelling of haemorrhoids
  Muscle spasm in leg
  Pain & swelling in knee
  Pain in leg & heel

Method of treatment
  Needle: 0.7 inch perpendicularly.
  Moxa: Warm heating, 2 minutes.
  Feeling: Ache and/or swelling.

Bl 58; *Fei-Yang*; 'Flying Up'

Location
  7 *cun* above Bl 60 on posterior border of fibula, 1 *cun* inferolateral to Bl 57.

Regional anatomy
  Gastrocnemius muscle;
  Soleus muscle;
  Lateral cutaneous nerve of calf.

Connecting point
  Luo-Connecting point.

Functions
  Regulates *Tai*-Yang Meridian energy flow;
  Relieves wind and damp in *Jing-Luo*.

Symptoms
  Pain & swelling of haemorrhoids
  Pain in knee, leg & little toe
  Blurred vision
  Headache
  Epistaxis

Method of treatment
  Needle: 0.3 inch perpendicularly.
  Moxa: Warm heating, 2 minutes.
  Feeling: Ache and/or swelling.

Bl 59; *Fu-Yang*; 'Yang in Instep'

Location
  3 *cun* above Bl 60.

Regional anatomy
  Long peroneal muscle;
  Small saphenous vein;
  Peroneal artery;
  Sural nerve.

Connecting point
  Xi-Cleft Point of Yang-*Qiao* Meridian.

Symptoms
  Muscle spasm
  Lower back pain
  Pain in thigh & leg
  Paralysis of lower limbs
  Heaviness & pain in head

Method of treatment
  Needle: 0.5 inch perpendicularly.
  Moxa: Warm heating, 2 minutes.
  Feeling: Ache and/or numbness.

Bl 60; *Kun-Lun*; 'Mountains of Kun-Lun'

Location
  In depression between external malleolus and calcaneal tendon.

FOURTEEN MERIDIANS AND ACUPUNCTURE POINTS

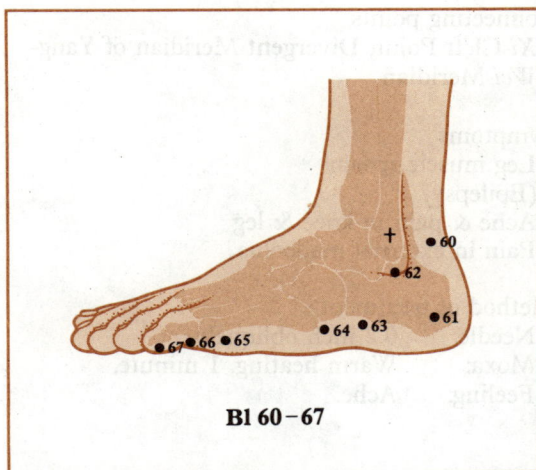

Bl 60–67

Clinical formula
  Bl 60 + GB 40 + Sp 5 + K 6 + Bl 61 = Pain in ankle and heel

Method of treatment
  Needle: 0.3 inch obliquely.
  Moxa: Warm heating, 2 minutes.
  Feeling: Ache and/or swelling.
  Warning: Needling is forbidden during pregnancy.

Bl 61; *Pu-Shen*; 'Visiting and Falling Down'

Location
  Posteroinferior to external malleolus directly below Bl 60 in calcaneal depression.

Regional anatomy
  External calcaneal branches of peroneal artery & vein;
  External calcaneal branch of sural nerve.

Connecting point
  Root of Yang-*Qiao* Meridian.

Symptoms
  Atrophy of leg & foot
  Pain in ankle & heel
  Muscle spasm
  Pain & swelling of knee

Method of treatment
  Needle: 0.3 inch obliquely.
  Moxa: Warm heating, 2 minutes.
  Feeling: Ache and/or swelling.

Bl 62; *Shen-Mai*; 'Information Vessel'

Location
  In depression directly below external malleolus.

Regional anatomy
  Short peroneal muscle;
  Small saphenous vein;
  Posteroexternal malleolar artery & vein;
  Sural nerve.

Connecting point
  Jing-River Point.

Functions
  Regulates *Tai*-Yang Meridian energy flow;
  Frees blood stasis in Uterus;
  Strengthens tendons;
  Dispels damp;
  Strengthens function of Kidneys.

Symptoms
  Lower back pain   Shortness of breath
  Epistaxis   Pain & swelling in
  Swelling of ankle & heel   genital region
  Stiff neck   Ophthalmalgia
  Headache   Sterility
  Coughing   Difficulty in labour

165

FOURTEEN MERIDIANS AND ACUPUNCTURE POINTS

Regional anatomy
External malleolar arterial network;
Sural nerve.

Connecting point
One of 'Eight Confluent Points' connecting to Yang-*Qiao* Meridian (which originates at this point).

Functions
Expels heat;
Relieves wind;
Creates quiet in mind and *Shen*;
Frees energy obstruction in tendons.

Symptoms
Dizziness   Fatigue
Migraine   Ache & pain in hip,
Lower back &   thigh, knee & leg
   leg pain   Premenstrual tension

Method of treatment
Needle: 0.3 inch obliquely.
Moxa: Warm heating, 1 minute.
Feeling: Ache and/or swelling.

Bl 63; *Jin-Men*; 'Door of Gold'

Location
Anteroinferior to Bl 62 in depression lateral to cuboid bone.

Regional anatomy
Tendon of long peroneal muscle;
Short extensor muscle of great toe;
Lateral plantar artery & vein;
Lateral dorsal cutaneous nerve of foot;
Lateral plantar nerve.

Connecting points
Xi-Cleft Point; Divergent Meridian of Yang-*Wei* Meridian.

Symptoms
Leg muscle spasm
(Epilepsy)
Ache & pain in knee & leg
Pain in external malleolus

Method of treatment
Needle: 0.2 inch obliquely.
Moxa: Warm heating, 1 minute.
Feeling: Ache.

Bl 64; *Jing-Gu*; 'Bone of Capital'

Location
On lateral side of dorsum of foot below tuberosity of fifth metatarsal bone.

Regional anatomy
Short extensor muscle of great toe;
Lateral plantar artery, vein & nerve;
Lateral dorsal cutaneous nerve of foot.

Connecting point
Yuan-Source Point.

Functions
Dispels wind;
Creates peace in Heart;
Clears brain.

Symptoms
Headache   Epistaxis
Lower back pain   Pain in thigh & foot
Blurred vision   Stiff neck
Fear   Cardiac pain
Muscle spasm

FOURTEEN MERIDIANS AND ACUPUNCTURE POINTS

Method of treatment
- Needle: 0.3 inch obliquely.
- Moxa: Warm heating, 1 minute.
- Feeling: Ache.

Bl 65; *Shu-Gu*; 'Thorny Bone'

Location
On lateral side of dorsum of foot, posteroinferior to head of fifth metatarsal bone.

Regional anatomy
Short extensor muscle of great toe;
Fourth common plantar digital artery, vein & nerve;
Lateral dorsal cutaneous nerve of foot.

Connecting point
Shu-Stream Point.

Symptoms
Pain in spine & lower back	Headache
Pain in thigh & popliteal fossa	Diarrhoea
Deafness	Stiff neck

Method of treatment
- Needle: 0.3 inch perpendicularly.
- Moxa: Warm heating, 1 minute.
- Feeling: Ache and/or numbness.

Bl 66; *Tong-Gu*; 'Through the Valley'

Location
In depression anteroinferior to fifth metatarsophalangeal joint.

Regional anatomy
Plantar digital artery & vein;
Proper plantar digital nerves;
Lateral dorsal cutaneous nerve of foot.

Connecting point
Ying-Spring Point.

Symptoms
Heaviness of head	Epistaxis
Dizziness	Stiff neck
Tension	Indigestion
Fear	Blurred vision

Method of treatment
- Needle: 0.2 inch perpendicularly.
- Moxa: Warm heating, 1 minute.
- Feeling: Ache and/or numbness.

Bl 67; *Zhi-Yin*; 'Arrival of Yin'

Location
On lateral side of small toe, 0.1 *cun* posterior to corner of nail.

Regional anatomy
Dorsal & plantar digital proprial arterial network;
Plantar digital proprial nerve;
Lateral dorsal cutaneous nerve of foot.

Connecting point
Jing-Well Point.

Functions
Disperses wind in vertex of head;
Dispels energy obstruction in Lower Heater.

Symptoms
Nasal obstruction	Dysuria
Heaviness of head	Incorrect fetal position during last month of pregnancy
Cold in little toe	
Restlessness	
Ophthalmalgia	

167

FOURTEEN MERIDIANS AND ACUPUNCTURE POINTS

Method of treatment
  Needle: 0.1 inch obliquely.
  Moxa: Warm heating, 2 minutes.
  Feeling: Pain.
  Warning: Needling is forbidden during pregnancy.
                Moxibustion may be applied for correcting fetal position, but this should only be done by, or under the direction of, an experienced practitioner.

8. Kidney Meridian of Foot Shao-Yin

This Meridian is characterized by high energy flow and low blood flow. The energy flow originates at K 1 and receives energy from the Bladder Meridian, Bl 67. Emerging from the plantar aspect of the tuberosity of the navicular bone, it travels behind the medial malleolus, round the heel and ascends the medial side of the leg to connect with Sp 6. From there it continues on to the medial side of the popliteal fossa, K 10, proceeding to the thigh (towards the vertebral column) to connect with GV 1, where it follows the spine to the Kidney and then connects with the Bladder. It also links with the Conception Vessel Meridian at CV 3 and CV 4. A branch from GV 1 goes to the abdomen, K 11, then ascends to the chest at K 27.

From the Kidney the main Meridian enters the Liver and passes through the diaphragm to ramify in the Lungs. A branch runs up the throat to terminate at the root of the tongue. From the Lung the main Meridian leads to the Heart, spreading its energy over the chest, and links with the Pericardium Meridian.

There are twenty-seven acupuncture points on each side of the Kidney Meridian.

Associated organs
   Belongs to Kidney;
- Related to Bladder;
- Directly connected with Liver, Lung and Heart.

Connecting points
- Sp 6 GV 1 CV 3 CV 4

Symptomatology
- Disorders along Meridian course
    Pain in back of spine   Dry mouth
    Lumbago   Pain in thigh,
    Cold feet   leg & heel
    Weak feet

- Disorders in organ
    Dizziness   Drowsiness
    Facial oedema   Restlessness
    Darkened complexion Diarrhoea
    Blurred vision   Abdominal
    Shortness of breath   distention
    Dyspnoea   Impotence

Acupuncture Points of Kidney Meridian

K 1; *Yong-Quan*; 'Well Spring'

Location
   On plantar surface of foot in centre of crease formed when toes are flexed.

Regional anatomy
   Tendons of long & short flexor muscles of toes;
   Lumbrical muscles of foot;
   Plantar interosseous muscle;
   Plantar arch;
   Second common plantar digital nerve.

Connecting point
   Jing-Well Point.

FOURTEEN MERIDIANS AND ACUPUNCTURE POINTS

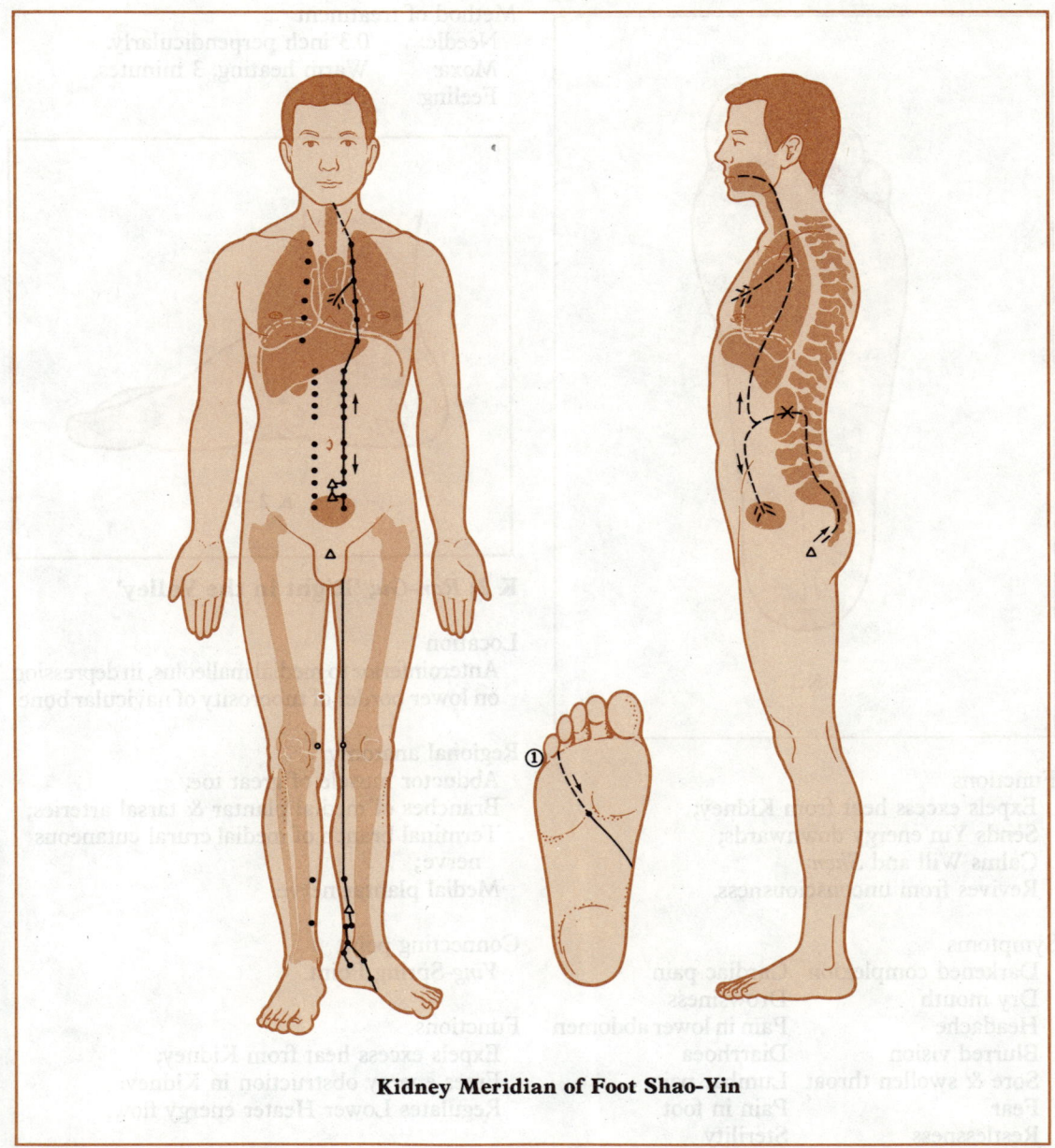

Kidney Meridian of Foot Shao-Yin

FOURTEEN MERIDIANS AND ACUPUNCTURE POINTS

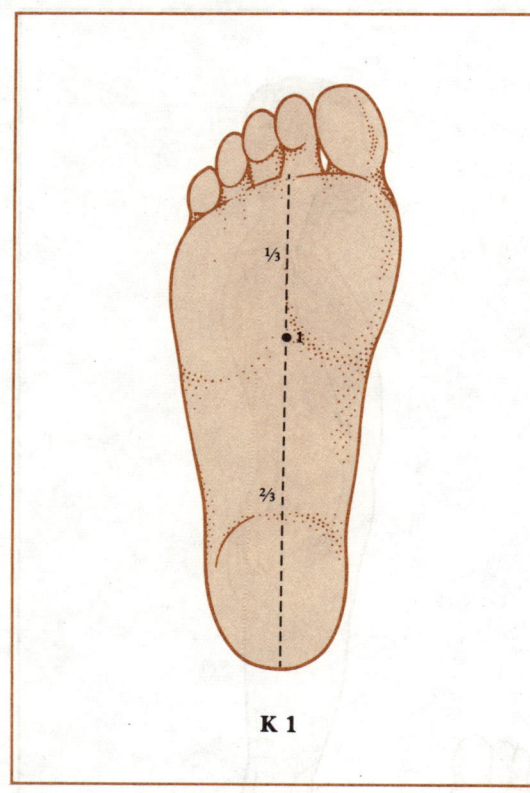

K 1

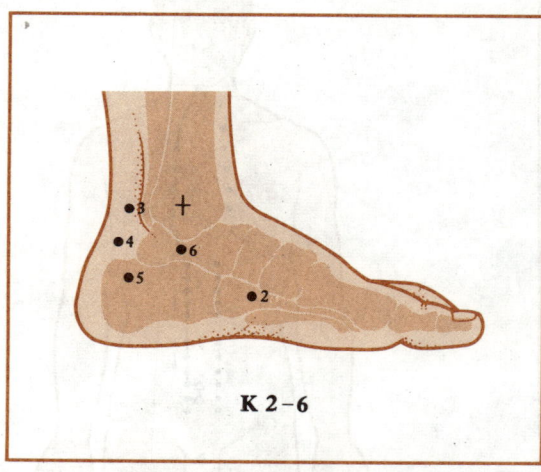

K 2–6

Method of treatment
- Needle: 0.3 inch perpendicularly.
- Moxa: Warm heating, 3 minutes.
- Feeling: Pain.

K 2; *Ran-Gu*; 'Right in the Valley'

Location
  Anteroinferior to medial malleolus, in depression on lower border of tuberosity of navicular bone.

Regional anatomy
  Abductor muscle of great toe;
  Branches of medial plantar & tarsal arteries;
  Terminal branch of medial crural cutaneous nerve;
  Medial plantar nerve.

Connecting point
  Ying-Spring Point.

Functions
  Expels excess heat from Kidney;
  Frees energy obstruction in Kidney;
  Regulates Lower Heater energy flow.

Functions
  Expels excess heat from Kidney;
  Sends Yin energy downwards;
  Calms Will and *Shen*;
  Revives from unconsciousness.

Symptoms
  Darkened complexion   Cardiac pain
  Dry mouth   Drowsiness
  Headache   Pain in lower abdomen
  Blurred vision   Diarrhoea
  Sore & swollen throat Lumbar pain
  Fear   Pain in foot
  Restlessness   Sterility

170

Symptoms
- Swelling of throat
- Shortness of breath
- Fear
- Swelling in foot & heel
- Lower abdominal distention
- Restlessness
- Sweating
- Diarrhoea
- Cardiac pain
- Seminal emission
- Sterility
- Irregular menstruation

Method of treatment
- Needle: 0.2 inch perpendicularly.
- Moxa: Warm heating, 2 minutes.
- Feeling: Ache and/or swelling.

K 3; *Tai-Xi*; 'Supreme Rivulet'

Location
At level of and in depression between eminence of medial malleolus and calcaneal tendon.

Regional anatomy
Posterior tibial artery & vein;
Medial crural cutaneous nerve on course of tibial nerve.

Connecting points
Shu-Stream and *Yuan*-Source Points.

Functions
Strengthens Kidney Yin;
Dispels heat;
Strengthens *Yuan* energy;
Harmonizes function of Uterus.

Symptoms
- Cardiac pain
- Cold hands & feet
- Dyspnoea
- Coughing
- Fever
- Swelling of throat
- Pain in chest & abdomen
- Drowsiness
- Pain & swelling in ankle

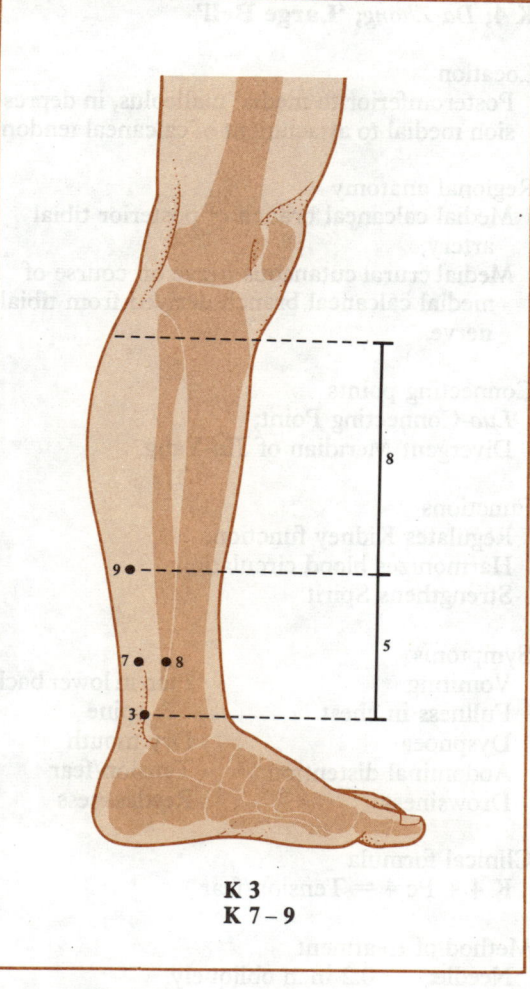

K 3
K 7–9

Clinical formula
Bl 60 + Bl 62 + K 3 = Pain & swelling in ankle

Method of treatment
- Needle: 0.3 inch obliquely.
- Moxa: Warm heating, 3 minutes.
- Feeling: Ache and/or numbness.

FOURTEEN MERIDIANS AND ACUPUNCTURE POINTS

K 4; *Da-Zhong*; 'Large Bell'

Location
  Posteroinferior to medial malleolus, in depression medial to attachment of calcaneal tendon.

Regional anatomy
  Medial calcaneal branch of posterior tibial artery;
  Medial crural cutaneous nerve on course of medial calcaneal branch derived from tibial nerve.

Connecting points
  Luo-Connecting Point;
  Divergent Meridian of *Tai*-Yang.

Functions
  Regulates Kidney function;
  Harmonizes blood circulation;
  Strengthens Spirit.

Symptoms
  Vomiting
  Fullness in chest
  Dyspnoea
  Abdominal distention
  Drowsiness
  Pain in lower back & spine
  Dry mouth
  Tension/fear
  Restlessness

Clinical formula
  K 4 + Pc 4 = Tension/fear

Method of treatment
  Needle: 0.2 inch obliquely.
  Moxa: Warm heating, 2 minutes.
  Feeling: Ache and/or numbness.

K 5; *Shui-Quan*; 'Water Source'

Location
  1 *cun* below K 3, in depression anterosuperior to medial side of tuberosity of calcaneum.

Regional anatomy
  Medial calcaneal branch of posterior tibial artery;
  Medial crural cutaneous nerve on course of medial calcaneal branch derived from tibial nerve.

Connecting point
  Xi-Cleft Point.

Functions
  Harmonizes blood and energy flows in Uterus;
  Dispels energy obstruction in Lower Heater.

Symptoms
  Blurred vision
  Dysmenorrhoea
  Pain & distention in abdomen

Method of treatment
  Needle: 0.2 inch obliquely.
  Moxa: Warm heating, 2 minutes.
  Feeling: Ache and/or numbness.

K 6; *Zhao-Hai*; 'Sea of Luminescence'

Location
  1 *cun* below medial malleolus.

Regional anatomy
  Abductor muscle of great toe;
  Posterior tibial artery & veins;
  Medial crural cutaneous nerve;
  Tibial nerve (posterior).

Connecting points
  Origin of Yin-*Qiao* Meridian; one of 'Eight Confluent Points' connecting with Yin-*Qiao* Meridian.

FOURTEEN MERIDIANS AND ACUPUNCTURE POINTS

Functions
Regulates Meridian energy flow;
Harmonizes blood circulation;
Expels excess heat;
Calms Will and *Shen*;
Frees energy obstruction in throat.

Symptoms
Dry mouth   Drowsiness
Sadness   Lower abdominal pain
Fatigue   Irregular menstruation

Method of treatment
Needle: 0.3 inch perpendicularly.
Moxa: Warm heating, 2 minutes.
Feeling: Ache and/or numbness.

K 7; *Fu-Liu*; 'Returning Current'

Location
2 *cun* above K 3 on anterior border of calcaneal tendon.

Regional anatomy
Soleus muscle;
Posterior tibial artery, vein & nerve;
Medial cutaneous nerve of calf;
Medial crural cutaneous nerve.

Connecting point
Jing-River Point.

Functions
Balances function of Bladder;
Dispels damp;
Clears blood stasis in Bladder;
Strengthens Kidney;
Expels heat.

Symptoms
Pain in lower back   Oedema
 & spine   Diarrhoea
Anger   Abdominal distention
Blurred vision   Hidrosis
Dry tongue   Frequency of
Weakness in legs   micturition

Clinical formula
K 7 + LI 4 = Hidrosis

Method of treatment
Needle: 0.3 inch perpendicularly.
Moxa: Warm heating, 3 minutes.
Feeling: Ache and/or numbness.

K 8; *Jiao-Xin*; 'Crossing Letters'

Location
2 *cun* above K 3, 0.5 *cun* anterior to K 7, posterior to medial border of tibia.

Regional anatomy
Long flexor muscle of toes;
Posterior tibial artery & vein;
Medial crural cutaneous nerve;
Tibial nerve.

Connecting point
Xi-Cleft Point of Yin-*Qiao* Meridian.

Symptoms
Pain in genital area;
Difficult bladder & bowel movements;
Excessive uterine bleeding;
Irregular menstruation;
Lower abdominal pain.

Method of treatment
Needle: 0.3 inch perpendicularly.
Moxa: Warm heating, 2 minutes.

173

FOURTEEN MERIDIANS AND ACUPUNCTURE POINTS

Feeling: Ache and/or numbness.

K 9; *Zhu-Bin*; 'Construction on the Shore'

Location
5 *cun* above K 3.

Regional anatomy
Gastrocnemius muscle;
Soleus muscle;
Posterior tibial artery & vein;
Medial cutaneous nerve of calf;
Medial crural cutaneous nerve;
Tibial nerve.

Connecting point
Xi-Cleft Point of Yin-*Wei* Meridian.

Symptoms
Irritability
Pain in leg

Method of treatment
Needle: 0.3 inch perpendicularly.
Moxa: Warm heating, 2 minutes.
Feeling: Ache and/or numbness.

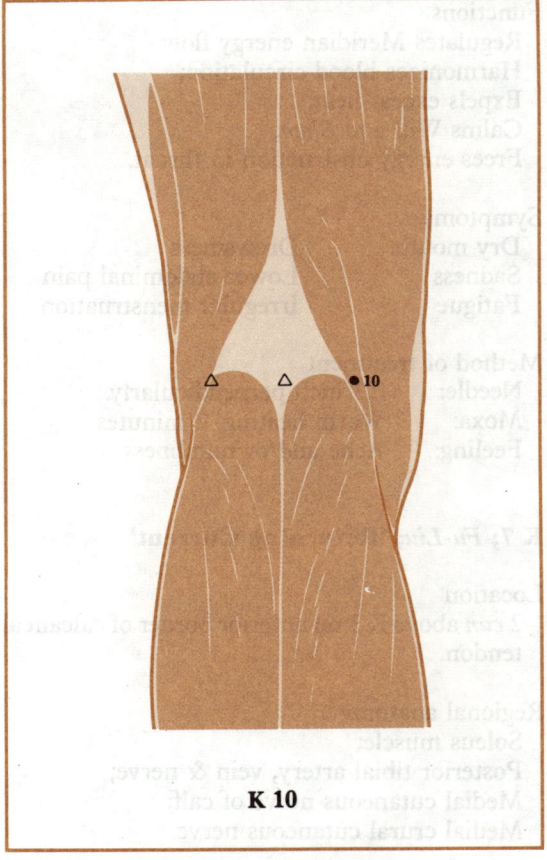

K 10; *Yin-Gu*; 'Valley of Yin'

Location
At medial side of popliteal fossa, level with Bl 40 between tendons of semitendinous and semimembranous muscles when knee is flexed.

Regional anatomy
Semitendinous muscle;
Semimembranous muscle;
Medial superior genicular artery & vein;
Medial femoral cutaneous nerve.

Connecting point
He-Sea Point.

Functions
Dispels damp;
Balances Bladder function;
Strengthens Kidney function;
Expels heat;
Eases pathogenic energy;
Harmonizes Lower Heater function.

FOURTEEN MERIDIANS AND ACUPUNCTURE POINTS

Symptoms
  Pain in medial aspect of popliteal fossa
  Dysuria
  Pain in genital areas
  Excessive uterine bleeding
  Abdominal distention

Method of treatment
  Needle: 0.4 inch perpendicularly.
  Moxa: Warm heating, 3 minutes.
  Feeling: Ache and/or numbness.

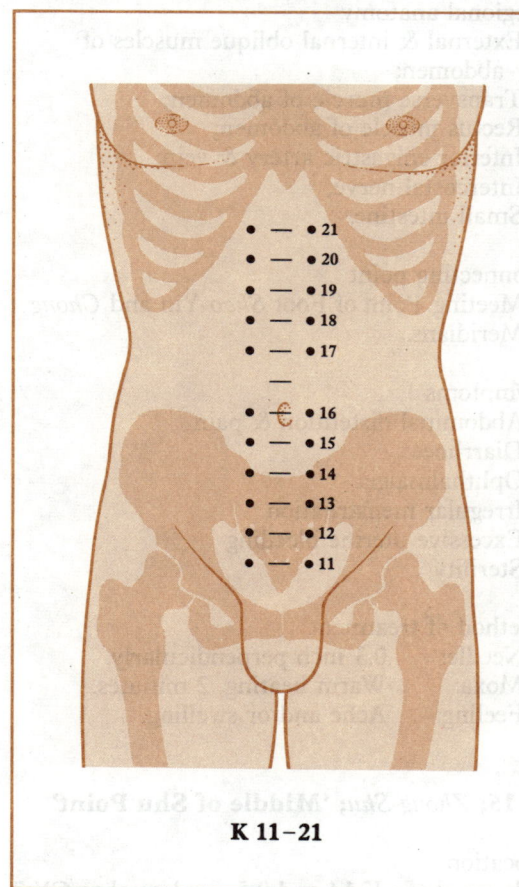

K 11–21

K 11; *Heng-Gu*; 'Horizontal Bone'

Location
  On superior border of pubic symphysis, 0.5 *cun* lateral to CV 2.

Regional anatomy
  External & internal oblique muscles of abdomen;
  Transverse muscle of abdomen;
  Rectus muscle of abdomen;
  Inferior epigastric artery;
  External pudendal artery;
  Iliohypogastric nerve;
  Small intestine;
  Bladder.

Connecting point
  Meeting Point of Foot *Shao*-Yin and *Chong* Meridians.

Symptoms
  Urine retention
  Fullness in lower abdomen
  Pain in external genitalia
  Loss of *Ching*

Method of treatment
  Needle: **Forbidden.**
  Moxa: Warm heating, 3 minutes.

K 12; *Da-He*; 'Great Conspicuousness'

Location
  1 *cun* above K 11 and 0.5 *cun* lateral to CV 3.

Regional anatomy
  External & internal oblique muscles of abdomen;
  Transverse muscle of abdomen;
  Rectus muscle of abdomen;
  Inferior epigastric artery & vein;

Subcostal nerve;
Iliohypogastric nerve;
Small intestine;
Bladder.

Symptoms
Fatigue
Loss of *Ching*
Ophthalmalgia
Leucorrhoea
Pain in external genitalia

Method of treatment
Needle: 0.3 inch perpendicularly.
Moxa: Warm heating, 3 minutes.
Feeling: Ache and/or swelling.
Warning: For urine retention, do not insert needle too deeply.

K 13; *Qi-Xue*; 'Energetic Point'

Location
1 *cun* above K 12 and 0.5 *cun* lateral to CV 4.

Regional anatomy
External & internal oblique muscles of abdomen;
Transverse muscle of abdomen;
Rectus muscle of abdomen;
Inferior epigastric artery & vein;
Subcostal nerve;
Small intestine.

Connecting point
Meeting Point of Foot *Shao*-Yin and *Chong* Meridians.

Symptoms
Abdominal pain
Ophthalmalgia
Pain in lower back & spine
Irregular menstruation
Diarrhoea

Method of treatment
Needle: 0.3 inch perpendicularly.
Moxa: Warm heating, 2 minutes.
Feeling: Ache and/or swelling.

K 14; *Si-Man*; 'Four Full Ones'

Location
1 *cun* above K 13 and 0.5 *cun* lateral to CV 5.

Regional anatomy
External & internal oblique muscles of abdomen;
Transverse muscle of abdomen;
Rectus muscle of abdomen;
Inferior epigastric artery & vein;
Intercostal nerve;
Small intestine.

Connecting point
Meeting Point of Foot *Shao*-Yin and *Chong* Meridians.

Symptoms
Abdominal distention & pain
Diarrhoea
Ophthalmalgia
Irregular menstruation
Excessive uterine bleeding
Sterility

Method of treatment
Needle: 0.3 inch perpendicularly.
Moxa: Warm heating, 2 minutes.
Feeling: Ache and/or swelling.

K 15; *Zhong-Shu*; 'Middle of Shu Point'

Location
1 *cun* above K 14 and 0.5 *cun* lateral to CV 7.

FOURTEEN MERIDIANS AND ACUPUNCTURE POINTS

Regional anatomy
  External & internal oblique muscles of abdomen;
  Transverse muscle of abdomen;
  Rectus muscle of abdomen;
  Inferior epigastric artery & vein;
  Intercostal nerve;
  Small intestine.

Connecting point
  Meeting Point of Foot *Shao*-Yin and *Chong* Meridians.

Symptoms
  Abdominal distention
  Constipation
  Pain lower back & spine
  Irregular menstruation

Method of treatment
  Needle: 0.8 inch perpendicularly.
  Moxa: Warm heating, 2 minutes.
  Feeling: Ache and/or swelling.

K 16; *Huang-Shu*; 'Shu Point of Vitals'

Location
  0.5 *cun* lateral to centre of umbilicus.

Regional anatomy
  External & internal oblique muscles of abdomen;
  Transverse muscle of abdomen;
  Rectus muscle of abdomen;
  Inferior epigastric artery & vein;
  Intercostal nerve;
  Small intestine.

Connecting point
  Meeting Point of Foot *Shao*-Yin and *Chong* Meridians.

Functions
  Expels heat from Kidneys;
  Dispels pathogenic energy;
  Harmonizes *Chong* Meridian function;
  Regulates Lower Heater energy flow.

Symptoms
  Abdominal pain   Abdominal distention
  Constipation   Ophthalmalgia

Method of treatment
  Needle: 0.8 inch perpendicularly.
  Moxa: Warm heating, 2 minutes.
  Feeling: Ache and/or swelling.

K 17; *Shang-Qu*; 'Merchant of Tunes'

Location
  2 *cun* above K 16 and 0.5 *cun* lateral to CV 10.

Regional anatomy
  Rectus muscle of abdomen;
  Branches of superior & inferior epigastric arteries & veins;
  Intercostal nerve;
  Stomach.

Connecting point
  Meeting Point of Foot *Shao*-Yin and *Chong* Meridians.

Symptoms
  Abdominal pain
  Indigestion

Method of treatment
  Needle: 0.5 inch perpendicularly.
  Moxa: Warm heating, 2 minutes.
  Feeling: Ache and/or swelling.

FOURTEEN MERIDIANS AND ACUPUNCTURE POINTS

K 18; *Shi-Guan*; 'Stone Gate'

Location
1 *cun* above K 17 and 0.5 *cun* lateral to CV 11.

Regional anatomy
Rectus muscle of abdomen;
Branches of superior epigastric artery & vein;
Intercostal nerve;
Stomach.

Connecting point
Meeting Point of Foot *Shao*-Yin and *Chong* Meridians.

Symptoms
Abdominal pain   Stiff spine
Constipation   Sterility

Method of treatment
Needle: 0.5 inch perpendicularly.
Moxa: Warm heating, 2 minutes.
Feeling: Ache and/or swelling.

K 19; *Yin-Du*; 'Capital of Yin'

Location
1 *cun* above K 18 and 0.5 *cun* lateral to CV 12.

Regional anatomy
Rectus muscle of abdomen;
Superior epigastric artery & vein;
Intercostal vein;
Liver;
Stomach.

Connecting point
Meeting Point of Foot *Shao*-Yin and *Chong* Meridians.

Symptoms
Abdominal distention & pain
Pain in rib

Method of treatment
Needle: 0.3 inch perpendicularly.
Moxa: Warm heating, 2 minutes.
Feeling: Ache and/or swelling.

K 20; *Tong-Gu*; 'Open Valley'

Location
1 *cun* above K 19 and 0.5 *cun* lateral to CV 13.

Regional anatomy
Rectus muscle of abdomen;
Superior epigastric artery & vein;
Intercostal nerve;
Liver.

Connecting point
Meeting Point of Foot *Shao*-Yin and *Chong* Meridians.

Symptoms
Facial paralysis   Fullness in chest
Vomiting   Fear
Indigestion

Method of treatment
Needle: 0.3 inch perpendicularly.
Moxa: Warm heating, 2 minutes.
Feeling: Ache and/or swelling.

K 21; *Yuo-Men*; 'The Pylorus'

Location
1 *cun* above K 20 and 0.5 *cun* lateral to CV 14.

FOURTEEN MERIDIANS AND ACUPUNCTURE POINTS

Regional anatomy
  Rectus muscle of abdomen;
  Superior epigastric artery & vein;
  Intercostal nerve;
  Liver.

Connecting point
  Meeting Point of Foot *Shao*-Yin and *Chong* Meridians.

Symptoms
  Lower abdominal distention   Pain in chest
  Restlessness   Diarrhoea

Method of treatment
  Needle: 0.3 inch perpendicularly.
  Moxa: Warm heating, 2 minutes.
  Feeling: Ache and/or swelling.

K 22; *Bu-Lang*; **'Walk to Corridor'**

Location
  2 *cun* lateral to Conception Vessel in fifth intercostal space.

Regional anatomy
  Greater pectoral muscle;
  External intercostal membrane;
  Internal intercostal muscle;
  Intercostal artery, vein & nerve;
  Anterior cutaneous branch of intercostal nerve;
  Lung;
  Liver;
  Heart.

Symptoms
  Fullness & pain in chest
  Nasal obstruction
  Shortness of breath

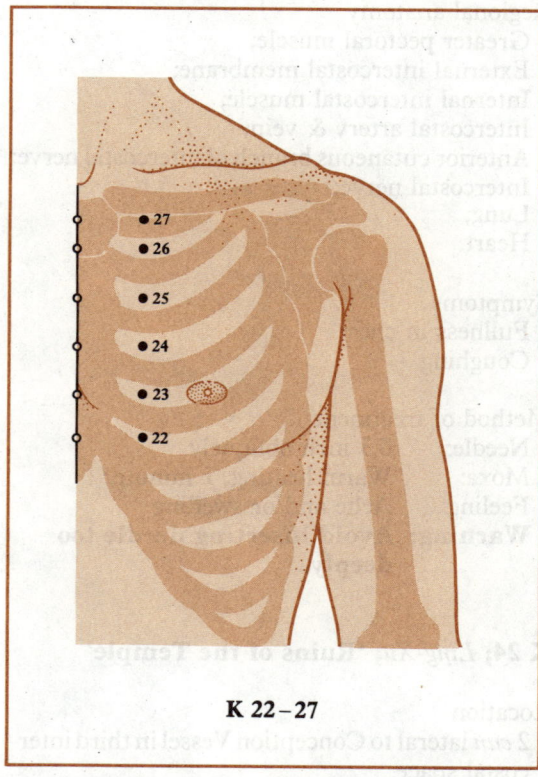

K 22–27

Method of treatment
  Needle: 0.3 inch obliquely.
  Moxa: Warm heating, 1 minute.
  Feeling: Ache and/or swelling.
  Warning: **Avoid inserting needle too deeply.**

K 23; *Shen-Feng*; **'Spiritual Seal'**

Location
  2 *cun* lateral to Conception Vessel in fourth intercostal space.

FOURTEEN MERIDIANS AND ACUPUNCTURE POINTS

Regional anatomy
  Greater pectoral muscle;
  External intercostal membrane;
  Internal intercostal muscle;
  Intercostal artery & vein;
  Anterior cutaneous branch of intercostal nerve;
  Intercostal nerve;
  Lung;
  Heart.

Symptoms
  Fullness in chest
  Coughing

Method of treatment
  Needle: 0.3 inch obliquely.
  Moxa: Warm heating, 1 minute.
  Feeling: Ache and/or swelling.
  Warning: Avoid inserting needle too deeply.

K 24; *Ling-Xu*; 'Ruins of the Temple'

Location
2 *cun* lateral to Conception Vessel in third intercostal space.

Regional anatomy
  Greater pectoral muscle;
  External intercostal membrane;
  Internal intercostal muscle;
  Intercostal artery & vein;
  Anterior cutaneous branch of intercostal nerve;
  Intercostal nerve;
  Lung.

Symptoms
  Fullness & pain in chest
  Shortness of breath
  Coughing

Method of treatment
  Needle: 0.3 inch obliquely.
  Moxa: Warm heating, 1 minute.
  Feeling: Ache and/or swelling.
  Warning: Avoid inserting needle too deeply.

K 25; *Shen-Cang*; 'Spirit Shelter'

Location
2 *cun* lateral to Conception Vessel in second intercostal space.

Regional anatomy
  Greater pectoral muscle;
  External intercostal membrane;
  Internal intercostal muscle;
  Intercostal artery & vein;
  Anterior cutaneous branch of intercostal nerve;
  Intercostal nerve;
  Lung.

Symptoms
  Vomiting
  Coughing
  Shortness of breath

Method of treatment
  Needle: 0.3 inch obliquely.
  Moxa: Warm heating, 1 minute.
  Feeling: Ache and/or swelling.
  Warning: Avoid inserting needle too deeply.

K 26; *Yu-Zhong*; 'Eventual Centre'

Location
2 *cun* lateral to Conception Vessel in first intercostal space.

Regional anatomy
  Greater pectoral muscle;
  External intercostal membrane;
  Internal intercostal muscle;
  Intercostal artery & vein;
  Anterior cutaneous branch of intercostal nerve;
  Medial supraclavicular nerve;
  Intercostal nerve;
  Lung.

Symptoms
  Coughing
  Dyspnoea
  Fullness in chest

Method of treatment
  Needle: 0.3 inch obliquely.
  Moxa: Warm heating, 1 minute.
  Feeling: Ache and/or swelling.
  Warning: Avoid inserting needle too deeply.

K 27; *Shu-Fu*; 'Shu Point of the Palace'

Location
2 *cun* lateral to Conception Vessel in depression on lower border of clavicle.

Regional anatomy
  Greater pectoral muscle;
  Anterior perforating branches of internal mammary artery & vein;
  Medial supraclavicular nerve.

Symptoms
  Coughing   Dyspnoea
  Abdominal distention   Pain in chest

Method of treatment
  Needle: 0.3 inch obliquely.
  Moxa: Warm heating, 1 minute.
  Feeling: Ache and/or swelling.
  Warning: Avoid inserting needle too deeply.

9. Pericardium Meridian of Hand Jue-Yin

This Meridian is characterized by low energy flow and high blood flow. The energy flow originates in the middle of the chest. Emerging from the Pericardium, it descends through the diaphragm to the abdomen, connecting successively with the Meridians of the Upper, Middle and Lower Heaters.

The Main Meridian from the chest continues on to Pc 1 and, via the axilla, follows the medial aspect of the upper arm, running between the Lung and Heart Meridians, to terminate at Pc 9 on the middle finger. From Pc 8 the Main Meridian continues down to the ring finger to TH 1, its link with the Three Heater Meridian.

There are nine acupuncture points on each side of the Pericardium Meridian.

Associated organs
- Belongs to Pericardium;
- Related to Three Heater.

Symptomatology
- Disorders along Meridian course
  Stiff neck
  Muscle spasm in upper limb
  Red complexion
  Ophthalmalgia
  Swelling in axillary region
  Pain & stiffness in arm, elbow & hand

- Disorders in organ
  Delirium   Fullness in chest
  Coma   Stiff tongue
  Restlessness   Cardiac pain
  Palpitations   Mania

FOURTEEN MERIDIANS AND ACUPUNCTURE POINTS

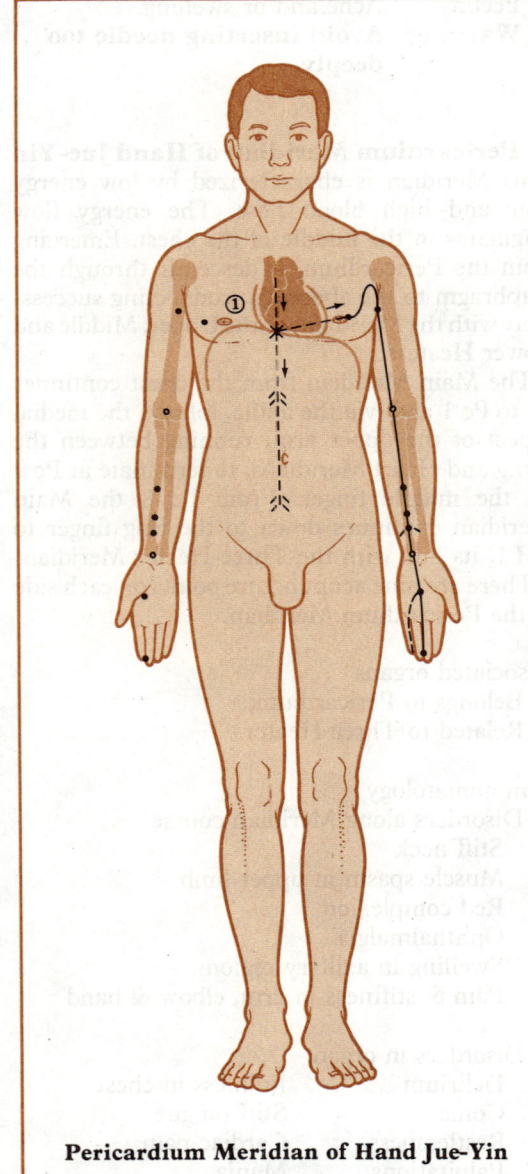

Pericardium Meridian of Hand Jue-Yin

Acupuncture Points of Pericardium Meridian

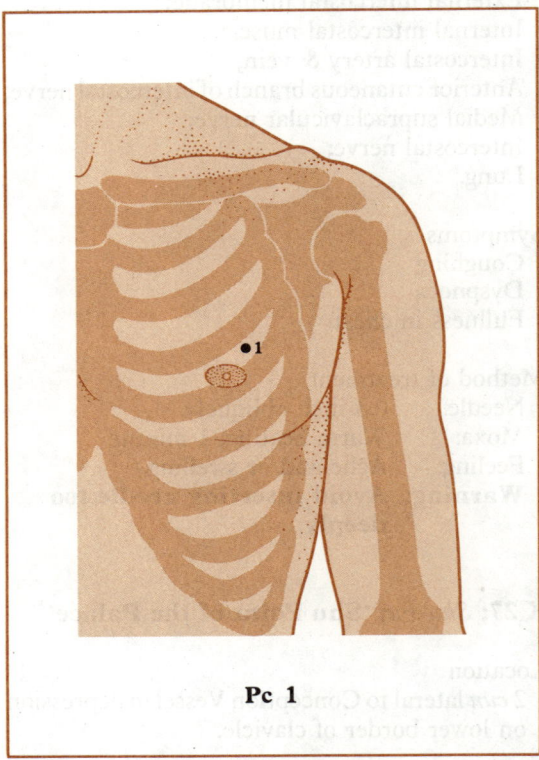

Pc 1

Pc 1; *Tian-Chi*; 'Celestial Bond'

Location
  1 *cun* lateral to nipple, in fourth intercostal space.

Regional anatomy
  Greater & smaller pectoral muscles;
  Thoracoepigastric vein;
  Branches of lateral thoracic artery & vein;
  Muscular branch of anterior thoracic nerve;
  Intercostal nerve;
  Lung.

FOURTEEN MERIDIANS AND ACUPUNCTURE POINTS

Connecting point
  Meeting Point of Hand *Jue*-Yin, Foot *Jue*-Yin and Foot *Shao*-Yang Meridians.

Symptoms
  Fullness in chest
  Pain in upper limbs
  Swelling in axillary region

Method of treatment
  Needle: 0.3 inch obliquely.
  Moxa: Warm heating, 1 minute.
  Feeling: Ache and/or numbness.
  Warning: Avoid inserting needle too deeply.

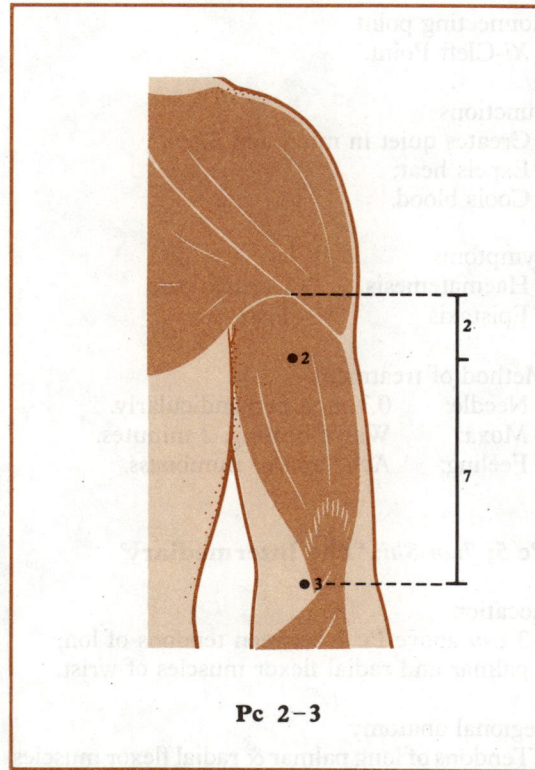

Pc 2–3

Pc 2; *Tian-Quan*; 'Celestial Source'

Location
  2 *cun* below end of anterior axillary fold, between two heads of biceps muscle of arm.

Regional anatomy
  Biceps muscle of arm;
  Muscular branches of brachial artery & vein;
  Medial cutaneous nerve of arm;
  Musculocutaneous nerve;
  Median nerve.

Symptoms
  Blurred vision   Fullness in chest
  Cardiac pain   Pain in arm & shoulder

Method of treatment
  Needle: 0.6 inch perpendicularly.
  Moxa: Warm heating, 2 minutes.
  Feeling: Ache and/or numbness.

Pc 3; *Qu-Ze*; 'Crooked Marsh'

Location
  On transverse cubital crease at ulnar side of tendon of biceps muscle of arm.

Regional anatomy
  Biceps muscle of arm;
  Brachial artery & vein;
  Medial nerve.

Connecting point
  He-Sea Point of Pericardium.

Functions
  Draws down pathogenic energy of
    Upper Heater;
  Clears Heart Fire;
  Expels excess heat from blood;
  Eases muscle spasm.

FOURTEEN MERIDIANS AND ACUPUNCTURE POINTS

Symptoms
Cardiac pain   Dry mouth
Fear   Pain in arm, elbow & wrist

Clinical formula
Pc 3 + Pc 6 + Pc 7 = Cardiac pain

Method of treatment
Needle: 0.3 inch perpendicularly.
Moxa: Warm heating, 1 minute.
Feeling: Ache and/or numbness.

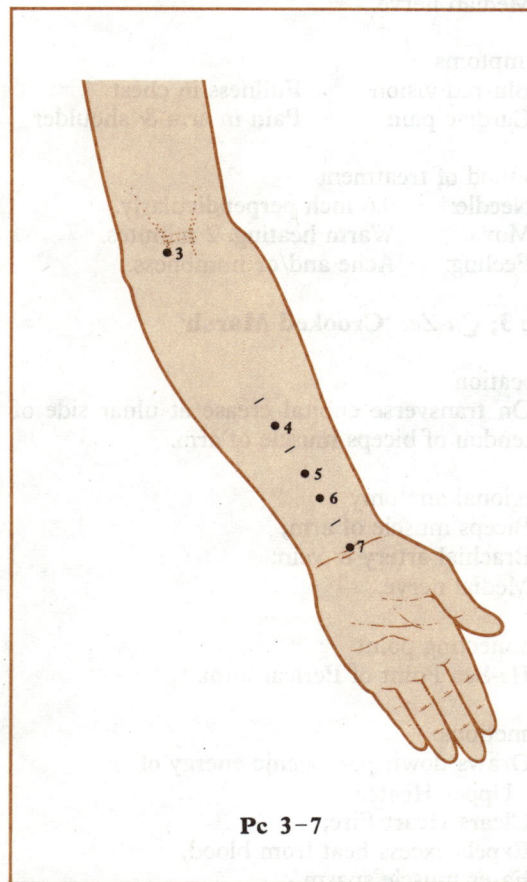

Pc 3–7

Pc 4; *Xi-Men*; 'Cleft Door'

Location
5 *cun* above Pc 7 between tendons of long palmar and radial flexor muscles of wrist.

Regional anatomy
Tendons of long palmar & radial flexor muscles of wrist;
Superficial & deep flexor muscles of fingers;
Medial artery & vein;
Anterior interosseous artery & vein;
Medial cutaneous nerve of forearm;
Median nerve;
Anterior interosseous nerve of forearm.

Connecting point
Xi-Cleft Point.

Functions
Creates quiet in mind and *Shen*;
Expels heat;
Cools blood.

Symptoms
Haematemesis   Cardiac pain
Epistaxis   Fear

Method of treatment
Needle: 0.3 inch perpendicularly.
Moxa: Warm heating, 2 minutes.
Feeling: Ache and/or numbness.

Pc 5; *Jian-Shi*; 'The Intermediary'

Location
3 *cun* above Pc 7 between tendons of long palmar and radial flexor muscles of wrist.

Regional anatomy
Tendons of long palmar & radial flexor muscles

FOURTEEN MERIDIANS AND ACUPUNCTURE POINTS

of wrist;
Superficial & deep flexor muscles of fingers;
Median artery & vein;
Medial & lateral cutaneous nerves of forearm;
Palmar cutaneous branch of median nerve;
Median nerve;
Anterior interosseous nerve of forearm.

Connecting point
  Jing-River Point.

Functions
  Regulates Heart energy;
  Clears mind and *Shen*;
  Dispels sputum stasis in chest;
  Expels pathogenic energy in *Jue*-Yin and *Shao*-Yang Meridians.

Symptoms
  Cardiac pain   Pain in axilla, elbow & forearm
  Loss of voice   Irregular menstruation

Clinical formula
  Pc 5 + LI 4 = Loss of voice

Method of treatment
  Needle: 0.5 inch perpendicularly.
  Moxa: Warm heating, 2 minutes.
  Feeling: Ache and/or numbness.

Pc 6; *Nei-Guan*; 'Inner Gate'

Location
  2 *cun* above Pc 6 between tendons of long palmar and radial flexor muscles of wrist.

Regional anatomy
  Tendons of long palmar & radial flexor muscles of wrist;
  Superficial & deep flexor muscles of fingers;
  Median artery & vein;
  Medial & lateral cutaneous nerves of forearm;
  Palmar cutaneous branch of median nerve;
  Median nerve;
  Anterior interosseous nerve of forearm.

Connecting points
  Luo-Connecting Point; one of 'Eight Confluent Points' connecting with Yin-*Wei* Meridian.

Functions
  Regulates Pericardium energy flow;
  Harmonizes Three Heater function;
  Calms *Shen*;
  Harmonizes Stomach function;
  Frees and harmonizes chest energy flow.

Symptoms
  Loss of will   Red eyes
  Cardiac pain   Pain in forearm

Method of treatment
  Needle: 0.5 inch perpendicularly.
  Moxa: Warm heating, 2 minutes.
  Feeling: Ache and/or numbness.

Pc 7; *Da-Ling*; 'Grand Mound'

Location
  In depression in middle of transverse crease of wrist, between tendons of long palmar and radial flexor muscles of wrist.

Regional anatomy
  Tendons of long palmar & radial flexor muscles of wrist;
  Long flexor muscle of thumb;
  Deep flexor muscle of fingers;
  Palmar arterial & venous network of wrist;
  Median nerve.

185

FOURTEEN MERIDIANS AND ACUPUNCTURE POINTS

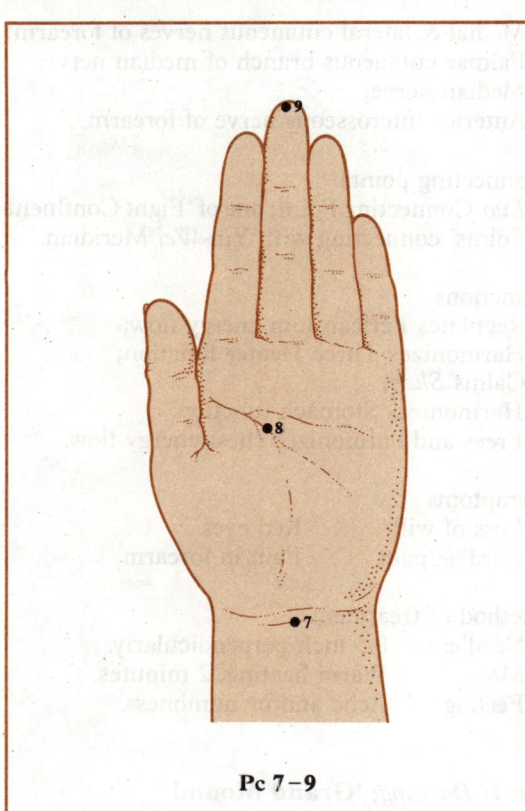

Pc 7–9

Restlessness Shortness of breath

Clinical formula
Pc 7 + Pc 6 + Pc 3 = Cardiac pain

Method of treatment
Needle: 0.3 inch obliquely.
Moxa: Warm heating, 2 minutes.
Feeling: Ache and/or numbness.

Pc 8.; *Lao-Gong*; 'Palace of Labour'

Location
Between tips of middle and ring fingers (between second and third metacarpal bones on radial side of third metacarpal bone) when fingers are clenched.

Regional anatomy
Fibrous digital sheath;
Lumbrical muscles of hand;
Tendons of superficial & deep flexor muscles of fingers;
Adductor muscle of thumb;
Palmar interosseous muscles;
Common palmar digital artery;
Second common palmar digital nerve of median nerve.

Connecting point
Ying-Spring Point.

Functions
Clears Heart Fire;
Expels damp and heat;
Dispels wind;
Cools blood;
Harmonizes Stomach function;
Calms *Shen*.

Connecting points
Shu-Stream and *Yuan*-Source Points.

Functions
Clears Heart Fire and calms *Shen*;
Balances chest and Stomach functions;
Clears *Jing* blood;
Cools blood.

Symptoms
Pain in forearm   Sadness
  & wrist   Cardiac pain
Fear   Dry mouth

Symptoms
- Apoplexy
- Anger
- Restlessness
- Pain in palm
- Pain in chest
- Epistaxis
- Foul breath

Method of treatment
- Needle: 0.2 inch perpendicularly.
- Moxa: Warm heating, 2 minutes.
- Feeling: Soreness.

Pc 9; *Zhong-Chong*; **'Middle of Thoroughfare'**

Location
In centre of tip of middle finger.

Regional anatomy
Arterial & venous network formed by palmar digital proprial artery & vein;
Palmar digital proprial nerve of median nerve.

Connecting point
Jing-Well Point.

Functions
Opens 'Gate of the Spirit';
Revives from unconsciousness;
Clears Heart Fire;
Expels heat.

Symptoms
- Restlessness
- Hot sensation in palm
- Cardiac pain
- Stiff tongue

Method of treatment
- Needle: 0.1 inch obliquely or prick with three-edged needle to cause bleeding.
- Moxa: Warm heating, 1 minute.
- Feeling: Pain.

10. Three Heater Meridian of Hand Shao-Yang

This Meridian is characterized by high energy flow and low blood flow. The energy flow originates at the tip of the ring finger, TH 1, and ascends the posterior surface of the arm between the two Yang Meridians to the shoulder at TH 14. From this point, it travels via SI 12 to TH 15 and from there to GV 14 via GB 21. It continues through the supraclavicular fossa and descends into the chest to connect with the Pericardium. After passing through the diaphragm into the abdomen, it links up with its three divisions, the Upper, Middle and Lower Heaters. From here, a branch travels downwards to connect with Bl 39, the Inferior *He*-Sea Point of the Three Heater.

The main Meridian emerges from the chest at the supraclavicular fossa, ascends to the neck and follows the posterior border of the ear to TH 20. From this point, it runs to the superior aspect of the ear, links up with GB 4, GB 6 and GB 3, and curves round the cheek to SI 18 to terminate in the infraorbital region.

The main Meridian passes through the retroauricular region at TH 17 and enters the ear, re-emerging in front of the ear at SI 19. From there it continues to TH 21 and to the outer canthus, TH 23, to link with the Gall Bladder Meridian at GB 1.

There are twenty-three acupuncture points on each side of the Three Heater Meridian.

Associated organs
- Belongs to Three Heater;
- Related to Pericardium.

Connecting points
SI 12 SI 18 SI 19 GB 1 GB 3 GB 4 GB 6
GB 21 GV 14

FOURTEEN MERIDIANS AND ACUPUNCTURE POINTS

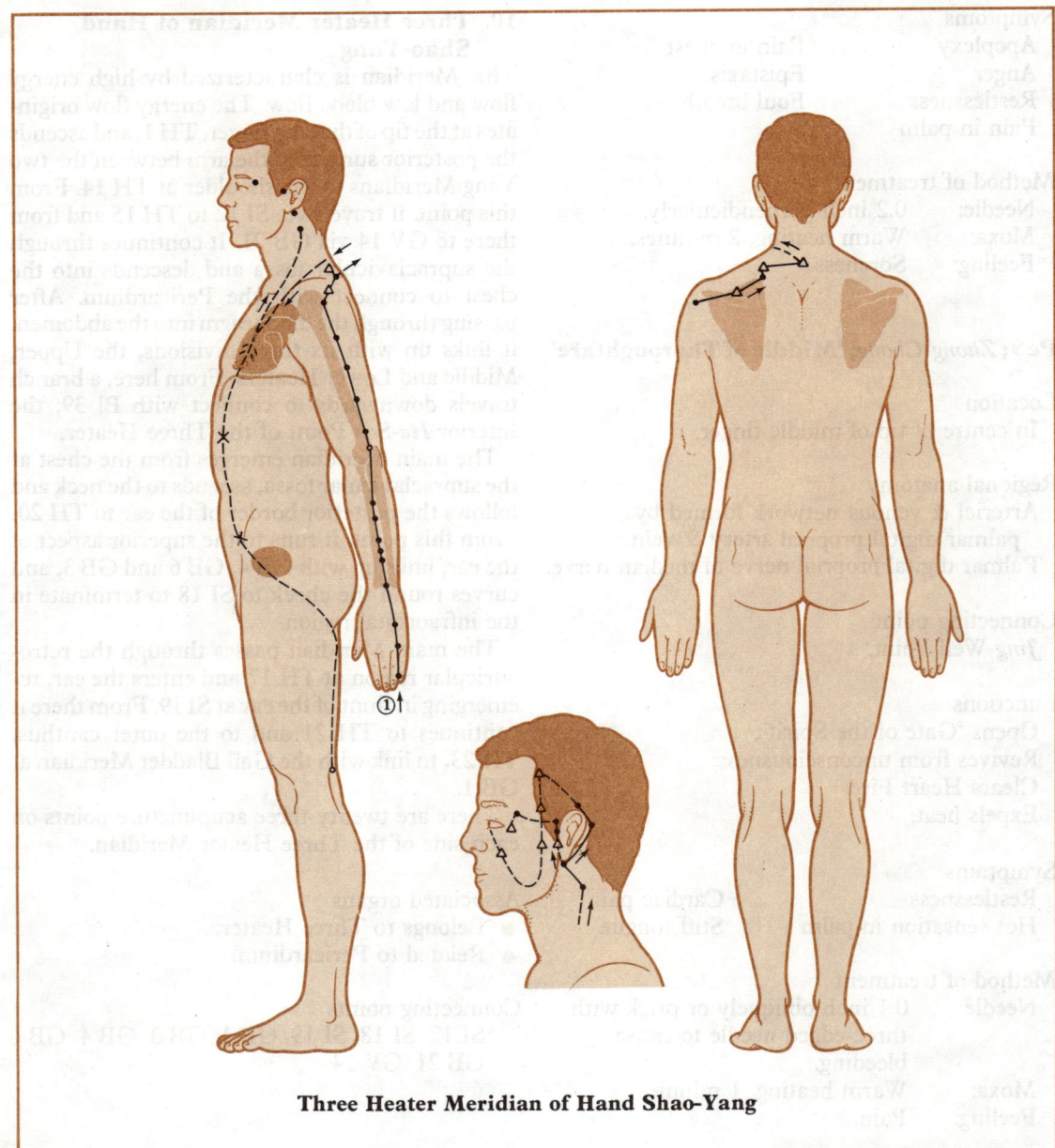

Three Heater Meridian of Hand Shao-Yang

FOURTEEN MERIDIANS AND ACUPUNCTURE POINTS

Symptomatology
  Disorders along Meridian course
    Pain & swelling of throat
    Deafness
    Pain in cheek
    Redness & pain in eye
    Pain behind ear & over mastoid
    Pain in shoulder & arm

  Disorders in organ
    Abdominal distention   Frequent urination
    Urine retention   (micturition)
    Oedema   Enuresis

Acupuncture Points of Three Heater Meridian

TH 1; *Guan-Chong*; 'Gate of Thoroughfare'

Location
0.1 *cun* posterior to corner of fourth fingernail (on side towards little finger).

Regional anatomy
  Arterial & venous network formed by palmar digital proprial artery & vein;
  Palmar digital proprial nerve derived from ulnar nerve.

Connecting point
  Jing-Well Point.

Functions
  Expels heat from *Jing-Luo*;
  Expels heat from Three Heater.

Symptoms
  Sore & swollen throat   Pain in arm & elbow
  Dry mouth   Blurred vision
  Headache

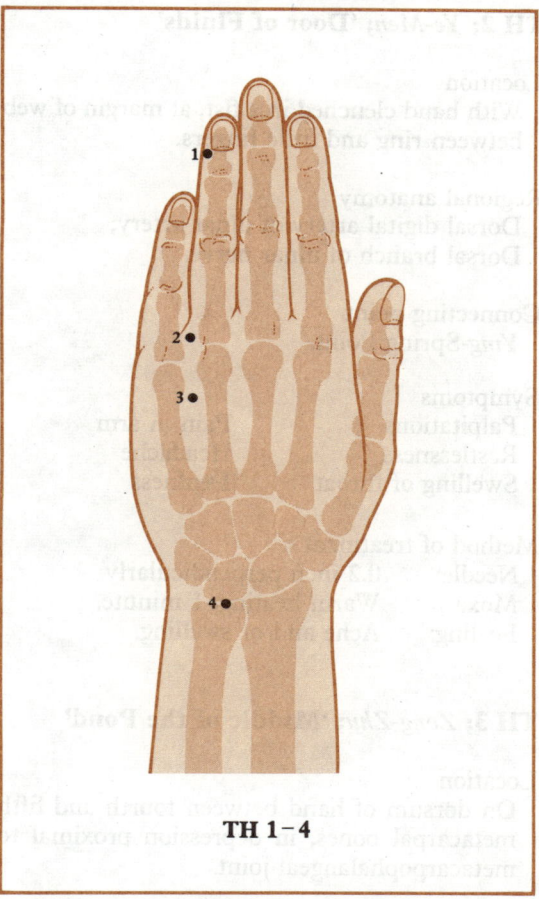

TH 1–4

Method of treatment
  Needle: 0.1 inch obliquely or prick with three-edged needle to cause bleeding.
  Moxa: Warm heating, 1 minute.
  Feeling: Pain.

189

FOURTEEN MERIDIANS AND ACUPUNCTURE POINTS

TH 2; *Ye-Men*; 'Door of Fluids'

Location
With hand clenched in a fist, at margin of web between ring and little fingers.

Regional anatomy
Dorsal digital artery of ulnar artery;
Dorsal branch of ulnar nerve.

Connecting point
Ying-Spring Point.

Symptoms
Palpitations	Pain in arm
Restlessness	Headache
Swelling of throat	Deafness

Method of treatment
Needle: 0.2 inch perpendicularly.
Moxa: Warm heating, 1 minute.
Feeling: Ache and/or swelling.

TH 3; *Zong-Zhu*; 'Middle of the Pond'

Location
On dorsum of hand between fourth and fifth metacarpal bones, in depression proximal to metacarpophalangeal joint.

Regional anatomy
Dorsal interosseous muscles of hand;
Dorsal venous network of hand;
Fourth dorsal metacarpal artery;
Dorsal branch of ulnar nerve.

Connecting point
Shu-Stream Point.

Functions
Regulates energy flow in *Shao*-Yang Meridian;
Expels excess heat from Three Heater.

Symptoms
Fever	Blurred vision
Headache	Swelling of throat
Dizziness	Pain in arm, elbow
Deafness	& fingers

Method of treatment
Needle: 0.3 inch perpendicularly.
Moxa: Warm heating, 1 minute.
Feeling: Ache and/or numbness.

TH 4; *Yang-Chi*; 'Pond of Yang'

Location
At junction of ulna and carpal bones, in depression lateral to tendon of extensor muscle of fingers.

Regional anatomy
Tendons of extensor muscles of fingers & of little finger;
Inferiorly, dorsal venous network of wrist;
Posterior carpal artery;
Dorsal branch of ulnar nerve;
Terminal branch of posterior cutaneous nerve of forearm.

Connecting point
Yuan-Source Point.

Functions
Expels excess heat from body;
Clears excess heat from Three Heater.

Symptoms
Dry mouth	Fever
Restlessness	Pain in arm & wrist

FOURTEEN MERIDIANS AND ACUPUNCTURE POINTS

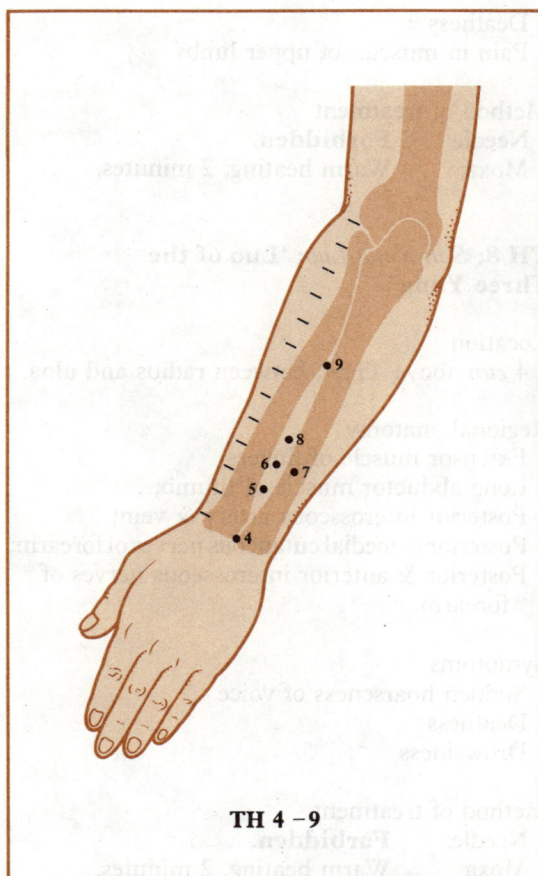

TH 4 – 9

Regional anatomy
   Extensor muscle of fingers;
   Long extensor muscle of thumb;
   Posterior & anterior interosseous arteries
      & veins;
   Posterior cutaneous nerve of forearm;
   Posterior interosseous branch of radial nerve;
   Anterior interosseous branch of median nerve.

Connecting points
   Luo-Connecting Point; one of 'Eight Confluent
   Points' connecting with Yang-*Wei* Meridian.

Functions
   Prevents attack to body by external causes of
      disease;
   Expels excess heat from Three Heater.

Symptoms
   Deafness
   Pain in arm, elbow & fingers

Method of treatment
   Needle: 0.3 inch perpendicularly.
   Moxa: Warm heating, 2 minutes.
   Feeling: Ache and/or numbness.

Note
Pc 6 is behind this point; when necessary, both
points may be needled together from TH 5.

TH 6; *Zhi-Gou*; **'Branch of Ditch'**

Location
   3 *cun* above TH 4, between radius and ulna.

Regional anatomy
   Extensor muscle of fingers;
   Long extensor muscle of thumb;
   Posterior & anterior interosseous arteries
      & veins;

Method of treatment
   Needle: 0.2 inch obliquely.
   Moxa: Warm heating, 1 minute.
   Feeling.   Ache.

TH 5; *Wai-Guan*; **'External Gate'**

Location
   2 *cun* above TH 4, between radius and ulna.

Posterior cutaneous nerve of forearm;
Posterior interosseous branch of radial nerve;
Anterior interosseous branch of median nerve.

Connecting point
Jing-River Point.

Functions
Clears pathogenic energy in Three Heater;
Regulates Fu energy flow;
Expels excess heat from Three Heater.

Symptoms
Fever   Restlessness
Ache in shoulder & arm   Cardiac pain
Pain in axilla region   Skin disorders

Method of treatment
Needle: 0.2 inch perpendicularly.
Moxa: Warm heating, 2 minutes.
Feeling: Ache and/or numbness.

TH 7; *Hui-Zong*; 'Reunion of Ancestors'

Location
At same level as and one finger-breadth lateral to TH 6, on radial side of ulna.

Regional anatomy
Ulnar extensor muscle of wrist;
Extensor muscles of little & index fingers;
Posterior interosseous artery & vein;
Posterior & medial cutaneous nerves of forearm;
Posterior & anterior interosseous nerves of forearm.

Connecting point
Xi-Cleft Point.

Symptoms
(Epilepsy)

Deafness
Pain in muscles of upper limbs

Method of treatment
Needle: **Forbidden.**
Moxa: Warm heating, 2 minutes.

TH 8; *San-Yang-Luo*; 'Luo of the Three Yang'

Location
4 *cun* above TH 4, between radius and ulna.

Regional anatomy
Extensor muscle of fingers;
Long abductor muscle of thumb;
Posterior interosseous artery & vein;
Posterior & medial cutaneous nerves of forearm;
Posterior & anterior interosseous nerves of forearm.

Symptoms
Sudden hoarseness of voice
Deafness
Drowsiness

Method of treatment
Needle: **Forbidden.**
Moxa: Warm heating, 2 minutes.

TH 9; *Si-Du*; 'Four Gutters'

Location
7 *cun* above TH 4, between radius and ulna.

Regional anatomy
Extensor muscle of fingers;
Ulnar extensor muscle of wrist;
Posterior interosseous artery & vein;
Posterior & medial cutaneous nerves of forearm;

FOURTEEN MERIDIANS AND ACUPUNCTURE POINTS

Posterior & anterior interosseous nerves of forearm.

Symptoms
Deafness
Toothache

Method of treatment
Needle: 0.6 inch perpendicularly.
Moxa: Warm heating, 2 minutes.
Feeling: Ache and/or swelling.

TH 10; *Tian-Jing*; 'Celestial Wells'

Location
With elbow flexed, in depression 1 *cun* superior to olecranon.

Regional anatomy
Tendon of triceps muscle of arm;
Arterial & venous network of elbow;
Posterior cutaneous nerve of arm;
Muscular branch of radial nerve.

Connecting point
He-Sea Point.

Functions
Dispels damp in *Jing-Luo*;
Expels excess heat from Three Heater.

Symptoms
Cardiac pain
Shortness of breath
Coughing
Palpitations
Drowsiness
Swelling & pain in mandibular region
Stiff neck
Pain in lumbar region & hip

Method of treatment
Needle: 0.3 inch obliquely.
Moxa: Warm heating, 2 minutes.

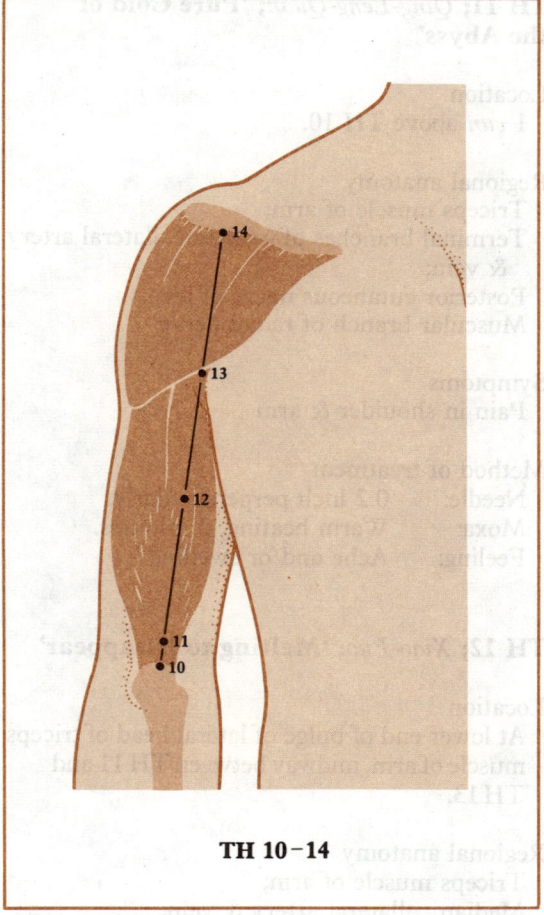

Feeling: Ache and/or swelling.

Note
Bl 39 is the main *He*-Sea Point of the Three Heater Meridian.

TH 10-14

193

FOURTEEN MERIDIANS AND ACUPUNCTURE POINTS

TH 11; *Qing-Leng-Quan*; 'Pure Cold of the Abyss'

Location
1 *cun* above TH 10.

Regional anatomy
Triceps muscle of arm;
Terminal branches of median collateral artery & vein;
Posterior cutaneous nerve of arm;
Muscular branch of radial nerve.

Symptoms
Pain in shoulder & arm

Method of treatment
Needle: 0.2 inch perpendicularly.
Moxa: Warm heating, 2 minutes.
Feeling: Ache and/or swelling.

TH 12; *Xiao-Luo*; 'Melting to Disappear'

Location
At lower end of bulge of lateral head of triceps muscle of arm, midway between TH 11 and TH 13.

Regional anatomy
Triceps muscle of arm;
Median collateral artery & vein;
Posterior cutaneous nerve of arm;
Muscular branch of radial nerve.

Symptoms
Pain in arm   Stiff neck
Headache   Mania

Method of treatment:
Needle: 0.5 inch perpendicularly.
Moxa: Warm heating, 2 minutes.
Feeling: Ache and/or swelling.

TH 13; *Nao-Hui*; 'Reunion of the Muscle'

Location
3 *cun* below TH 14 on posterior border of deltoid muscle.

Regional anatomy
Triceps muscle of arm;
Median collateral artery & vein;
Posterior cutaneous nerve of arm;
Muscular branch of radial nerve;
Radial nerve.

Connecting point
Meeting Point of Hand *Shao*-Yang and Yang-*Wei* Meridians.

Symptoms
Ache & pain in arm
Swelling & pain in shoulder

Method of treatment
Needle: 0.5 inch perpendicularly.
Moxa: Warm heating, 3 minutes.
Feeling: Ache and/or swelling.

TH 14; *Jian-Liao*; 'Shoulder Bone'

Location
In depression between acromion and greater tubercle of humerus. With arm in passive horizontal abduction, in posterior of two depressions formed. (LI 15 is located in anterior depression.)

Regional anatomy
Deltoid muscle;
Muscular branch of posterior circumflex humeral artery;

FOURTEEN MERIDIANS AND ACUPUNCTURE POINTS

Muscular branch of axillary nerve.

Functions
Dispels wind and damp in *Jing-Luo*;
Regulates blood and energy flows.

Symptoms
Pain in arm & shoulder

Method of treatment
Needle: 0.7 inch obliquely.
Moxa: Warm heating, 3 minutes.
Feeling: Ache.

TH 15; *Tian-Liao*; 'Celestial Bone'

Location
Midway between GB 21 and SI 13 on superior angle of scapula.

Regional anatomy
Trapezius muscle;
Supraspinous muscle;
Descending branch of transverse cervical artery;
Muscular branch of suprascapular artery;
Accessory nerve;
Branch of suprascapular nerve.

Connecting point
Meeting Point of Hand and Foot *Shao*-Yang and Yang-*Wei* Meridians.

Symptoms
Restlessness
Fullness in chest
Ache & pain in shoulder & arm
Pain in supraclavicular fossa
Stiff neck

Method of treatment
Needle: 0.5 inch perpendicularly.

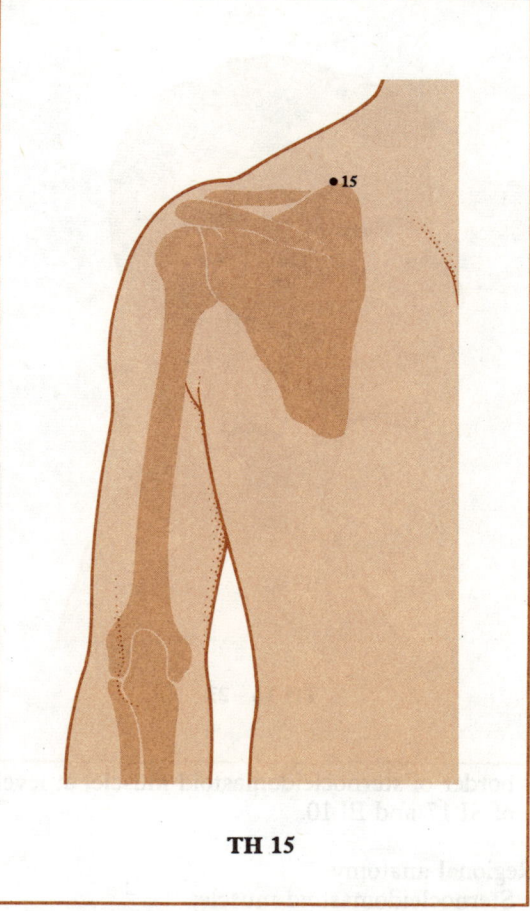

TH 15

Moxa: Warm heating, 2 minutes.
Feeling: Ache.
Warning: Avoid inserting needle too deeply.

TH 16; *Tian-You*; 'Window to the Sky'

Location
Posteroinferior to mastoid process on posterior

195

FOURTEEN MERIDIANS AND ACUPUNCTURE POINTS

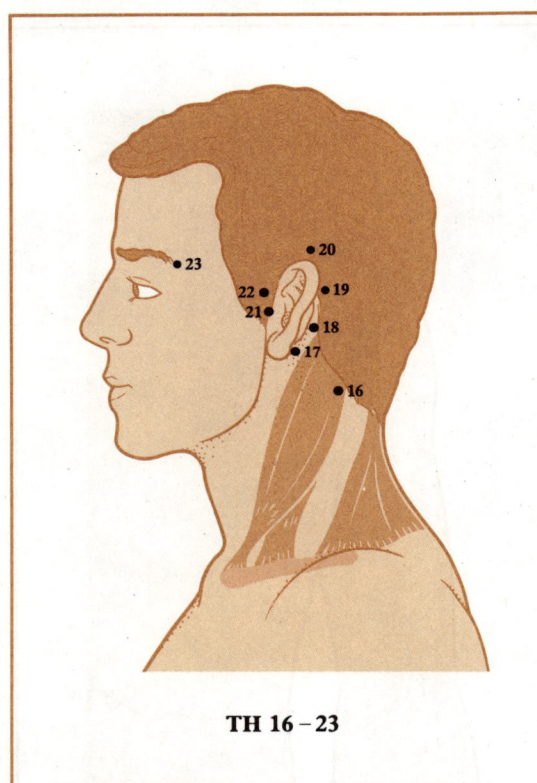

TH 16 – 23

border of sternocleidomastoid muscle, at level of SI 17 and Bl 10.

Regional anatomy
  Sternocleidomastoid muscle;
  Posterior auricular artery;
  Lesser occipital nerve.

Symptoms
  Blurred vision   Headache
  Ophthalmalgia   Facial swelling
  Bad dreams   Stiff neck
  Restlessness

Method of treatment
  Needle: 0.5 inch perpendicularly.
  Moxa: **Forbidden.**
  Feeling: Ache.
  Warning: **Avoid inserting needle too deeply.
              Moxibustion with moxa cones causes facial swelling.**

TH 17; *Yi-Feng*; 'Wind and Nebula'

Location
  Posterior to lobule of ear in depression between mandible and mastoid process.

Regional anatomy
  Posterior auricular artery & vein;
  External jugular vein;
  Great auricular nerve;
  Facial nerve.

Connecting point
  Meeting Point of Hand and Foot *Shao*-Yang Meridians.

Functions
  Harmonizes energy flow of Three Heater Meridian;
  Opens 'Gate of the Ear';
  Eases wind and heat in Meridian.

Symptoms
  Tinnitus aurium   Trismus
  Deafness   Swelling of cheek
  Facial paralysis

Clinical formula
  TH 17 + LI 4 + St 7 = Acute mumps (epidemic parotitis)

FOURTEEN MERIDIANS AND ACUPUNCTURE POINTS

Method of treatment
　Needle:　　0.3 inch obliquely.
　Moxa:　　　Warm heating, 2 minutes.
　Feeling:　　Ache and/or swelling.
　Warning:　To treat deafness, the needle may be inserted to a depth of about 1 inch, but the practitioner must be experienced in this technique.

TH 18; *Qi-Mai*; 'Nourishment of the Vessels'

Location
　Posterior to ear, about one-third of distance from TH 17 along curve formed by TH 17 to TH 20.

Regional anatomy
　Posterior auricular muscle;
　Posterior auricular artery & vein;
　Posterior auricular branch of great auricular nerve.

Symptoms
　Headache
　Tinnitus aurium
　Fear

Method of treatment
　Needle:　　0.1 inch obliquely or prick with three-edged needle to cause bleeding.
　Moxa:　　　Warm heating, 1 minute.
　Feeling:　　Soreness.

TH 19; *Lu-Xi*; 'Rest of the Head'

Location
　Posterior to ear, about two-thirds of distance from TH 17 along curve formed by TH 17 and TH 20.

Regional anatomy
　Posterior auricular muscle;
　Posterior auricular artery & vein;
　Anastomotic branch of great auricular & lesser occipital nerves.

Symptoms
　Tinnitus aurium
　Headache
　Swelling & pain in ear

Method of treatment
　Needle:　　Prick with three-edged needle to cause bleeding.
　Moxa:　　　Warm heating, 1 minute.
　Feeling:　　Soreness.
　Warning:　Bleed only one drop of blood.

TH 20; *Jiao-Sun*; 'Apex of the Ear'

Location
　Above apex of ear within hairline of temple.

Regional anatomy
　Posterior auricular muscle;
　Branches of superficial temporal artery & vein;
　Branches of auriculotemporal nerve.

Connecting point
　Meeting Point of Hand and Foot *Shao*-Yang and Hand Yang-*Ming* Meridians.

Symptoms
　Blurred vision
　Stiff neck
　Stiff jaw

FOURTEEN MERIDIANS AND ACUPUNCTURE POINTS

Method of treatment
  Needle: 0.2 inch horizontally.
  Moxa: Warm heating, 1 minute.
  Feeling: Ache and/or numbness.

TH 21; *Er-Men*; 'Gate of the Ear'

Location
  0.5 *cun* above SI 19, in depression anterior to supratragic notch and slightly superior to condyle of mandible.

Regional anatomy
  Superficial temporal artery & vein;
  Branches of auriculotemporal & facial nerves.

Functions
  Frees energy flow;
  Expels excess heat;
  Opens 'Gate of the Ear'.

Symptoms
  Tinnitus aurium
  Deafness
  Stiff jaw

Method of treatment
  Needle: 0.3 inch obliquely.
  Moxa: Warm heating, 1 minute.
  Feeling: Soreness and/or swelling.
  Warnings: To treat deafness, the needle may be inserted to a depth of about 1 inch, but the practitioner must be experienced in this technique. If there is pus in the ear, do not apply needles or moxibustion.

TH 22; *He-Liao*; 'Harmony of the Ear Bone'

Location
  Anterosuperior to TH 21 at level of root of helix, within hairline.

Regional anatomy
  Temporal muscle;
  Superficial temporal artery & vein;
  Branch of auriculotemporal nerve;
  On course of temporal branch of facial nerve.

Connecting point
  Meeting Point of Hand and Foot *Shao*-Yang and Hand *Tai*-Yang Meridians.

Symptoms
  Headache
  Stiff jaw
  Swelling in mandibular region
  Tinnitus aurium
  Runny nose

Method of treatment
  Needle: 0.2 inch obliquely.
  Moxa: Not to be used as it affects the eyes.
  Feeling: Swelling and/or numbness.
  Warning: Avoid inserting needle too deeply.

TH 23; *Si-Zhu-Kong*; 'Hollow Bamboo'

Location
  In depression at lateral end of eyebrow.

Regional anatomy
  Orbicular muscle of eye;
  Frontal branches of superficial temporal artery & vein;
  Zygomatic branch of facial nerve;
  Branch of auriculotemporal nerve;

Supraorbital nerve.

Functions
- Dispels wind;
- Relieves pain in eyes;
- Expels heat;
- Regulates and harmonizes energy flow in Three Heater Meridian.

Symptoms
Headache	Blurred vision
Dizziness	Restlessness
Mania	Migraine headache

Method of treatment
Needle:	0.3 inch horizontally.
Moxa:	**Forbidden.**
Feeling:	Swelling.

11. Gall Bladder Meridian of Foot Shao-Yang

This Meridian is characterized by high energy flow and low blood flow. The energy flow originates at the outer canthus, GB 1, and runs up to the corner of the forehead, St 8, then curves down at GB 4 to the ear at GB 7 to connect with TH 21 and TH 20. It winds round behind the ear to GB 12, then returns to the forehead at GB 14. From this point it ascends to GB 17, links up with GV 20 and continues on to GB 18. After running down to the neck, GB 20, and then to SI 17, it passes in front of the Three Heater Meridian to the shoulder to connect with GV 14. From here it turns back to GB 21 and (via SI 12) on to the supraclavicular fossa.

A branch from GB 20 proceeds to TH 17 and enters the ear, emerges at GB 2, connects with SI 19, St 7 and GB 3, then returns to GB 1. It then continues down to St 5 where it divides into two branches: one ascends to the infraorbital region; the other descends to St 6 and down to the supraclavicular fossa, where it meets up with the Main Meridian.

At the supraclavicular fossa the Main Meridian gives off a branch which descends into the chest and passes through the diaphragm to connect with the Liver and Gall Bladder. It then travels inside the hypochondriac region, descends into the lower abdomen, follows along the margin of the pubic hair and enters, transversely, the hip region, GB 30.

The Main Meridian itself descends in front of the axilla, Pc 1, continues along the lateral aspect of the chest and runs through the ribs at Liv 13 to the groin. It flows via GB 29 and Bl 31 and Bl 34, then back to the hip region, GB 30, where it meets up with its branch. From GB 30, the Main Meridian descends to the thigh, knee and lower leg; from the anterior aspect of the external malleolus, it follows the dorsum of the foot, terminating at the tip of the fourth toe, GB 44. From GB 41, the Main Meridian runs between the first and second metatarsal bones to the great toe, where it links up with the Liver Meridian at Liv 1.

There are forty-four acupuncture points on each side of the Gall Bladder Meridian.

Associated organs
- Belongs to Gall Bladder;
- Related to Liver;
- Directly connected with Heart.

Connecting points
- St 8 St 7 TH 17 TH 20 TH 21 SI 12 SI 17 SI 19 GV 14 Liv 13 Bl 31 Bl 34 Pc 1

Symptomatology
- Disorders along Meridian course

Heat & cold	Swelling in axilla region
Headache	Deafness
Ophthalmalgia	Pain in hip, thigh, leg
Pain in cheek	& knee

FOURTEEN MERIDIANS AND ACUPUNCTURE POINTS

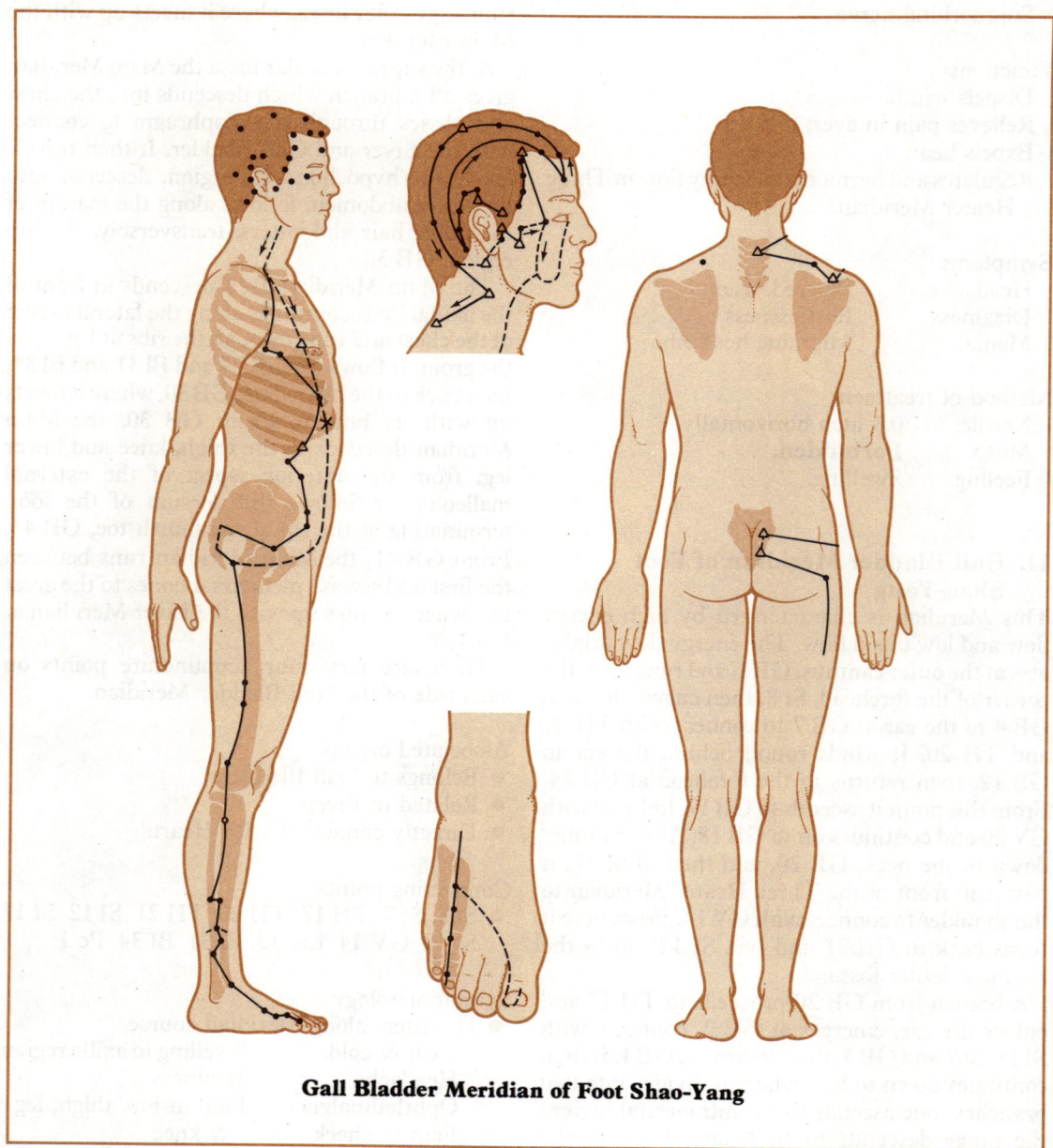

Gall Bladder Meridian of Foot Shao-Yang

FOURTEEN MERIDIANS AND ACUPUNCTURE POINTS

Disorders in organ
    Pain in hypochondriac region
    Vomiting
    Bitter taste in mouth
    Pain in chest
    Fear

Acupuncture Points of Gall Bladder Meridian

GB 1; *Tong-Zi-Liao*; 'Bone of the Eye'

Location
    Lateral to outer canthus, in depression on lateral side of orbit.

Regional anatomy
    Orbicular muscle of eye;
    Zygomaticoorbital artery & vein;
    Zygomaticofacial & zygomaticotemporal nerves;
    Temporal branch of facial nerve.

Connecting point
    Meeting Point of Hand *Tai*-Yang, and Hand and Foot *Shao*-Yang Meridians.

Functions
    Dispels wind and heat;
    Regulates blood and energy flows;
    Relieves pain in eyes;
    Strengthens eye function.

Symptoms
    Itchy eyes   Red eyes
    Blurred vision   Headache
    Lacrimation

Method of treatment
    Needle: 0.3 inch horizontally.

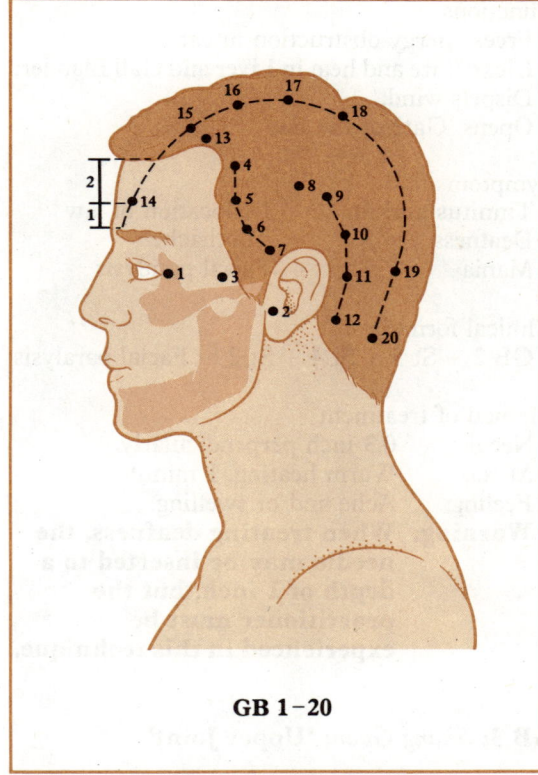

GB 1–20

Moxa: Warm heating, 1 minute.
Feeling: Ache and/or swelling.

GB 2; *Ting-Hui*; 'Reunion of Hearing'

Location
    Anterior to intertragic notch, below SI 19, at posterior border of condyle of mandible, located with mouth slightly open.

Regional anatomy
    Superficial temporal artery;
    Great auricular & facial nerves.

FOURTEEN MERIDIANS AND ACUPUNCTURE POINTS

Functions
  Frees energy obstruction in ear;
  Clears Fire and heat in Liver and Gall Bladder;
  Dispels wind;
  Opens 'Gate of the Ear'.

Symptoms
  Tinnitus aurium   Dislocation of jaw
  Deafness   Toothache
  Mania   Facial paralysis

Clinical formula
  GB 2 + St 5 + St 4 + St 2 = Facial paralysis

Method of treatment
  Needle: 0.3 inch perpendicularly.
  Moxa: Warm heating, 1 minute.
  Feeling: Ache and/or swelling.
  Warning: When treating deafness, the needle may be inserted to a depth of 1 inch, but the practitioner must be experienced in this technique.

GB 3; *Shang-Guan*; 'Upper Joint'

Location
  On superior border of zygomatic arch, in depression directly above St 7.

Regional anatomy
  Temporal muscle;
  Zygomaticoorbital artery & vein;
  Zygomatic branch of facial nerve & zygomaticofacial nerve.

Connecting point
  Meeting point of Hand and Foot *Shao*-Yang and Foot Yang-*Ming* Meridians.

Symptoms
  Stiff jaw   Trigeminal neuralgia
  Facial paralysis   Tinnitus aurium
  Blurred vision   Deafness

Method of treatment
  Needle: 0.3 inch perpendicularly.
  Moxa: Warm heating, 1 minute.
  Feeling: Ache and/or swelling.
  Warning: Avoid inserting needle too deeply.

GB 4; *Han-Yan*; 'Accept or Reject'

Location
  At hairline of temporal region, one-quarter of distance between St 8 and GB 7.

Regional anatomy
  Superior & anterior auricular muscles;
  Temporal muscle;
  Superficial temporal artery & vein;
  Auriculotemporal nerve.

Connecting point
  Meeting Point of Hand and Foot *Shao*-Yang and Foot Yang-*Ming* Meridians.

Symptoms
  Migraine   Pain in wrist
  Headache   Tinnitus aurium
  Dizziness   Stiff neck

Method of treatment
  Needle: 0.3 inch horizontally.
  Moxa: Warm heating, 1 minute.
  Feeling: Ache and/or numbness.

GB 5; *Xuan-Lu*; 'Suspended Head'

Location
Within hairline of temporal region, halfway between St 8 and GB 7.

Regional anatomy
Superior & anterior auricular muscles;
Temporal muscle;
Superficial temporal artery & vein;
Auriculotemporal nerve.

Connecting point
Meeting Point of Hand and Foot *Shao*-Yang and Foot Yang-*Ming* Meridians.

Symptoms
Headache   Facial swelling
Toothache   Blurred vision
Migraine

Method of treatment
Needle: 0.3 inch horizontally.
Moxa: Warm heating, 1 minute.
Feeling: Ache and/or swelling.
Warning: Avoid inserting needle too deeply as it will affect the hearing.

GB 6; *Xuan-Li*; 'Suspended a Fraction'

Location
Within hairline, inferior to corner of temporal region, halfway between GB 5 and GB 7.

Regional anatomy
Superior & anterior auricular muscles;
Temporal muscle;
Superficial temporal artery & vein;
Auriculotemporal nerve.

Connecting point
Meeting Point of Hand and Foot *Shao*-Yang and Foot Yang-*Ming* Meridians.

Symptoms
Facial swelling   Pain in outer canthus
Migraine   Restlessness

Method of treatment
Needle: 0.3 inch horizontally.
Moxa: Warm heating, 1 minute.
Feeling: Ache and/or swelling.

GB 7; *Qu-Bin*; 'Twisted Hair on the Temples'

Location
Within hairline, anterosuperior to ear, level with eyebrow.

Regional anatomy
Superior & anterior auricular muscles;
Temporal muscle;
Superficial temporal artery & vein;
Auriculotemporal nerve.

Connecting point
Meeting Point of Foot *Shao*-Yang and Foot *Tai*-Yang Meridians.

Symptoms
Swelling & pain in cheek & submandibular region
Stiff neck
Pain in temporal region

Method of treatment
Needle: 0.3 inch horizontally.
Moxa: Warm heating, 1 minute.
Feeling: Ache and/or swelling.

FOURTEEN MERIDIANS AND ACUPUNCTURE POINTS

GB 8; *Shuai-Gu*; 'Straight to the Valley'

Location
Superior to apex of ear, 1.5 *cun* within hairline.

Regional anatomy
Temporal muscle;
Parietal branches of superficial temporal artery & vein;
Anastomotic branch of auriculotemporal nerve & greater occipital nerve.

Connecting point
Meeting Point of Foot *Shao*-Yang and Foot *Tai*-Yang Meridians.

Symptoms
Pain in diaphragm   Pain in temporal region
Heaviness of head   Vomiting

Method of treatment
Needle: 0.3 inch horizontally.
Moxa: Warm heating, 1 minute.
Feeling: Ache and/or swelling.

GB 9; *Tian-Chong*; 'Thoroughfare of Heaven'

Location
Posterosuperior to ear, 0.5 *cun* posterior to GB 8 and 2 *cun* within hairline.

Regional anatomy
Posterior auricular muscle;
Posterior auricular artery & vein;
Branch of greater occipital nerve.

Connecting point
Meeting Point of Foot *Shao*-Yang and Foot *Tai*-Yang Meridians.

Symptoms
(Epilepsy)   Swollen gums
Headache   Fear

Method of treatment
Needle: 0.3 inch horizontally.
Moxa: Warm heating, 1 minute.
Feeling: Ache and/or swelling.

GB 10; *Fu-Bai*; 'Floating Whiteness'

Location
About 1 *cun* inferoposterior to GB 9, level with upper border of root of ear, 1 *cun* within hairline.

Regional anatomy
Posterior auricular muscle;
Posterior auricular artery & vein;
Branch of greater occipital nerve.

Connecting point
Meeting Point of Foot *Shao*-Yang and Foot *Tai*-Yang Meridians.

Symptoms
Paralysis in lower limbs
Tinnitus aurium
Deafness
Pain & fullness in chest
Pain in shoulder & arm
Stiff neck

Method of treatment
Needle: 0.3 inch horizontally.
Moxa: Warm heating, 1 minute.
Feeling: Ache and/or numbness.

FOURTEEN MERIDIANS AND ACUPUNCTURE POINTS

GB 11; Head *Qiao-Yin*; 'Inspiration of Yin'

Location
  Posterosuperior to mastoid process, 1 *cun* posterior to GB 10 and 1 *cun* lateral to root of ear.

Regional anatomy
  Posterior auricular muscle;
  Branches of posterior auricular artery & vein;
  Anastomotic branch of greater & lesser occipital nerves.

Connecting point
  Meeting Point of Foot *Tai*-Yang, and Hand and Foot *Shao*-Yang Meridians.

Symptoms
  Muscle spasm in lower limbs
  Ophthalmalgia
  Tinnitus aurium
  Stiff tongue

Method of treatment
  Needle: 0.3 inch horizontally.
  Moxa: Warm heating, 1 minute.
  Feeling: Ache and/or swelling.

GB 12; *Wan-Gu*; 'Complete Bone'

Location
  In depression posteroinferior to mastoid process.

Regional anatomy
  Posterior auricular muscle;
  Posterior auricular artery & vein;
  Lesser occipital nerve.

Connecting point
  Meeting Point of Foot *Shao*-Yang and Foot *Tai*-Yang Meridians.

Symptoms
  Paralysis of lower limbs   Headache & pain in
  Restlessness   back of ear
  Swelling of face   Facial paralysis
  Stiff neck

Method of treatment
  Needle: 0.3 inch obliquely.
  Moxa: Warm heating, 1 minute.
  Feeling: Ache and/or swelling.

GB 13; *Ben-Shen*; 'Original Spirit'

Location
  0.5 *cun* within hairline of forehead, 3 *cun* lateral to GV 24.

Regional anatomy
  Frontal muscle;
  Frontal branches of superficial temporal artery & vein;
  Lateral branches of frontal artery & vein;
  Lateral branch of frontal nerve.

Connecting point
  Meeting Point of Foot *Shao*-Yang and Yang-*Wei* Meridians.

Symptoms
  (Epilepsy)   Dizziness
  Stiff neck   Pain in chest

Method of treatment
  Needle: 0.3 inch horizontally.
  Moxa: Warm heating, 1 minute.
  Feeling: Ache and/or swelling.

FOURTEEN MERIDIANS AND ACUPUNCTURE POINTS

GB 14; *Yang-Bai*; 'White Yang'

Location
On forehead, 1 *cun* above midpoint of eyebrow.

Regional anatomy
Frontal muscle;
Lateral branches of frontal artery & vein;
On lateral branch of frontal nerve.

Connecting point
Meeting Point of Hand and Foot Yang-*Ming*, Hand and Foot *Shao*-Yang, and Yang-*Wei* Meridians.

Functions
Dispels wind and Fire;
Strengthens eye function.

Symptoms
Itchiness & pain in eyes
Blurred vision
Feeling of coldness in back

Method of treatment
Needle: 0.3 inch horizontally.
Moxa: Warm heating, 1 minute.
Feeling: Ache and/or swelling.

GB 15; Head *Lin-Qi*; 'On the Point of Tears'

Location
Directly above GB 14, 0.5 *cun* within hairline.

Regional anatomy
Frontal muscle;
Frontal artery & vein;
Anastomotic branch of medial & lateral branches of frontal nerve.

Connecting point
Meeting Point of Foot *Shao*-Yang, Foot *Tai*-Yang and Yang-*Wei* Meridians.

Symptoms
Dizziness
Lacrimation
Headache
Nasal obstruction
Pain in outer canthus

Clinical formula
GB 15 + St 8 + LI 4 = Lacrimation

Method of treatment
Needle: 0.3 inch horizontally.
Moxa: Warm heating, 1 minute.
Feeling: Ache and/or swelling.

GB 16; *Mu-Chuang*; 'Window of the Eyes'

Location
1.5 *cun* posterior to GB 15.

Regional anatomy
Epicranial aponeurosis;
Frontal branches of superficial temporal artery & vein;
Anastomotic branch of medial & lateral branches of frontal nerve.

Connecting point
Meeting Point of Foot *Shao*-Yang and Yang-*Wei* Meridians.

Symptoms
Ophthalmalgia
Blurred vision
Dizziness
Head & facial swelling

Clinical formula
GB 16 + Pc 7 = Ophthalmalgia

Method of treatment
  Needle: 0.3 inch horizontally.
  Moxa: Warm heating, 1 minute.
  Feeling: Ache and/or swelling.

GB 17; *Zheng-Ying*; 'Vital Nutrition'

Location
  1 *cun* posterior to GB 16.

Regional anatomy
  Epicranial aponeurosis;
  Anastomosis of parietal branches of superficial temporal artery & vein;
  Occipital artery & vein;
  Anastomotic branch of frontal & greater occipital nerves.

Connecting point
  Meeting Point of Foot *Shao*-Yang and Yang-*Wei* Meridians.

Symptoms
  Dizziness   Toothache
  Migraine   Stiff jaw

Method of treatment
  Needle: 0.3 inch horizontally.
  Moxa: Warm heating, 1 minute.
  Feeling: Ache and/or swelling.
  Warning: Do not overmanipulate this point.

GB 18; *Cheng-Ling*; 'Supporting the Spirit'

Location
  1.5 *cun* posterior to GB 17.

Regional anatomy
  Epicranial aponeurosis;
  Branches of occipital artery & vein;
  Branch of greater occipital nerve.

Connecting point
  Meeting Point of Foot *Shao*-Yang and Yang-*Wei* Meridians.

Symptoms
  Headache   Nasal obstruction
  Epistaxis   Dyspnoea

Method of treatment
  Needle: **Forbidden.**
  Moxa: Warm heating, 1 minute.

Note
In spite of Dr Yang's *Compendium of Acupuncture and Moxibustion* (1601) forbidding needle insertion, modern books on acupuncture make no mention of this injunction.

GB 19; *Nao-Kong*; 'Hollow Brain'

Location
  Directly above GB 20 (at level of GV 17) and 1.5 *cun* posterior to GB 18.

Regional anatomy
  Occipital muscle;
  Occipital artery & vein;
  Greater occipital nerve.

Connecting point
  Meeting Point of Foot *Shao*-Yang and Yang-*Wei* Meridians.

Symptoms
  Fatigue   Dizziness
  Stiff neck   Palpitations
  Severe headache

FOURTEEN MERIDIANS AND ACUPUNCTURE POINTS

Clinical formula
 GB 19 + GB 20 = Severe headache

Method of treatment
 Needle: 0.4 inch horizontally.
 Moxa: Warm heating, 1 minute.
 Feeling: Ache and/or swelling.

GB 20; *Feng-Chi*; 'Wind Pond'

Location
 In posterior aspect of neck below occipital bone, in depression between upper portion of sternocleidomastoid muscle and trapezius muscle.

Regional anatomy
 Sternocleidomastoid muscle;
 Trapezius muscle;
 Splenius muscle of head;
 Branches of occipital artery & vein;
 Branch of lesser occipital nerve.

Connecting point
 Meeting Point of Hand and Foot *Shao*-Yang and Yang-*Wei* Meridians.

Functions
 Eliminates wind and expels heat;
 Strengthens function of eyes;
 Regulates blood and energy flows.

Symptoms
Common cold	Lacrimation
Dizziness	Ophthalmalgia
Migraine	Tension
Headache	Pain in back & lower back
Stiff neck	

Clinical formula
 GB 20 + GV 12 + Bl 12 = Preventing common cold

Method of treatment
 Needle: 0.4 inch obliquely.
 Moxa: Warm heating, 1 minute.
 Feeling: Ache.
 Warning: Skilled needle technique is very important at this point; great care must be taken to avoid inserting too deeply and in the wrong direction. Needle insertion here is better than moxa.

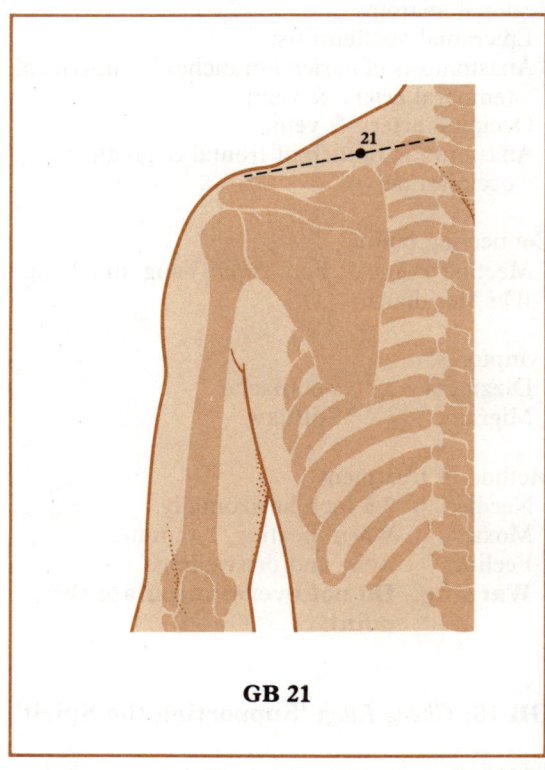

GB 21

GB 21; *Jian-Jing*; 'Well of the Shoulder'

Location
 Midway on a line from GV 14 to acromion.

FOURTEEN MERIDIANS AND ACUPUNCTURE POINTS

Regional anatomy
  Deltoid muscle;
  Trapezius muscle;
  Levator muscle of scapula;
  Supraspinous muscle;
  Transverse cervical artery & vein;
  Lateral branch of supraclavicular nerve;
  Accessory nerve.

Connecting point
  Meeting Point of Hand and Foot *Shao*-Yang, Foot Yang-*Ming*, and Yang-*Wei* Meridians.

Symptoms
  Apoplexy   Stiff neck
  Headache   Pain in shoulder & arm
  Difficult labour   Tension

Clinical formula
  GB 21 + GB 20 + LI 15 = Shoulder pain

Method of treatment
  Needle: 0.5 inch perpendicularly.
  Moxa: Warm heating, 2 minutes.
  Feeling: Ache.
  **Warning: Avoid inserting needle too deeply.
  Needling is forbidden in pregnancy.
  Overly strong manipulation of the needle causes fainting; in this case, the practitioner must quickly withdraw the needle and gently insert it at St 36.**

GB 22; *Yuan-Ye*; 'Profound Well-Head'

Location
  3 *cun* below axilla on midaxillary line.

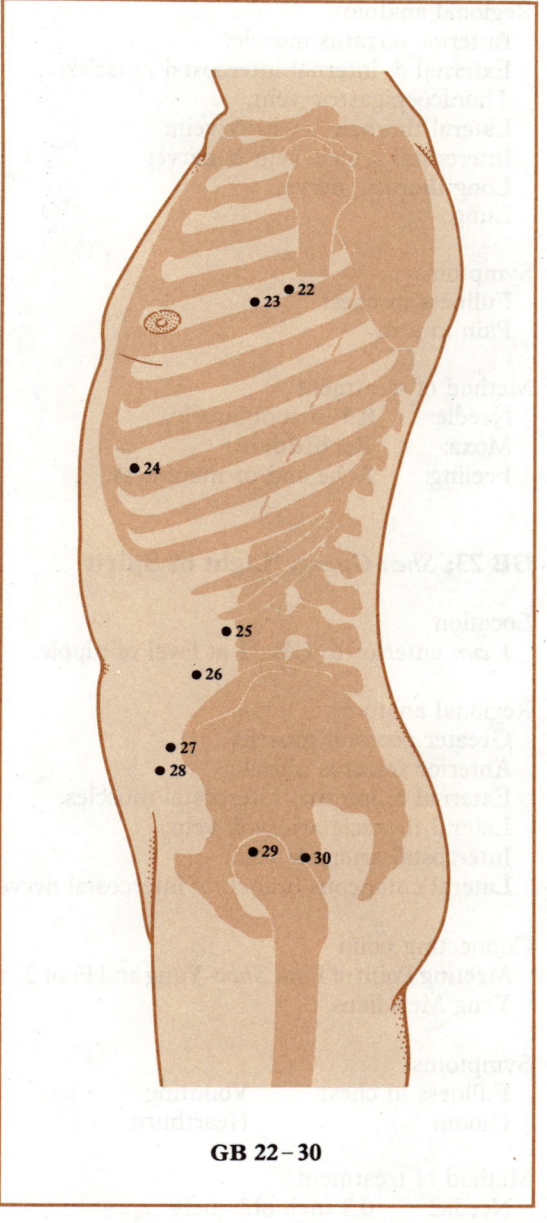

GB 22 – 30

209

Regional anatomy
  Anterior serratus muscle;
  External & internal intercostal muscles;
  Thoracoepigastric vein;
  Lateral thoracic artery & vein;
  Intercostal artery, vein & nerve;
  Long thoracic nerve;
  Lung.

Symptoms
  Fullness in chest
  Pain in arm

Method of treatment
  Needle: 0.3 inch obliquely.
  Moxa: **Forbidden.**
  Feeling: Ache and/or numbness.

GB 23; *Shen-Guang*; 'Light of Spirit'

Location
  1 *cun* anterior to GB 22 at level of nipple.

Regional anatomy
  Greater pectoral muscle;
  Anterior serratus muscle;
  External & internal intercostal muscles;
  Lateral thoracic artery & vein;
  Intercostal artery & vein;
  Lateral cutaneous branch of intercostal nerve.

Connecting point
  Meeting Point of Foot *Shao*-Yang and Foot *Tai*-Yang Meridians.

Symptoms
  Fullness in chest   Vomiting
  Gloom   Heartburn

Method of treatment
  Needle: 0.3 inch obliquely.

  Moxa: Warm heating, 2 minutes.
  Feeling: Ache and/or numbness.
  Warning: Avoid inserting needle perpendicularly and too deeply.

GB 24; *Ri-Yue*; 'Sun and Moon'

Location
  Between cartilages of seventh and eighth ribs, one rib below Liv 14.

Regional anatomy
  External & internal oblique muscles of abdomen;
  Transverse muscle of abdomen;
  Intercostal artery, vein & nerve;
  Gall bladder;
  Transverse colon.

Connecting points
  Meeting Point of Foot *Tai-Yin*, Foot *Shao*-Yang and Yang-*Wei* Meridians; Front-*Mu* point of Gall Bladder.

Functions
  Regulates Gall Bladder energy flow;
  Dispels damp and heat;
  Harmonizes function of Middle Heater.

Symptoms
  Gloom
  Feeling of heat in lower abdomen

Method of treatment
  Needle: 0.3 inch obliquely.
  Moxa: Warm heating, 2 minutes.
  Feeling: Ache and/or numbness.
  Warning: Avoid inserting needle too deeply.

GB 25; *Jing-Men*; 'Door of the Capital'

Location
At lower border of free end of twelfth rib.

Regional anatomy
External & internal oblique muscles of abdomen;
Transverse muscle of abdomen;
Intercostal artery, vein & nerve;
Kidney;
Large intestine.

Connecting point
Front-*Mu* point of Kidney.

Functions
Removes cold in Kidney;
Warms Kidney;
Dispels damp in Kidney and regulates its water metabolism;
Draws down pathogenic energy of Stomach.

Symptoms
Pain in small intestine
Lumbar pain
Pain in shoulder & back
Oedema
Abdominal distention

Method of treatment
Needle: 0.3 inch perpendicularly.
Moxa: Warm heating, 3 minutes.
Feeling: Ache and/or numbness.
Warning: Avoid inserting needle too deeply.

GB 26; *Dai-Mai*; 'Girdle Vessel'

Location
Directly below Liv 13 at level of umbilicus.

Regional anatomy
External & internal oblique muscles of abdomen;
Transverse muscle of abdomen;
Subcostal artery, vein & nerve.

Connecting point
Meeting Point of Foot *Shao*-Yang Meridian and Girdle Vessel.

Functions
Binds Girdle Vessel;
Harmonizes *Jing* blood function;
Strengthens Liver and Kidney functions;
Regulates Lower Heater energy.

Symptoms
Stiffness in lower back & lower abdomen
Lower abdominal pain
Irregular menstruation
Diarrhoea
Leucorrhoea

Method of treatment
Needle: 0.6 inch perpendicularly.
Moxa: Warm heating, 3 minutes.
Feeling: Ache and/or numbness.

Note
This point has been used for lower abdominal anaesthesia under acupuncture.

GB 27; *Wu-Shu*; 'Five Pivots'

Location
On lateral side of abdomen, in front of anterior superior iliac spine at level of CV 4.

Regional anatomy
External & internal oblique muscles of abdomen;

Transverse muscle of abdomen;
Superficial & deep circumflex iliac arteries
 & veins;
Iliohypogastric nerve.

Connecting point
Meeting Point of Foot *Shao*-Yang Meridian and Girdle Vessel.

Symptoms
Pain in lower abdomen
Leucorrhoea
Pain in groin

Method of treatment
Needle: 0.8 inch perpendicularly.
Moxa: Warm heating, 3 minutes.
Feeling: Ache and/or swelling.

GB 28; *Wei-Dao*; 'The Path of Maintenance'

Location
Anteroinferior to anterior superior iliac spine, 0.5 *cun* anterior to GB 27.

Regional anatomy
External & internal oblique muscles of abdomen;
Transverse muscle of abdomen;
Superficial & deep circumflex iliac arteries & veins;
Ilioinguinal nerve.

Connecting point
Meeting Point of Foot *Shao*-Yang Meridian and Girdle Vessel.

Functions
Regulates energy flow;
Balances functions of both Intestines;
Binds Girdle Vessel.

Symptoms
Vomiting
Oedema
Loss of appetite
Imbalance of Three Heater function
Pain in groin, lower back & hip joint

Method of treatment
Needle: 0.8 inch perpendicularly.
Moxa: Warm heating, 3 minutes.
Feeling: Ache and/or swelling.

GB 29; *Ju-Liao*; 'Lodgement of Bone'

Location
Midway between anterior superior iliac spine and greater trochanter, in lateral recumbent position.

Regional anatomy
Tensor muscle of fascia lata;
Lateral vastus muscle;
Branches of superficial circumflex iliac artery & vein;
Descending branches of lateral circumflex femoral artery & vein;
Lateral femoral cutaneous nerve.

Connecting point
Meeting Point of Foot *Shao*-Yang and Yang-*Qiao* Meridians.

Symptoms
Pain in lower back & lower abdomen
Pain in shoulder, chest & arm

Method of treatment
Needle: 0.8 inch obliquely.
Moxa: Warm heating, 3 minutes.
Feeling: Ache and/or swelling.

FOURTEEN MERIDIANS AND ACUPUNCTURE POINTS

GB 30; *Huan-Tiao;* 'Active Circle'

Location
  One-third of distance between greater trochanter and hiatus of sacrum (GV 2) in lateral recumbent position.

Regional anatomy
  Gluteus maximus muscle;
  Piriform muscle;
  Inferior gluteal artery & vein;
  Inferior cluneal cutaneous nerve;
  Inferior gluteal nerve;
  Sciatic nerve.

Connecting point
  Meeting Point of Foot *Shao*-Yang and Foot *Tai*-Yang Meridians.

Functions
  Dispels wind and damp in *Jing-Luo*;
  Frees energy obstruction in lumbar and hip regions.

Symptoms
  Pain in lumbar & hip regions
  Pain & weakness of lower extremities
  Hemiplegia

Clinical formula
  GB 30 + GB 34 + GB 38 + St 37 = Sciatica

Method of treatment
  Needle: 1.5 inch perpendicularly.
  Moxa: Warm heating, 3 minutes.
  Feeling: Ache and/or numbness.
  Warning: If necessary, the needle may be inserted to more than 1.5 inches, but strong manipulation should be avoided.

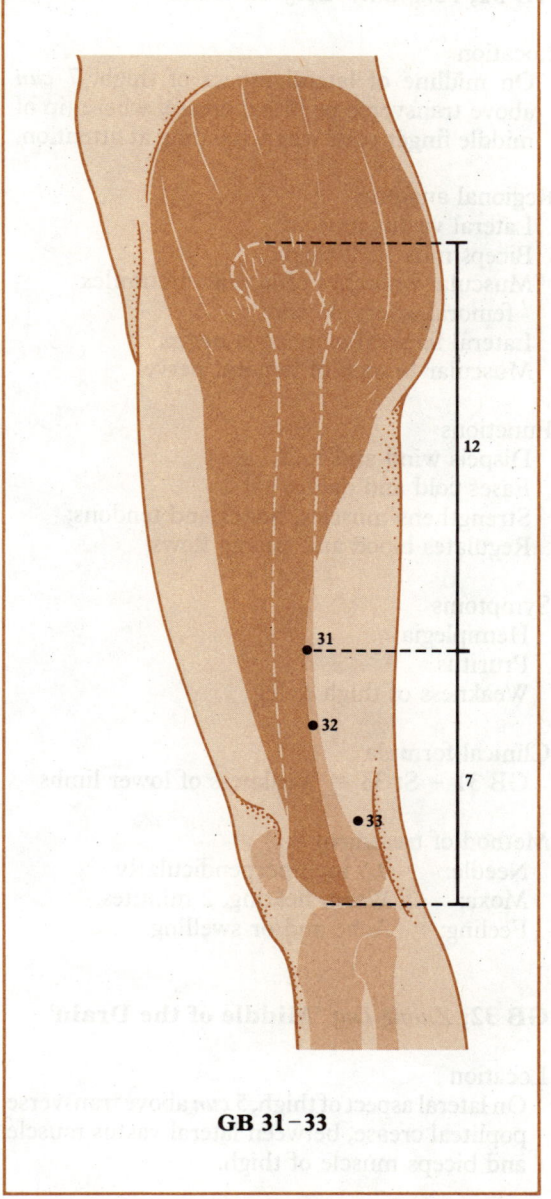

GB 31–33

FOURTEEN MERIDIANS AND ACUPUNCTURE POINTS

GB 31; *Feng-Shi*; 'City of Wind'

Location
On midline of lateral aspect of thigh, 7 *cun* above transverse popliteal crease, where tip of middle finger rests when standing at attention.

Regional anatomy
Lateral vastus muscle;
Biceps muscle of thigh;
Muscular branches of lateral circumflex femoral artery & vein;
Lateral femoral cutaneous nerve;
Muscular branch of femoral nerve.

Functions
Dispels wind and cold;
Eases cold and damp;
Strengthens muscles, bones and tendons;
Regulates blood and energy flows.

Symptoms
Hemiplegia
Pruritus
Weakness of thigh & leg

Clinical formula
GB 31 + St 33 = Weakness of lower limbs

Method of treatment
Needle: 0.6 inch perpendicularly.
Moxa: Warm heating, 2 minutes.
Feeling: Ache and/or swelling.

GB 32; *Zhong-Du*; 'Middle of the Drain'

Location
On lateral aspect of thigh, 5 *cun* above transverse popliteal crease, between lateral vastus muscle and biceps muscle of thigh.

Regional anatomy
Lateral vastus muscle;
Biceps muscle of thigh;
Muscular branches of lateral circumflex femoral artery & vein;
Lateral femoral cutaneous nerve;
Muscular branch of femoral nerve.

Symptoms
Pain & weakness of lower limbs

Method of treatment
Needle: 0.5 inch perpendicularly.
Moxa: Warm heating, 2 minutes.
Feeling: Ache and/or swelling.

GB 33; *Xi-Yang-Guan*; 'Gate of Yang'

Location
With knee flexed, in depression between tendon of biceps muscle of thigh and femur.

Regional anatomy
Tendon of biceps muscle of thigh;
Superior lateral genicular artery & vein;
Terminal branch of lateral femoral cutaneous nerve.

Symptoms
Pain in knee
Muscle & tendon contraction in popliteal fossa & leg

Method of treatment
Needle: 0.3 inch perpendicularly.
Moxa: **Forbidden.**
Feeling: Ache and/or swelling.

FOURTEEN MERIDIANS AND ACUPUNCTURE POINTS

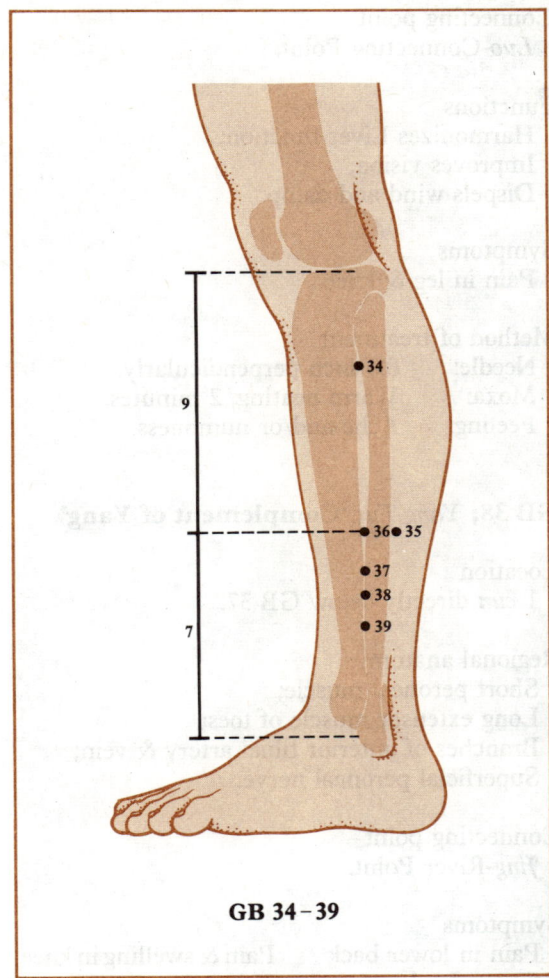

GB 34–39

Superficial & deep peroneal nerves.

Connecting points
He-Sea Point; one of 'Eight Influential Points' dominating tendons.

Functions
Regulates function of tendons;
Expels heat from Gall Bladder;
Dispels wind and damp in knee and leg;
Eases energy obstruction in *Jing-Luo*.

Symptoms
Pain in knee & thigh
Hemiplegia
Cold & bad circulation in lower limbs
Head & facial swelling

Method of treatment
Needle: 0.6 inch perpendicularly.
Moxa: Warm heating, 2 minutes.
Feeling: Ache and/or numbness.

GB 35; *Yang-Jiao*; 'Crossing Yang'

Location
7 *cun* above tip of external malleolus on posterior border of fibula at level of GB 36 and Bl 58.

Regional anatomy
Long & short peroneal muscles;
Long extensor muscle of toes;
Branches of peroneal artery & vein;
Lateral cutaneous nerve of calf.

Connecting point
Xi-Cleft Point of Yang-*Wei* Meridian.

Symptoms
Fullness in chest   Pain in leg & knee
Facial swelling

GB 34; *Yang-Ling-Quan*; 'Yang Hill Rivulet'

Location
In depression anteroinferior to head of fibula.

Regional anatomy
Short & long peroneal muscles;
Inferior lateral genicular artery & vein;

215

FOURTEEN MERIDIANS AND ACUPUNCTURE POINTS

Method of treatment
  Needle: 0.6 inch perpendicularly.
  Moxa: Warm heating, 2 minutes.
  Feeling: Ache and/or numbness.

GB 36; *Wai-Qiu*; 'External Region'

Location
  7 *cun* above tip of external malleolus on anterior border of fibula.

Regional anatomy
  Long peroneal muscle;
  Branches of anterior tibial artery & vein;
  Superficial peroneal nerve.

Connecting point
  Xi-Cleft Point.

Symptoms
  Fullness in chest
  Stiff neck

Method of treatment
  Needle: 0.3 inch perpendicularly.
  Moxa: Warm heating, 2 minutes.
  Feeling: Ache and/or numbness.

GB 37; *Guang-Ming*; 'Bright Light'

Location
  5 *cun* above tip of external malleolus on anterior border of fibula.

Regional anatomy
  Short peroneal muscle;
  Long extensor muscle of toes;
  Branches of anterior tibial artery & vein;
  Superficial peroneal nerve.

Connecting point
  Luo-Connecting Point.

Functions
  Harmonizes Liver function;
  Improves vision;
  Dispels wind and damp.

Symptoms
  Pain in leg & knee

Method of treatment
  Needle: 0.6 inch perpendicularly.
  Moxa: Warm heating, 2 minutes.
  Feeling: Ache and/or numbness.

GB 38; *Yang-Fu*; 'Complement of Yang'

Location
  1 *cun* directly below GB 37.

Regional anatomy
  Short peroneal muscle;
  Long extensor muscle of toes;
  Branches of anterior tibial artery & vein;
  Superficial peroneal nerve.

Connecting point
  Jing-River Point.

Symptoms
  Pain in lower back   Pain & swelling in knee
  General aches & pain Headache

Method of treatment
  Needle: 0.3 inch perpendicularly.
  Moxa: Warm heating, 2 minutes.
  Feeling: Ache.

FOURTEEN MERIDIANS AND ACUPUNCTURE POINTS

GB 39; *Xuan-Zhong*; 'Suspended Bell'

Location
2 *cun* directly below GB 37.

Regional anatomy
Short peroneal muscle;
Long extensor muscle of toes;
Branches of anterior tibial artery & vein;
Superficial peroneal nerve.

Connecting point
One of 'Eight Influential Points' dominating Bone Marrow.

Functions
Dispels Gall Bladder Fire;
Expels heat in Marrow;
Eases wind and damp in *Jing-Luo*.

Symptoms
Fullness in chest	Depression
Stiff neck	Pain & weakness in
Abdominal distention	lower limbs

Method of treatment
Needle: 0.6 inch perpendicularly.
Moxa: Warm heating, 2 minutes.
Feeling: Ache and/or swelling.

GB 40; *Qiu-Xu*; 'Hill of Ruins'

Location
Anteroinferior to external malleolus, in depression on lateral side of tendon of long extensor muscle of toes.

Regional anatomy
Tendon of long extensor muscle of toes;
Branch of anterolateral malleolar artery;

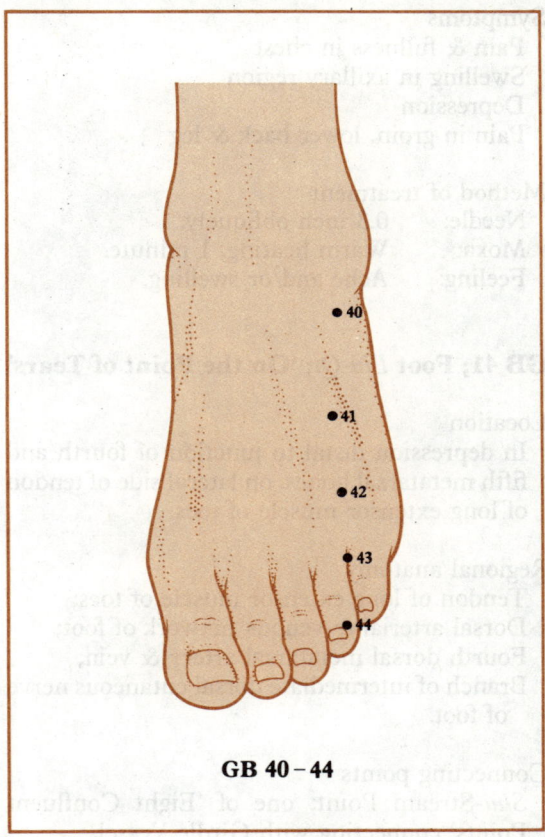

GB 40 – 44

Branches of intermediate dorsal cutaneous & superficial peroneal nerves.

Connecting point
Yuan-Source Point.

Functions
Dispels wind and heat in area between internal and superficial regions of body;
Expels damp and heat;
Balances functions of Liver and Gall Bladder;
Clears pathogenic energy.

FOURTEEN MERIDIANS AND ACUPUNCTURE POINTS

Symptoms
  Pain & fullness in chest
  Swelling in axillary region
  Depression
  Pain in groin, lower back & leg

Method of treatment
  Needle: 0.3 inch obliquely.
  Moxa: Warm heating, 1 minute.
  Feeling: Ache and/or swelling.

GB 41; Foot *Lin-Qi*; 'On the Point of Tears'

Location
  In depression distal to junction of fourth and fifth metatarsal bones, on lateral side of tendon of long extensor muscle of toes.

Regional anatomy
  Tendon of long extensor muscle of toes;
  Dorsal arterial & venous network of foot;
  Fourth dorsal metatarsal artery & vein;
  Branch of intermediate dorsal cutaneous nerve of foot.

Connecting points
  Shu-Stream Point; one of 'Eight Confluent Points' connecting with Girdle Vessel.

Functions
  Dispels wind and Fire;
  Improves hearing and vision;
  Eases energy obstruction in Liver and Gall Bladder;
  Eliminates heat and sputum.

Symptoms
  Fullness in chest   Dizziness
  General ache & pain   Irregular
  Ache & pain in foot   menstruation

Method of treatment
  Needle: 0.2 inch perpendicularly.
  Moxa: Warm heating, 1 minute.
  Feeling: Ache.

GB 42; *Di-Wu-Hui*; 'Five Terrestrial Reunions'

Location
  Between fourth and fifth metatarsal bones, on medial side of tendon of long extensor muscle of toes.

Regional anatomy
  Tendon of long extensor muscle of toes;
  Dorsal arterial & venous network of foot;
  Fourth dorsal metatarsal artery & vein;
  Branch of intermediate dorsal cutaneous nerve of foot.

Symptoms
  Pain in axillary region
  Pain & swelling of foot

Method of treatment
  Needle: 0.2 inch perpendicularly.
  Moxa: **Forbidden.**
  Feeling: Ache.

GB 43; *Xia-Xi*; Narrow Stream'

Location
  Between fourth and fifth toes, proximal to margin of web.

Regional anatomy
  Dorsal digital artery, vein & nerve.

Connecting point
  Ying-Spring Point.

Functions
Expels heat;
Dispels wind;
Relieves pain.

Symptoms
Fullness in chest
Dizziness
Swelling in mandibular region
Deafness
Pain in chest

Method of treatment
Needle: 0.3 inch perpendicularly.
Moxa: Warm heating, 1 minute.
Feeling: Ache and/or swelling.

GB 44; Foot *Qiao-Yin*; 'Inspiration of Yin'

Location
On lateral side of fourth toe, 0.1 *cun* posterior to corner of nail.

Regional anatomy
Arterial & venous network formed by dorsal digital artery & vein, & plantar digital artery & vein;
Dorsal digital nerve.

Connecting point
Jing-Well Point.

Functions
Clears wind in Liver Yang;
Regulates functions of Liver and Gall Bladder;
Expels heat.

Symptoms
Pain in hypochondriac region
Headache
Dry mouth
Stiff tongue
Bad dreams
Restlessness
Ophthalmalgia

Method of treatment
Needle: 0.1 inch obliquely.
Moxa: Warm heating, 1 minute.
Feeling: Painful.

12. Liver Meridian of Foot Jue-Yin

This Meridian is characterized by low energy flow and high blood flow. The energy flow originates in the big toe at Liv 1. It travels along the dorsum of the foot, passes through Sp 6, runs between the two Yin Meridians of the foot and continues upwards along the medial aspect of the thigh to Liv 11. It then connects with Sp 12 and Sp 13, and returns to Liv 12 at the groin. From here it curves around the external genitalia, ascends to the lower abdomen and links with CV 2, CV 3 and CV 4.

From the lower abdomen, the energy flow runs to Liv 13 where it divides into two branches: one branch circles around the Stomach to enter the Liver and connect with the Gall Bladder; the other branch runs to Liv 14, passing through the diaphragm to ascend, via the costal and hypochondriac regions, to the throat and nasopharynx, and enters the eye, from where it continues upwards to the vertex. A branch from the eye descends to the cheek to curve around the mouth within the lips.

The main Meridian from the Liver passes through the diaphragm, flows into the Lungs and links with the Lung Meridian to begin again the recycling of the Twelve Main Meridian Energy Flows.

There are fourteen acupuncture points on each side of the Liver Meridian.

Associated organs
- Belongs to Liver;
- Related to Gall Bladder;

FOURTEEN MERIDIANS AND ACUPUNCTURE POINTS

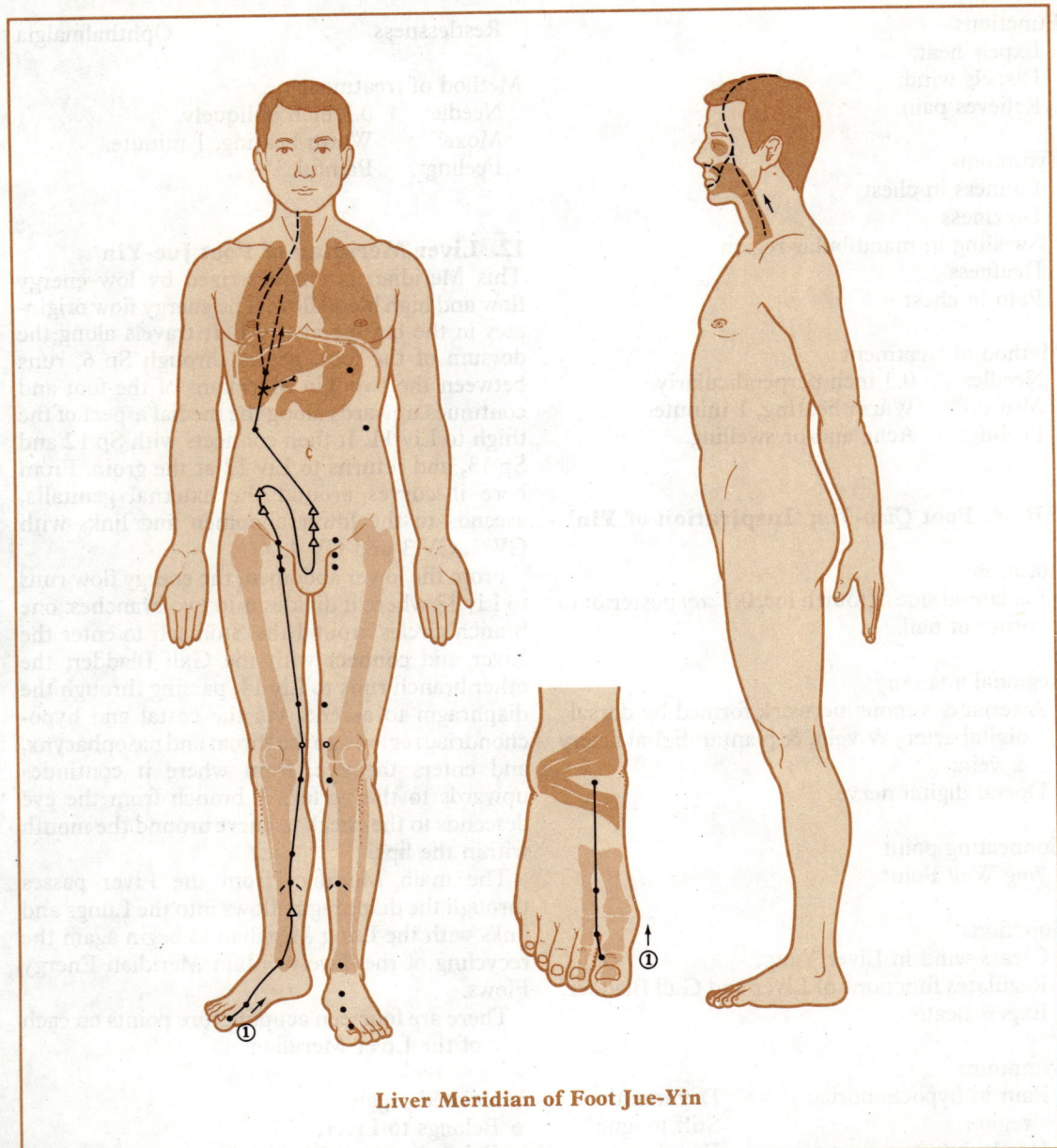

Liver Meridian of Foot Jue-Yin

FOURTEEN MERIDIANS AND ACUPUNCTURE POINTS

- Directly connected to Lung, Stomach, Kidney and Brain.

Connecting points
- Sp 6   Sp 12   Sp 13   CV 2   CV 3   CV 4

Symptomatology
- Disorders along Meridian course
  - Headache
  - Dizziness
  - Blurred vision
  - Tinnitus aurium
  - Fever
  - Spasm in extremities

- Disorders in organ
  - Fullness & pain in hypochondriac region
  - Fullness in chest & stomach
  - Vomiting
  - Abdominal pain
  - Jaundice icterus
  - Diarrhoea
  - Enuresis
  - Bad temper

Acupuncture Points of Liver Meridian

Liv 1; *Da-Dun*; 'Great Toe'

Location
On lateral side of dorsum of terminal phalanx of great toe, between lateral corner of nail and interphalangeal joint.

Regional anatomy
Dorsal digital artery & vein;
Dorsal digital nerve from deep peroneal nerve.

Connecting point
Jing-Well Point.

Functions
Dispels pathogenic energy;
Balances *Jing* blood;
Balances Meridian energy flow;
Regulates function of Lower Heater;

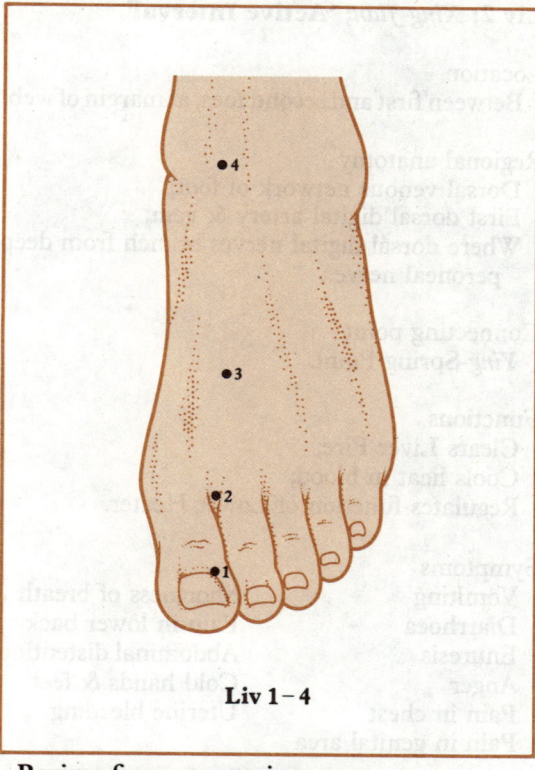

Liv 1-4

Revives from unconsciousness;
Clears mind and *Shen*.

Symptoms
Enuresis
Pain in genital region
Abdominal pain & distention
Depression
Uterine bleeding

Method of treatment
Needle: 0.1 inch obliquely.
Moxa: Warm heating, 1 minute.
Feeling: Painful.
Warning: Moxibustion is forbidden during pregnancy and for a month after childbirth.

221

FOURTEEN MERIDIANS AND ACUPUNCTURE POINTS

Liv 2; *Xing-Jian*; 'Active Interval'

Location
Between first and second toes, at margin of web.

Regional anatomy
Dorsal venous network of foot;
First dorsal digital artery & vein;
Where dorsal digital nerves branch from deep peroneal nerve.

Connecting point
Ying-Spring Point.

Functions
Clears Liver Fire;
Cools heat in blood;
Regulates function of Lower Heater.

Symptoms
Vomiting	Shortness of breath
Diarrhoea	Pain in lower back
Enuresis	Abdominal distention
Anger	Cold hands & feet
Pain in chest	Uterine bleeding
Pain in genital area	

Method of treatment
Needle: 0.3 inch obliquely.
Moxa: Warm heating, 1 minute.
Feeling: Ache and/or swelling.

Liv 3; *Tai-Chong*; 'Supreme Thoroughfare'

Location
In depression distal to junction of first and second metatarsal bones.

Regional anatomy
Tendon of long extensor muscle of toes;
Dorsal venous network of foot;
First dorsal metatarsal artery;
Branch of deep peroneal nerve.

Connecting points
Shu-Stream and *Yuan*-Source Points.

Functions
Clears excess Liver Fire and Liver Yang;
Dispels heat and damp in Lower Heater.

Symptoms
Cardiac pain	Pain in genital area
Oedema	Enuresis
Uterine bleeding	Pain in groin
Pain in lower back & lower abdomen	Pain in ankle

Clinical formula
Liv 3 + Sp 6 = Uterine bleeding

Method of treatment
Needle: 0.3 inch perpendicularly.
Moxa: Warm heating, 1 minute.
Feeling: Ache and/or swelling.

Liv 4; *Zhong-Feng*; 'Middle Seal'

Location
1 *cun* anterior to medial malleolus, in depression on medial side of tendon of anterior tibial muscle.

Regional anatomy
Tendon of anterior tibial muscle;
Dorsal venous network of foot;
Anterior medial malleolar artery;
Branch of medial dorsal cutaneous nerve of foot;
Saphenous nerve.

Connecting point
  Jing-River Point.

Symptoms
  Pain & swelling in lower abdomen
  Urine retention
  Pain in lower back
  Cold feet
  Pain in genital area

Method of treatment
  Needle: 0.4 inch obliquely.
  Moxa: Warm heating, 1 minute.
  Feeling: Ache and/or swelling.

Liv 5; *Li-Gou*; 'Shin Drain'

Location
  5 *cun* above tip of medial malleolus and near medial border of tibia.

Regional anatomy
  Great saphenous vein posteriorly;
  Branch of saphenous nerve.

Connecting point
  Luo-Connecting Point.

Symptoms
  Pain in groin
  Shortness of breath
  Lower abdominal distention
  Fear
  Ache & pain in lower extremities
  Depression
  Irregular menstruation
  Leucorrhoea
  Pain in testicles

Method of treatment
  Needle: 0.2 inch obliquely.
  Moxa: Warm heating, 2 minutes.
  Feeling: Ache and/or swelling.

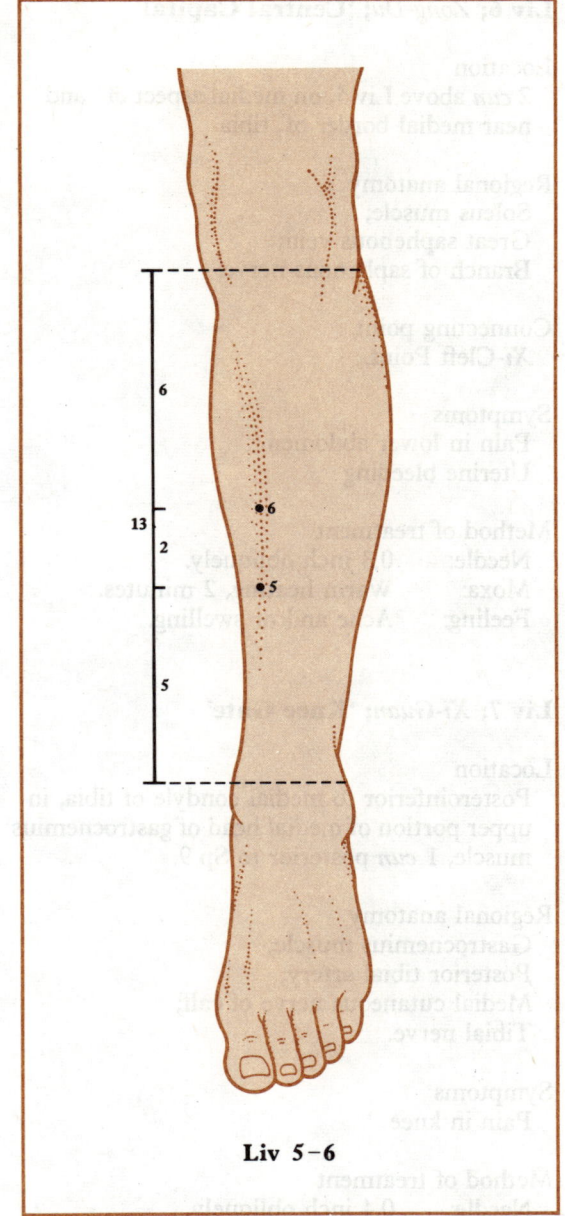

Liv 5–6

FOURTEEN MERIDIANS AND ACUPUNCTURE POINTS

Liv 6; *Zong-Du*; 'Central Capital'

Location
2 *cun* above Liv 5, on medial aspect of, and near medial border of, tibia.

Regional anatomy
Soleus muscle;
Great saphenous vein;
Branch of saphenous nerve.

Connecting point
Xi-Cleft Point.

Symptoms
Pain in lower abdomen
Uterine bleeding

Method of treatment
Needle: 0.3 inch obliquely.
Moxa: Warm heating, 2 minutes.
Feeling: Ache and/or swelling.

Liv 7; *Xi-Guan*; 'Knee Gate'

Location
Posteroinferior to medial condyle of tibia, in upper portion of medial head of gastrocnemius muscle, 1 *cun* posterior to Sp 9.

Regional anatomy
Gastrocnemius muscle;
Posterior tibial artery;
Medial cutaneous nerve of calf;
Tibial nerve.

Symptoms
Pain in knee

Method of treatment
Needle: 0.4 inch obliquely.

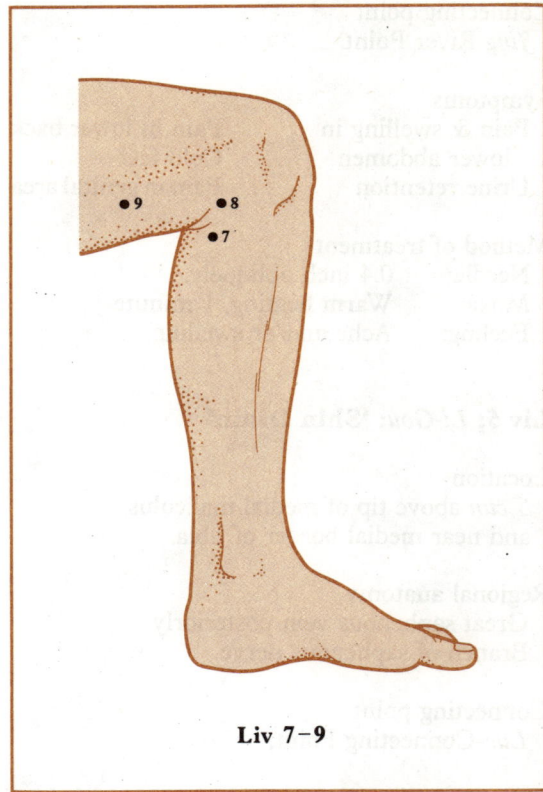

Liv 7-9

Moxa: Warm heating, 2 minutes.
Feeling: Ache and/or swelling.

Liv 8; *Qu-Quan*; 'Crooked Well'

Location
On medial aspect of knee joint. With knee flexed, above medial end of transverse popliteal crease, posterior to medial condyle of tibia and on anterior border of insertion of semi-membranous and semitendinous muscles.

FOURTEEN MERIDIANS AND ACUPUNCTURE POINTS

Regional anatomy
  Semimembranous muscle;
  Semitendinous muscle;
  Sartorius muscle;
  Great saphenous vein;
  Genu suprema artery;
  Saphenous nerve.

Connecting point
  He-Sea Point.

Functions
  Dispels heat and damp;
  Regulates function of Bladder;
  Clears Fire in Liver;
  Regulates Lower Heater function.

Symptoms
  Pain in groin
  Abdominal distention
  Dysuria
  Dizziness
  Pain in knee
  Pain & swelling in external genitalia

Clinical formula
  Liv 8 + Liv 2 = Pain in external genitalia

Method of treatment
  Needle: 0.4 inch perpendicularly.
  Moxa: Warm heating, 2 minutes.
  Feeling: Ache and/or swelling.

Liv 9; *Yin-Bao*; 'Envelope of Yin'

Location
  4 *cun* above medial epicondyle of femur, between medial vastus and sartorius muscles.

Regional anatomy
  Medial vastus muscle;
  Sartorius muscle;
  Long & short adductor muscles;
  Femoral artery & vein;
  Medial circumflex femoral artery;
  Anterior femoral cutaneous nerve;
  Obturator nerve.

Symptoms
  Pain in lower back & lower abdomen
  Enuresis
  Irregular menstruation

Method of treatment
  Needle: 0.6 inch perpendicularly.
  Moxa: Warm heating, 2 minutes.
  Feeling: Ache and/or swelling.

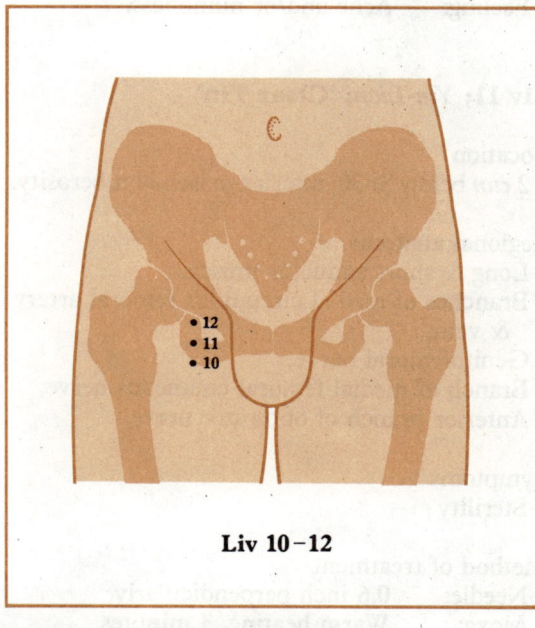

Liv 10–12

Liv 10; *Wu-Li*; 'Five Miles'

Location
  3 *cun* below St 30 on long adductor muscle.

FOURTEEN MERIDIANS AND ACUPUNCTURE POINTS

Regional anatomy
Long & short adductor muscles;
Medial circumflex femoral artery & vein;
Genitofemoral nerve;
Anterior femoral cutaneous nerve;
Anterior branch of obturator nerve.

Symptoms
Abdominal distention
Drowsiness

Method of treatment
Needle: 0.6 inch perpendicularly.
Moxa: Warm heating, 2 minutes.
Feeling: Ache and/or numbness.

Liv 11; *Yin-Lian*; 'Clear Yin'

Location
2 *cun* below St 30, inferior to ischial tuberosity.

Regional anatomy
Long & short adductor muscles;
Branches of medial circumflex femoral artery & vein;
Genitofemoral nerve;
Branch of medial femoral cutaneous nerve;
Anterior branch of obturator nerve.

Symptoms
Sterility

Method of treatment
Needle: 0.6 inch perpendicularly.
Moxa: Warm heating, 3 minutes.
Feeling: Ache and/or swelling.

Liv 12; *Ji-Mai*; 'Hurried Pulse'

Location
Inferolateral to pubic spine, 2.5 *cun* lateral to anterior midline at inguinal groove, lateral and 0.5 *cun* inferior to St 30.

Regional anatomy
Round ligament of uterus;
Branches of external pudendal artery & vein;
Pubic branches of inferior epigastric artery & vein;
Femoral vein;
Ilioinguinal nerve;
Anterior branch of obturator nerve inferiorly.

Symptoms
Pain in external genitalia
Lower abdominal pain

Method of treatment
Needle: **Forbidden.**
Moxa: Warm heating, 3 minutes.

Liv 13; *Zang-Men*; 'Door of Regulation'

Location
At lateral side of abdomen on free end of eleventh floating rib.

Regional anatomy
External & internal oblique muscles of abdomen;
Transverse muscle of abdomen;
Intercostal artery & nerve;
Liver;
Spleen.

Connecting points
Front-*Mu* Point of Spleen; one of 'Eight Influential Points' dominating Zang organs.

FOURTEEN MERIDIANS AND ACUPUNCTURE POINTS

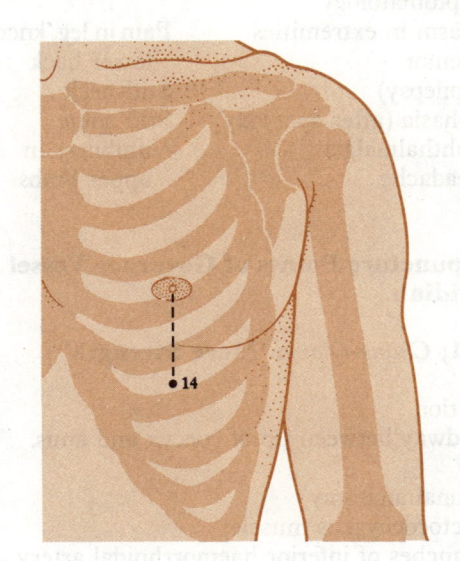

Functions
Eases cold in five Zang;
Dispels energy obstruction in Middle Heater;
Clears sputum;
Increases functions of digestion and absorption.

Symptoms
Indigestion   Gastric pain
Pain in chest & rib   Pain in lower back
Dry mouth   Abdominal distention
Loss of appetite   Fatigue
Vomiting   Fear

Method of treatment
Needle: 0.3 inch perpendicularly.
Moxa: Warm heating, 3 minutes.
Feeling: Ache and/or numbness.
Warning: Avoid inserting needle too deeply as vital organs (Liver and Spleen) are found beneath this point.

Liv 14; *Qi-Men*; 'Door of Expectation'

Location
On mammillary line in sixth intercostal space.

Regional anatomy
External & internal oblique muscles of abdomen;
Transverse muscle of abdomen;
Intercostal artery, vein & nerve;
Liver;
Stomach;
Transverse colon.

Connecting points
Front-*Mu* Point of Liver; Meeting Point of Foot *Tai*-Yin, Foot *Jue*-Yin and Yin-*Wei* Meridians.

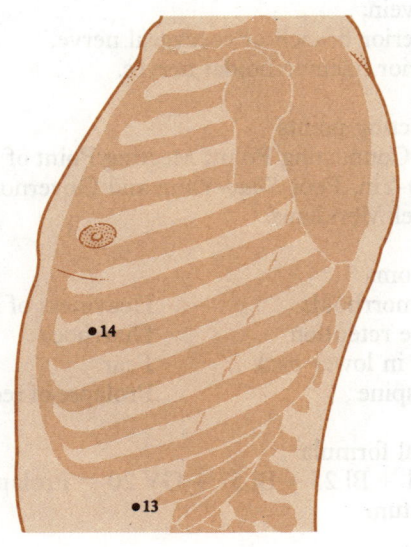

Liv 13–14

FOURTEEN MERIDIANS AND ACUPUNCTURE POINTS

Functions
  Expels heat in blood;
  Dispels cold in body;
  Frees blood and sputum stases in Lung;
  Regulates Liver function;
  Harmonizes energy flow.

Symptoms
  Abdominal distention & pain
  Dyspnoea
  Fullness & pain in chest
  Gastric pain

Method of treatment
  Needle: 0.3 inch obliquely.
  Moxa: Warm heating, 2 minutes.
  Feeling: Ache and/or numbness.
  Warning: Avoid inserting needle too deeply.

13. Governor Vessel Meridian (Du Mai)

This Meridian is recognized as the 'Sea of all Yang Meridians' as it unifies the Yang energy of the entire body. The energy flow originates at GV 1. It descends to emerge at the perineum and links up with CV 1. The Main Meridian moves its energy upwards posteriorly along the interior of the spinal column to connect with Bl 12 (both sides) at GV 12. It then turns back to GV 13 and proceeds to GV 16 where it enters the Brain. From GV 16 the Meridian ascends to the vertex, travels over the forehead and nose, curls round the upper lip and terminates at the gum between the incisor teeth at GV 28.

There are twenty-eight acupuncture points in the Governor Vessel Meridian.

Connecting points
• Bl 12   CV 1

Symptomatology
  Spasm in extremities   Pain in leg, knee &
  Tremor   lower back
  (Epilepsy)   Stiff neck
  Aphasia (after apoplexy)   Stiff spine
  Ophthalmalgia   Numbness in
  Headache   upper limbs

Acupuncture Points of Governor Vessel Meridian

GV 1; *Chang-Qiang*; 'More Strength'

Location
  Midway between tip of coccyx and anus.

Regional anatomy
  Rectococcygeus muscle;
  Branches of inferior haemorrhoidal artery & vein;
  Posterior branch of coccygeal nerve;
  Inferior haemorrhoidal nerves.

Connecting points
  Luo-Connecting Point; Meeting Point of Foot *Shao*-Yin, Foot *Shao*-Yang and Governor Vessel Meridians.

Symptoms
  Haemorrhoids   Heaviness of head
  Urine retention   Diarrhoea
  Pain in lower back   Fear
    & spine   Prolapse of rectum

Clinical formula
  GV 1 + Bl 25 + Bl 57 + GV 20 = Prolapse of rectum

Method of treatment
  Needle: 0.6 inch obliquely.
  Moxa: Warm heating, 2 minutes.

FOURTEEN MERIDIANS AND ACUPUNCTURE POINTS

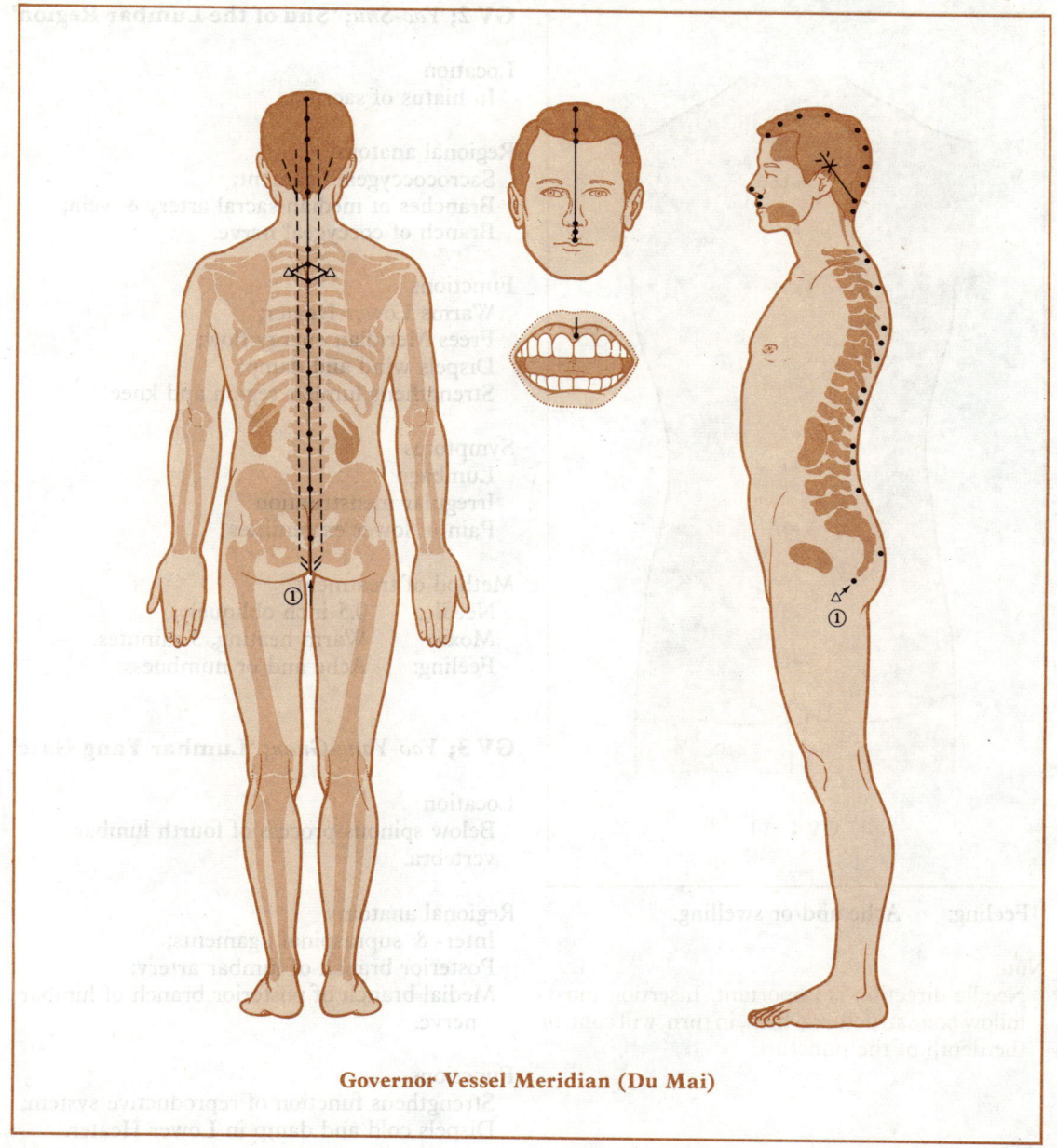

Governor Vessel Meridian (Du Mai)

FOURTEEN MERIDIANS AND ACUPUNCTURE POINTS

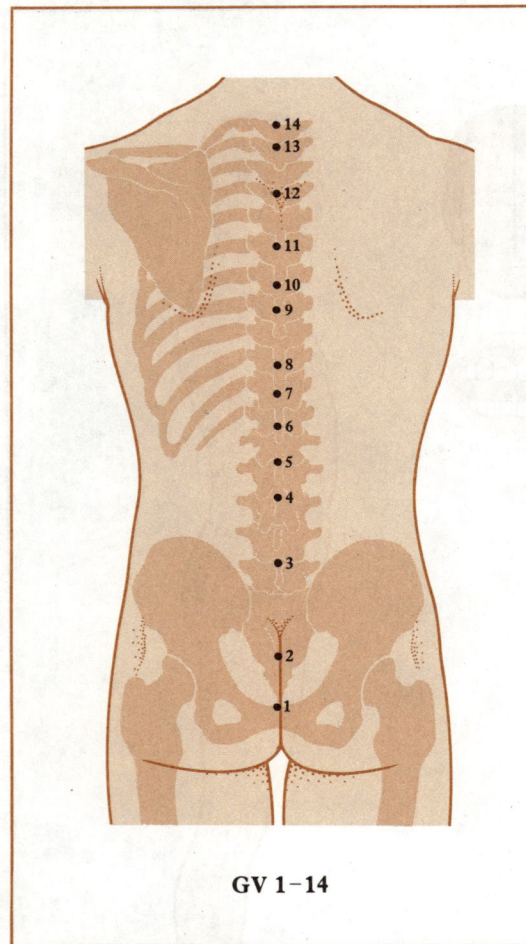

GV 1–14

Feeling: Ache and/or swelling.

Note
Needle direction is important. Insertion must follow bone structure which, in turn, will control the depth of the puncture.

GV 2; *Yao-Shu*; 'Shu of the Lumbar Region'

Location
  In hiatus of sacrum.

Regional anatomy
  Sacrococcygeal ligament;
  Branches of median sacral artery & vein;
  Branch of coccygeal nerve.

Functions
  Warms Lower Heater;
  Frees Meridian energy flow;
  Dispels wind and damp;
  Strengthens lumbar region and knee.

Symptoms
  Lumbago
  Irregular menstruation
  Pain in lower extremities

Method of treatment
  Needle: 0.5 inch obliquely.
  Moxa: Warm heating, 3 minutes.
  Feeling: Ache and/or numbness.

GV 3; *Yao-Yang-Guan*; 'Lumbar Yang Gate'

Location
  Below spinous process of fourth lumbar vertebra.

Regional anatomy
  Inter- & supraspinal ligaments;
  Posterior branch of lumbar artery;
  Medial branch of posterior branch of lumbar nerve.

Functions
  Strengthens function of reproductive system;
  Dispels cold and damp in Lower Heater.

FOURTEEN MERIDIANS AND ACUPUNCTURE POINTS

Symptoms
Difficulty in knee joint movement
Pain & muscle spasm in lower extremities

Method of treatment
Needle: 0.4 inch obliquely.
Moxa: Warm heating, 3 minutes.
Feeling: Ache and/or numbness.
Warning: Avoid movement of body after needle insertion as needles will bend or break.

GV 4; *Ming-Men*; 'Vital Gate'

Location
Below spinous process of second lumbar vertebra.

Regional anatomy
Inter- & supraspinal ligaments;
Posterior branch of lumbar artery;
Medial branch of posterior branch of lumbar nerve.

Functions
Strengthens Kidney *Ching* function;
Strengthens function of reproductive system;
Frees function of tendon;
Harmonizes blood circulation;
Regulates Meridian energy flow.

Symptoms
Headache   Enuresis
Fever   Pain in lower back & spine

Clinical formula
GV 4 + Bl 23 = Enuresis

Method of treatment
Needle: 0.4 inch obliquely.
Moxa: Warm heating, 3 minutes.
Feeling: Swelling.

GV 5; *Xuan-Shu*; 'Suspended Pivot'

Location
Below spinous process of first lumbar vertebra.

Regional anatomy
Inter- & supraspinal ligaments;
Posterior branch of lumbar artery;
Medial branch of posterior branch of lumbar nerve.

Symptoms
Stiff lower back & spine
Abdominal distention
Diarrhoea

Method of treatment
Needle: 0.3 inch obliquely.
Moxa: Warm heating, 2 minutes.
Feeling: Ache and/or numbness.

GV 6; *Ji-Zhong*; 'Middle of the Spine'

Location
Below spinous process of eleventh thoracic vertebra.

Regional anatomy
Inter- & supraspinal ligaments;
Dorsal branch of posterior intercostal artery;
Posterior branch of thoracic nerve.

Symptoms
(Epilepsy)
Diarrhoea
Abdominal distention

Method of treatment
Needle: 0.3 inch obliquely.

FOURTEEN MERIDIANS AND ACUPUNCTURE POINTS

Moxa: **Forbidden.**
Feeling: Ache and/or numbness.
Warning: **Avoid inserting needle too deeply.**

GV 7; *Zhong-Shu*; 'Central Pivot'

Location
  Below spinous process of tenth thoracic vertebra.

Regional anatomy
  Inter- & supraspinal ligaments;
  Dorsal branch of posterior intercostal artery;
  Posterior branch of thoracic nerve.

Symptoms
  Vomiting
  Abdominal distention
  Pain in lower back

Method of treatment
  Needle: 0.3 inch obliquely.
  Moxa: Warm heating, 2 minutes.
  Feeling: Ache and/or numbness.

GV 8; *Jin-Suo*; 'Muscle and Tendon Retraction'

Location
  Below spinous process of ninth thoracic vertebra.

Regional anatomy
  Inter- & supraspinal ligaments;
  Dorsal branch of posterior intercostal artery;
  Posterior branch of thoracic nerve.

Symptoms
  (Epilepsy)   Stiff spine
  Restlessness   Gastric pain

Method of treatment
  Needle: 0.3 inch obliquely.
  Moxa: Warm heating, 2 minutes.
  Feeling: Ache and/or numbness.

GV 9; *Zhi-Yang*; 'Arrival of Yang'

Location
  Below spinous process of seventh thoracic vertebra.

Regional anatomy
  Inter- & supraspinal ligaments;
  Dorsal branch of posterior intercostal artery;
  Posterior branch of thoracic nerve.

Symptoms
  Pain in lumbar region & spine
  Pain in stomach
  Fullness in chest
  Abdominal distention
  Heaviness of extremities

Method of treatment
  Needle: 0.3 inch obliquely.
  Moxa: Warm heating, 2 minutes.
  Feeling: Ache and/or swelling.

GV 10; *Ling-Tai*; 'Temple of the Soul'

Location
  Below spinous process of sixth thoracic vertebra.

Regional anatomy
  Inter- & supraspinal ligaments;
  Dorsal branch of posterior intercostal artery;
  Posterior branch of thoracic nerve.

Symptoms
  Asthma
  Furuncles

Method of treatment
  Needle: **Forbidden.**
  Moxa: Warm heating, 3 minutes.

Note
  This is a good point for treating asthma. According to Dr. Yang's *Compendium of Acupuncture and Moxibustion*, needle insertion is **forbidden**.

GV 11; *Shen-Dao*; 'Divine Path'

Location
  Below spinous process of fifth thoracic vertebra.

Regional anatomy
  Inter- & supraspinal ligaments;
  Dorsal branch of posterior intercostal artery;
  Posterior branch of thoracic nerve.

Symptoms
  Headache   Depression
  Poor memory   Palpitations
  Gloom

Method of treatment
  Needle: **Forbidden.**
  Moxa: Warm heating, 3 minutes.

Note
  In Dr. Yang's *Compendium of Acupuncture and Moxibustion*, needle insertion is **forbidden**.

GV 12; *Shen-Zhu*; 'Column'

Location
  Below spinous process of third thoracic vertebra.

Regional anatomy
  Inter- & supraspinal ligaments;
  Dorsal branch of posterior intercostal artery;
  Posterior branch of thoracic nerve.

Functions
  Dispels heat in body;
  Calms mind and Will;
  Strengthens Lung function;
  Tones *Jing* blood.

Symptoms
  Pain in lower back & spine
  Hysterical mania

Method of treatment
  Needle: 0.3 inch obliquely.
  Moxa: Warm heating, 3 minutes.
  Feeling: Ache and/or swelling.

GV 13; *Tao-Dao*; 'Path of Contentment'

Location
  Below spinous process of first thoracic vertebra.

Regional anatomy
  Inter- & supraspinal ligaments;
  Dorsal branch of posterior intercostal artery;
  Posterior branch of thoracic nerve.

Connecting point
  Meeting Point of Foot *Tai*-Yang and Governor Vessel Meridians.

FOURTEEN MERIDIANS AND ACUPUNCTURE POINTS

Functions
Expels excess heat from Lungs;
Tones body.

Symptoms
Fever	Restlessness
Stiff spine	Headache

Method of treatment
Needle: 0.3 inch obliquely.
Moxa: Warm heating, 2 minutes.
Feeling: Ache.

GV 14; *Da-Zhui*; 'Large Vertebra'

Location
Between spinous processes of seventh cervical vertebra and first thoracic vertebra.

Regional anatomy
Inter- & supraspinal ligaments;
Deep cervical artery & vein;
Posterior branch of thoracic nerve.

Connecting point
Meeting Point of all Yang (three Foot and three Hand) Meridians and Governor Vessel Meridian.

Functions
Dispels heat in three Yang Meridians;
Regulates energy flows of all Yang Meridians;
Clears mind and *Shen*.

Symptoms
Fullness in chest	Fatigue
Vomiting	Stiff neck & shoulder
Fever	

Method of treatment
Needle: 0.3 inch obliquely.
Moxa: Warm heating, 2 minutes.
Feeling: Ache and/or numbness.

GV 15; *Ya-Men*; 'Door of Mutism'

Location
At midpoint of nape, in depression 0.5 *cun* within hairline, between first and second cervical vertebrae.

Regional anatomy
Branches of occipital artery, vein & nerve.

Connecting point
Meeting Point of Governor Vessel and Yang-*Wei* Meridians.

Functions
Frees 'Gate of the Voice';
Clears mind and *Shen*;
Regulates energy flow in Brain.

Symptoms
Stiff tongue	Epistaxis
Fever	Stiff spine
Post-apoplexy aphasia	

Method of treatment
Needle: 0.4 inch perpendicularly.
Moxa: **Forbidden.**
Feeling: Ache and/or swelling.
Warning: In China, this point has been used to treat deaf mutes. The needle depth is over 1 inch; without experience, puncturing to this depth is very dangerous. Skill in needle technique is essential.

FOURTEEN MERIDIANS AND ACUPUNCTURE POINTS

GV 16; *Feng-Fu*; 'Wind Palace'

Location
On posterior midline directly below external occipital protuberance.

Regional anatomy
Branches of occipital artery, vein & nerve; Greater occipital nerve.

Connecting point
Meeting Point of Foot *Tai*-Yang, Yang-*Wei* and Governor Vessel Meridians.

Functions
Dispels wind;
Expels heat;
Regulates energy flow in Brain;
Clears mind and *Shen*.

Symptoms
Apoplexy	Hemiplegia
Post-apoplexy aphasia	Epistaxis
Stiff neck	Mental disorders
Headache	

Method of treatment
Needle: 0.3 inch perpendicularly.
Moxa: **Forbidden.**
Feeling: Ache and/or swelling.
Warning: It is dangerous to insert needle too deeply. Avoid manipulation of needle after insertion.

GV 17; *Nao-Hu*; 'Door of the Brain'

Location
1.5 *cun* above GV 16, superior to external occipital protuberance.

GV 15–27

235

FOURTEEN MERIDIANS AND ACUPUNCTURE POINTS

Regional anatomy
Branches of occipital arteries & veins on both sides;
Branch of greater occipital nerve.

Connecting point
Meeting Point of Foot *Tai*-Yang and Governor Vessel Meridians.

Symptoms
Facial pain
Heaviness & swelling of head

Method of treatment
Needle: **Forbidden.**
Moxa: **Forbidden.**

Note
Neither needle insertion nor moxa is advised. Massage is the correct treatment.

GV 18; *Qiang-Jian*; 'Middle Strength'

Location
1.5 *cun* above GV 17, on crossline between sagittal and lambdoid sutures.

Regional anatomy
Branches of occipital arteries & veins on both sides;
Branch of greater occipital nerve.

Symptoms
Headache   Stiff neck
Dizziness   Restlessness
Vomiting

Method of treatment
Needle: 0.2 inch horizontally.
Moxa: Warm heating, 1 minute.
Feeling: Ache and/or swelling.

GV 19; *Hou-Ding*; 'Posterior Summit'

Location
1.5 *cun* above GV 18.

Regional anatomy
Branches of occipital arteries & veins on both sides;
Branch of greater occipital nerve.

Symptoms
Stiff neck
Dizziness
Mania

Method of treatment
Needle: 0.2 inch horizontally.
Moxa: Warm heating, 1 minute.
Feeling: Ache and/or swelling.

GV 20; *Bai-Hui*; 'One Hundred Meetings'

Location
On midline of head, halfway on line connecting apices of both ears.

Regional anatomy
Anastomotic network of superficial temporal arteries & veins;
Branch of greater occipital nerve.

Connecting point
Meeting Point of all Foot and Hand Yang Meridians and Governor Vessel Meridian.

Functions
Dispels 'Liver wind';
Eases excess Liver Yang;
Clears mind and *Shen*;
Revives from coma;
Promotes Yang energy;

FOURTEEN MERIDIANS AND ACUPUNCTURE POINTS

Expels excess heat from Yang Meridians.

Symptoms
Apoplexy	Fatigue
Hemiplegia	Prolapse of rectum
Stiff jaw	(Epilepsy)
Restlessness	Headache
Palpitations	Vertigo
Poor memory	

Clinical formula
GV 20 + GV 1 = Prolapse of rectum

Method of treatment
- Needle: 0.2 inch horizontally.
- Moxa: Warm heating, 1 minute.
- Feeling: Ache and/or swelling.
- **Warning: Only when absolutely necessary should moxa be used on top of the head.**

GV 21; *Qian-Ding*; 'Anterior Summit'

Location
1.5 *cun* anterior to GV 20.

Regional anatomy
Anastomotic network of right & left superficial temporal arteries & veins;
On side connecting branch of frontal nerve with branch of greater occipital nerve.

Symptoms
Headache	Red & swollen face
Vertigo	Rhinorrhoea
Oedema	

Method of treatment
- Needle: 0.2 inch horizontally.
- Moxa: Warm heating, 1 minute.
- Feeling: Ache and/or swelling.

GV 22; *Xin-Hui*; 'Door to the Brain'

Location
1.5 *cun* anterior to GV 21, at junction of sagittal and coronal sutures.

Regional anatomy
Anastomotic network of superficial temporal artery & vein with frontal artery & vein;
Branch of frontal nerve.

Symptoms
Headache	Nasal obstruction
Epistaxis	Loss of sense of smell
Red & swollen face	
Vertigo	Palpitations

Method of treatment
- Needle: 0.2 inch horizontally.
- Moxa: Warm heating, 1 minute.
- Feeling: Ache and/or swelling.
- **Warning: It is forbidden to use needle or moxa on children under eight years old, as the frontal and parietal bones of their skulls are not yet completely joined.**

GV 23; *Shang-Xing*; 'Superior Star'

Location
1 *cun* within anterior hairline on midline of head.

Regional anatomy
Frontal muscle;
Branches of frontal artery, vein & nerve;
Branches of superficial temporal artery & vein.

Functions
Expels excess heat (in face and head) from all Yang Meridians.

FOURTEEN MERIDIANS AND ACUPUNCTURE POINTS

Symptoms
- Red & swollen face
- Swollen scalp
- Headache
- Nasal obstruction
- Vertigo
- Ophthalmalgia
- Rhinitis

Clinical formula
GV 23 + LI 20 + LI 4 + St 36 = Rhinitis (hypertrophic)

Method of treatment
- Needle: 02. inch horizontally.
- Moxa: Warm heating, 1 minute.
- Feeling: Pain and/or swelling.
- **Warning: Avoid overheating with moxa.**

GV 24; *Shen-Ting*; 'Divine Temple'

Location
On midsagittal line of head, 0.5 *cun* within anterior hairline.

Regional anatomy
Frontal muscle;
Branches of frontal artery, vein & nerve.

Connecting point
Meeting Point of Foot *Tai*-Yang, Foot Yang-*Ming* and Governor Vessel Meridians.

Symptoms
- Mania (Epilepsy)
- Headache
- Rhinorrhoea
- Ophthalmalgia
- Vertigo
- Palpitations
- Vomiting

Method of treatment
- Needle: **Forbidden.**
- Moxa: Warm heating, 1 minute.
- **Warning: Great care must be taken if needle is used.**

Note
In the ancient Chinese book, *A Classic of Acupuncture and Moxibustion* (AD 265), needle insertion is **forbidden**.

GV 25; *Pi-Jien*; 'Tip of the Nose'

Location
At tip of nose.

Regional anatomy
Lateral nasal branches of facial artery & vein;
External nasal branch of anterior ethmoidal nerve.

Symptoms
- Nasal obstruction
- Epistaxis
- Dyspnoea
- Rosacea

Clinical formula
GV 25 + LI 20 + LI 4 = Acne rosacea

Method of treatment
- Needle: 0.1 inch obliquely.
- Moxa: **Forbidden.**
- Feeling: Pain and/or swelling.

GV 26; *Shui-Gou*; 'Water Drain'

Location
Below nose, just above midpoint of philtrum.

Regional anatomy
Orbicular muscle of mouth;
Superior labial artery & vein;
Buccal branch of facial nerve;
Branch of infraorbital nerve.

Connecting point
Meeting Point of Hand and Foot Yang-*Ming*

FOURTEEN MERIDIANS AND ACUPUNCTURE POINTS

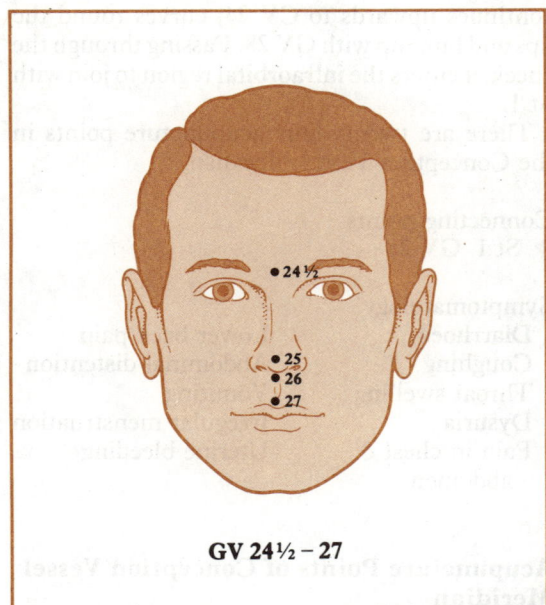

GV 24½ – 27

Meridians and Governor Vessel Meridian.

Functions
Revives from unconsciousness;
Clears mind;
Dispels wind and heat;
Harmonizes Yin and Yang energy flows.

Symptoms
General oedema	Facial paralysis
Mania	Pain & stiffness in
Apoplexy	lower back
(Epilepsy)	

Clinical formula
GV 26 + Pc 9 + LI 4 = Apoplexy

Method of treatment
Needle: 0.2 inch obliquely.
Moxa: Warm heating, 1 minute.

Feeling: Pain.

Note
Needle is better than moxa.

GV 27; *Dui-Duan*; 'Change of Point'

Location
On median tubercle of upper lip at junction with philtrum.

Regional anatomy
Superior labial artery & vein;
Buccal branch of facial nerve;
Branch of infraorbital nerve.

Symptoms
(Epilepsy)	Stiff lip
Dry throat	Aphthae on lips & in mouth
Epistaxis	

Method of treatment
Needle: 0.1 inch obliquely.
Moxa: Warm heating, 1 minute.
Feeling: Pain.

GV 28; *Yin-Jiao*; 'Meeting Point of Gum and Lip'

Location
Between upper lip and labial gingiva in frenulum of upper lip.

Regional anatomy
Superior labial artery & vein;
Branch of superior alveolar nerve.

Connecting point
Meeting Point of Conception Vessel, Governor Vessel and Foot Yang-*Ming* Meridians.

239

FOURTEEN MERIDIANS AND ACUPUNCTURE POINTS

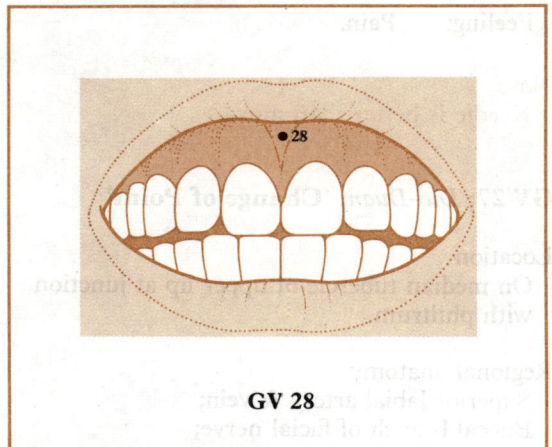

GV 28

Symptoms
  Nasal obstruction   Ophthalmalgia
  Stiff neck   Restlessness
  Painful & swollen gums

Method of treatment
  Needle: 0.1 inch obliquely or prick with three-edged needle to cause bleeding.
  Moxa: **Forbidden.**
  Feeling: Pain.

14. Conception Vessel Meridian (Ren Mai)

The Conception Vessel Meridian is recognized as the 'Sea of the Yin Meridians', as the three lower Yin Meridians, the Yin-*Qiao* Meridian and the *Chong* Meridian all join it. The energy flow originates in the lower abdomen (beneath CV 3) and emerges at CV 1. A branch runs backwards, connecting to the Governor Vessel Meridian, then travels upwards along the spine.

The main Meridian, arising at CV 1, flows anteriorly to the pubic region, then turns towards the centre of the abdomen, passes through CV 4 and follows the front midline to the throat. It continues upwards to CV 24, curves round the lips and links up with GV 28. Passing through the cheek, it enters the infraorbital region to join with St 1.

There are twenty-four acupuncture points in the Conception Vessel Meridian.

Connecting points
• St 1 GV 28

Symptomatology
  Diarrhoea   Lower back pain
  Coughing   Abdominal distention
  Throat swelling   Vomiting
  Dysuria   Irregular menstruation
  Pain in chest &   Uterine bleeding
    abdomen

Acupuncture Points of Conception Vessel Meridian

CV 1; *Hui-Yin*; 'Meeting of Yin'

Location
  In centre of perineum, between anus and scrotum in males, and anus and posterior labial commissure in females.

Regional anatomy
  Superficial & deep transverse muscles of perineum;
  External sphincter muscle of anus;
  Branches of perineal artery, vein & nerve.

Connecting point
  Meeting Point of Conception Vessel, Governor Vessel and *Chong* Meridians (all of which originate from this point).

Symptoms
  Pruritus vulvae

FOURTEEN MERIDIANS AND ACUPUNCTURE POINTS

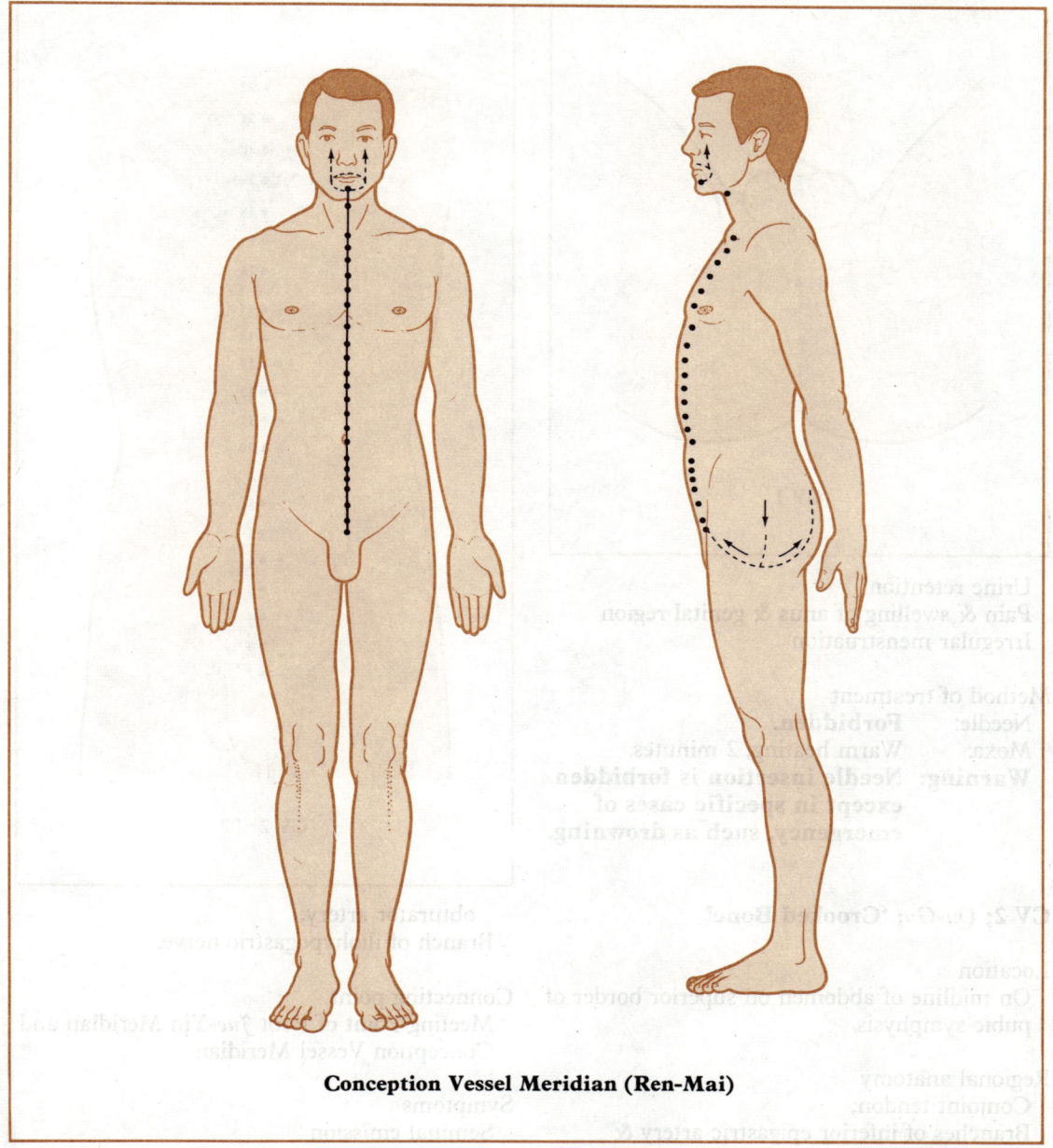

Conception Vessel Meridian (Ren-Mai)

FOURTEEN MERIDIANS AND ACUPUNCTURE POINTS

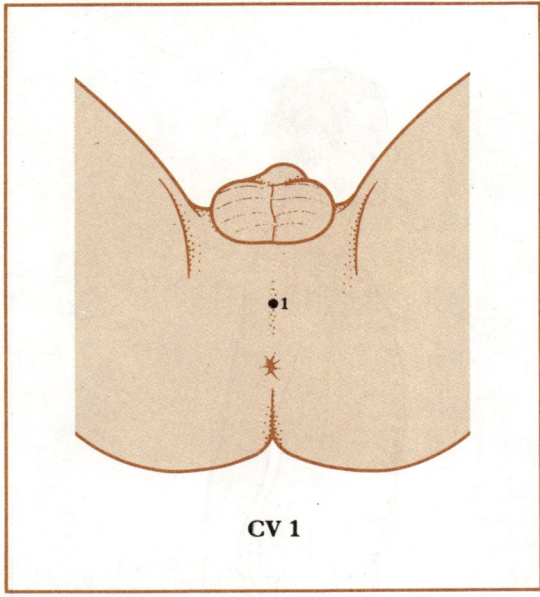

CV 1

Urine retention
Pain & swelling of anus & genital region
Irregular menstruation

Method of treatment
  Needle: **Forbidden.**
  Moxa: Warm heating, 2 minutes.
  Warning: Needle insertion is forbidden except in specific cases of emergency, such as drowning.

CV 2–22

CV 2; *Qu-Gu*; 'Crooked Bone'

Location
  On midline of abdomen on superior border of pubic symphysis.

Regional anatomy
  Conjoint tendon;
  Branches of inferior epigastric artery & obturator artery;
  Branch of iliohypogastric nerve.

Connecting point
  Meeting Point of Foot *Jue*-Yin Meridian and Conception Vessel Meridian.

Symptoms
  Seminal emission

FOURTEEN MERIDIANS AND ACUPUNCTURE POINTS

Weakness of Zang organs
Pain & distention of lower abdomen
Urine retention
Leucorrhoea

Method of treatment
Needle: 0.3 inch perpendicularly.
Moxa: Warm heating, 2 minutes.
Feeling: Ache and/or swelling.

CV 3; *Zhong-Ji*; 'Middle Pole'

Location
On midline of abdomen, 1 *cun* superior to CV 2 and 4 *cun* below umbilicus.

Regional anatomy
Branches of superficial & inferior epigastric arteries & veins;
Branch of iliohypogastric nerve;
Bladder.

Connecting points
Front-*Mu* Point of Bladder;
Meeting Point of three Foot Yin Meridians and Conception Vessel Meridian.

Functions
Strengthens function of reproductive system;
Frees function of Bladder;
Regulates Lower Heater function.

Symptoms
Abdominal distention
Loss of Kidney *Ching*
Swelling of external genitalia
Frequency of micturition
Sterility
Irregular menstruation

Method of treatment
Needle: 0.6 inch perpendicularly.
Moxa: Warm heating, 3 minutes.
Feeling: Ache and/or swelling.
Warning: Moxa is forbidden during pregnancy.

CV 4; *Guan-Yuan*; 'Gate of Yuan Energy'

Location
On midline of abdomen, 3 *cun* below umbilicus.

Regional anatomy
Branches of superficial & inferior epigastric arteries & veins;
Anterior cutaneous branch of subcostal nerve;
Small intestine.

Connecting points
Front-*Mu* Point of Small Intestine; Meeting Point of three Foot Yin Meridians and Conception Vessel Meridian.

Functions
Strengthens Kidney function;
Tones *Yuan* energy;
Promotes Yang energy;
Strengthens function of reproductive system;
Dispels cold and damp in lower abdomen;
Balances Bladder and Small Intestine functions;
Strengthens physical body to prevent attack by disease.

Symptoms
Fatigue   Loss of Kidney *Ching*
Pain around umbilicus Urine retention
Abdominal pain &   Irregular menstruation
  distention   Leucorrhoea
Headache   Sterility

FOURTEEN MERIDIANS AND ACUPUNCTURE POINTS

Method of treatment
- Needle: 0.6 inch obliquely.
- Moxa: Warm heating, 3 minutes.
- Feeling: Ache and/or swelling.
- **Warning: Needling is forbidden during pregnancy.**

CV 5; *Shi-Men*; 'Door of Stone'

Location
On midline of abdomen, 2 *cun* below umbilicus.

Regional anatomy
Branches of superficial & inferior epigastric arteries & veins;
Anterior cutaneous branch of intercostal nerve;
Small intestine.

Connecting point
Front-*Mu* Point of Three Heater.

Symptoms
Urine retention	Oedema
Lower abdominal pain	Vomiting
Diarrhoea	Indigestion
Abdominal distention	Uterine bleeding

Method of treatment
- Needle: 0.6 inch perpendicularly.
- Moxa: Warm heating, 2 minutes.
- Feeling: Ache and/or swelling.

Note
Acupuncture and moxibustion applied here may cause sterility in some women, particularly those who have never given birth.

CV 6; *Qi-Hai*; 'Energy Centre'

Location
On midline of abdomen, 1.5 *cun* below umbilicus.

Regional anatomy
Branches of superficial & inferior epigastric arteries & veins;
Anterior cutaneous branch of intercostal nerve;
Small intestine.

Functions
Harmonizes body energy flow;
Promotes *Yuan* energy flow;
Strengthens Kidney function;
Tones body;
Harmonizes *Jing* blood function;
Harmonizes Girdle Vessel function;
Strengthens Lower Heater function;
Dispels damp.

Symptoms
Abdominal distention	Irregular menstruation
Loss of energy	Leucorrhoea
General weakness after chronic illness	Lower back pain
	Enuresis
Fatigue	

Method of treatment
- Needle: 0.6 inch perpendicularly.
- Moxa: Warm heating, 3 minutes.
- Feeling: Ache and/or swelling.
- **Warning: Both acupuncture and moxibustion are forbidden during pregnancy.**

Note
This is an important point for strengthening body energy flow.

FOURTEEN MERIDIANS AND ACUPUNCTURE POINTS

CV 7; *Yin-Jiao*; 'Meeting of Yin'

Location
  On midline of abdomen, 1 *cun* below umbilicus.

Regional anatomy
  Branches of superficial & inferior epigastric arteries & veins;
  Anterior cutaneous branch of intercostal nerve;
  Small intestine.

Connecting point
  Meeting Point of Conception Vessel Meridian, Foot *Shao*-Yin Meridian and *Chong* Meridian.

Symptoms
  Abdominal pain & distention
  Pruritus vulvae
  Uterine bleeding
  Irregular menstruation
  Urine retention

Method of treatment
  Needle: 0.6 inch perpendicularly.
  Moxa: Warm heating, 2 minutes.
  Feeling: Ache and/or swelling.
  Warning: Moxibustion is forbidden during pregnancy.

CV 8; *Qi-Zhong*; 'Centre of Umbilicus'

Location
  In centre of umbilicus.

Regional anatomy
  Inferior epigastric artery & vein;
  Anterior cutaneous branch of intercostal nerve;
  Small intestine.

Functions
  Strengthens *Yuan* energy flow;
  Revives from coma;
  Improves Stomach and Intestine functions;
  Dispels cold and damp.

Symptoms
  Apoplexy   Oedema
  Diarrhoea   Abdominal pain & distention

Clinical formula
  CV 8 + Sp 6 = Diarrhoea

Method of treatment
  Needle: **Forbidden.**
  Moxa: Warm heating, 3 minutes.

CV 9; *Shui-Fen*; 'Division of Water'

Location
  On midline of abdomen, 1 *cun* above umbilicus.

Regional anatomy
  Inferior epigastric artery & vein;
  Anterior cutaneous branches of intercostal nerves;
  Small intestine.

Functions
  Strengthens Spleen function;
  Dispels damp;
  Improves water metabolism.

Symptoms
  Oedema
  Abdominal pain & distention
  Stiff spine & lower back

Clinical formula
  CV 9 + St 28 = Oedema

Method of treatment
  Needle: 0.6 inch perpendicularly.

245

FOURTEEN MERIDIANS AND ACUPUNCTURE POINTS

Moxa: Warm heating, 2 minutes.
Feeling: Ache and/or swelling.

Note
Ancient Chinese literature suggests that needling is insuitable. Moxa is preferable and produces good results.

CV 10; *Xia-Wan*; 'Lower Portion of Stomach'

Location
On midline of abdomen, 2 *cun* above umbilicus.

Regional anatomy
Inferior epigastric artery & vein;
Anterior cutaneous branch of intercostal nerve;
Transverse mesocolon.

Connecting point
Meeting Point of Conception Vessel and Foot *Tai*-Yin Meridians.

Functions
Increases digestion and absorption;
Frees energy obstruction in Stomach and Small Intestine.

Symptoms
Abdominal distention & pain
Anorexia
Indigestion
Loss of appetite

Method of treatment
Needle: 0.6 inch perpendicularly.
Moxa: Warm heating, 2 minutes.
Feeling: Pain and/or swelling.
Warning: Moxa is forbidden during pregnancy.

CV 11; *Jian-Li*; 'Distance of a Mile'

Location
On midline of abdomen, 3 *cun* above umbilicus.

Regional anatomy
Branches of superior & inferior epigastric arteries;
Anterior cutaneous branch of intercostal nerve;
Transverse mesocolon.

Functions
Strengthens Spleen function;
Harmonizes Stomach function;
Improves digestion;
Dispels damp;
Frees Middle Heater energy flow.

Symptoms
Abdominal distention & pain   Gastric pain
Oedema   Vomiting

Method of treatment
Needle: 0.5 inch perpendicularly.
Moxa: Warm heating, 2 minutes.
Feeling: Pain and/or swelling.
Warning: Moxa is forbidden during pregnancy.

CV 12; *Zhong-Wan*; 'Middle of the Stomach'

Location
On midline of abdomen, 4 *cun* above umbilicus.

Regional anatomy
Superior epigastric artery & vein;
Anterior cutaneous branch of intercostal nerve;
Stomach.

Connecting points
Front-*Mu* Point of Stomach; one of 'Eight

Influential Points' dominating Fu organs;
Meeting Point of Conception Vessel, Hand *Tai*-Yang, Hand *Shao*-Yang and Foot Yang-*Ming* Meridians.

Functions
Harmonizes Stomach energy flow;
Dispels damp;
Balances Middle Heater function;
Balances energy flow in Stomach and Small Intestine.

Symptoms
Dyspnoea   Gastric pain
Abdominal distention   Indigestion
Anorexia   Morning sickness

Clinical formula
CV 12 + CV 13 + TH 4 = Morning sickness

Method of treatment
Needle: 0.6 inch perpendicularly.
Moxa: Warm heating, 2 minutes.
Feeling: Pain and/or swelling.
Warning: Moxa is forbidden during pregnancy.

CV 13; *Shang-Wan*; 'Upper Portion of Stomach'

Location
On midline of abdomen, 5 *cun* above umbilicus.

Regional anatomy
Superior epigastric artery & vein;
Anterior cutaneous branch of intercostal nerve;
Liver;
Stomach.

Connecting point
Meeting Point of Conception Vessel, Foot Yang-*Ming* and Hand *Tai*-Yang Meridians.

Functions
Balances functions of Spleen and Stomach;
Dispels sputum in chest;
Regulates Meridian energy flow;
Calms mind and *Shen*.

Symptoms
Abdominal pain & distention   Gastric pain
Indigestion   Palpitations
Vomiting

Method of treatment
Needle: 0.6 inch perpendicularly.
Moxa: Warm heating, 2 minutes.
Feeling: Ache and/or swelling.
Warning: Moxa is forbidden during pregnancy.

CV 14; *Ju-Que*; 'A Big Fault'

Location
On midline of abdomen, 6 *cun* above umbilicus.

Regional anatomy
Superior epigastric artery & vein;
Anterior cutaneous branch of intercostal nerve;
Liver;
Stomach.

Connecting point
Front-*Mu* Point of Heart.

FOURTEEN MERIDIANS AND ACUPUNCTURE POINTS

Functions
Dispels sputum in chest;
Eases damp in Middle Heater;
Clears mind and *Shen*;
Harmonizes Middle Heater energy flow.

Symptoms
Dyspnoea
Coughing
Shortness of breath
Pain in chest & back
Gastric pain
Palpitations
Abdominal pain & distension

Method of treatment
Needle: 0.4 inch perpendicularly.
Moxa: Warm heating, 2 minutes.
Feeling: Ache and/or swelling.
Warning: Avoid inserting needle too deeply.

CV 15; *Jiu-Wei*; 'Tail of the Dove'

Location
7 *cun* above umbilicus and below xiphoid process.

Regional anatomy
Superior epigastric artery & vein;
Anterior cutaneous branch of intercostal nerve;
Liver;
Stomach.

Connecting point
Luo-Connecting Point.

Symptoms
Migraine headache
Dyspnoea
Fullness in chest
Coughing
Mania
Palpitations
Fatigue

Method of treatment
Needle: 0.3 inch obliquely, downwards.
Moxa: Warm heating, 1 minute.
Feeling: Ache and/or swelling.
Warning: Avoid inserting needle too deeply. Do not overheat with moxa.

CV 16; *Zhong-Ting*; 'Middle of the Front Yard'

Location
On midline of sternum at level of fifth intercostal space.

Regional anatomy
Sternum;
Perforating branches of internal mammary artery & vein;
Anterior cutaneous branch of intercostal nerve;
Pericardium;
Heart.

Symptoms
Fullness in chest
Vomiting

Method of treatment
Needle: 0.3 inch horizontally.
Moxa: Warm heating, 1 minute.
Feeling: Pain and/or swelling.
Warning: Needling should be gentle at all points in the sternum.

CV 17; *Shan-Zhong*; 'Middle of the Chest'

Location
On midline of sternum, between nipples at level of fourth intercostal space.

FOURTEEN MERIDIANS AND ACUPUNCTURE POINTS

Regional anatomy
 Sternum;
 Perforating branches of internal mammary artery & vein;
 Anterior cutaneous branch of intercostal nerve;
 Pericardium;
 Heart.

Connecting points
 Front-*Mu* Point of Pericardium; one of 'Eight Influential Points' dominating energy; Meeting Point of Conception Vessel, Foot *Tai*-Yin, Foot *Shao*-Yin, Hand *Tai*-Yang and Hand *Shao*-Yang Meridians.

Functions
 Regulates energy flow;
 Sends pathogenic energy downwards;
 Regulates Lung function;
 Dispels sputum;
 Frees energy flow in chest and diaphragm.

Symptoms
Dyspnoea	Fullness in chest
Shortness of breath	Cardiac pain
Coughing	Lactation deficiency

Method of treatment
 Needle: **Forbidden.**
 Moxa: Warm heating, 2 minutes.

Note
 The *Compendium of Acupuncture and Moxibustion* (1601) forbids needling this point.

CV 18; *Yu-Tang*; 'Jade Palace'

Location
 On midline of sternum at level of third intercostal space.

Regional anatomy
 Sternum;
 Perforating branches of internal mammary artery & vein;
 Anterior cutaneous branch of intercostal nerve;
 Pericardium;
 Heart.

Symptoms
Chest pain	Fullness in chest
Restlessness	Dyspnoea
Coughing	

Method of treatment
 Needle: 0.3 inch horizontally.
 Moxa: Warm heating, 2 minutes.
 Feeling: Ache and/or swelling.

CV 19; *Zi-Gong*; 'Violet Palace'

Location
 On midline of sternum at level of second intercostal space.

Regional anatomy
 Sternum;
 Perforating branches of internal mammary artery & vein;
 Anterior cutaneous branch of intercostal nerve;
 Pericardium;
 Heart.

Symptoms
Fullness in chest	Coughing
Chest pain	Restlessness

Method of treatment
 Needle: 0.3 inch horizontally.
 Moxa: Warm heating, 2 minutes.
 Feeling: Ache and/or swelling.

FOURTEEN MERIDIANS AND ACUPUNCTURE POINTS

CV 20; *Hua-Gai*; 'Cover of Splendour'

Location
On midline of sternum at level of first intercostal space.

Regional anatomy
Sternum;
Perforating branches of internal mammary artery & vein;
Anterior cutaneous branch of intercostal nerve;
Thymus;
Trachea.

Symptoms
Dyspnoea
Coughing
Sore throat
Fullness in chest

Method of treatment
Needle: 0.3 inch horizontally.
Moxa: Warm heating, 2 minutes.
Feeling: Ache and/or swelling.

CV 21; *Xuan-Ji*; 'Rotorcraft'

Location
On midline of sternum, halfway between CV 22 and CV 20.

Regional anatomy
Sternum;
Perforating branches of internal mammary artery & vein;
Medial supraclavicular nerve;
Anterior cutaneous branch of intercostal nerve;
Thymus;
Trachea.

Symptoms
Fullness in chest
Dyspnoea
Sore throat

Method of treatment
Needle: 0.3 inch horizontally.
Moxa: Warm heating, 2 minutes.
Feeling: Pain and/or swelling.

CV 22; *Tian-Tu*; 'Celestial Prominence'

Location
In centre of suprasternal fossa.

Regional anatomy
Jugular notch;
Sternocleidomastoid & sternothyroid muscles;
Jugular venous arch;
Inferior thyroid vein;
Brachiocephalic trunk;
Medial supraclavicular nerve;
Thymus;
Trachea.

Connecting point
Meeting Point of Yin-*Wei* and Conception Vessel Meridians.

Functions
Strengthens Lung function;
Dispels sputum;
Frees energy obstruction in throat.

Symptoms
Dyspnoea
Coughing
Hoarseness of voice
Swelling in throat & neck
Pain in chest & back
Vomiting

Method of treatment
Needle: 0.4 inch obliquely towards posteroinferior aspect of sternum.
Moxa: Warm heating, 2 minutes.
Feeling: Pain and/or swelling.
Warning: It is very dangerous to puncture too deeply.

FOURTEEN MERIDIANS AND ACUPUNCTURE POINTS

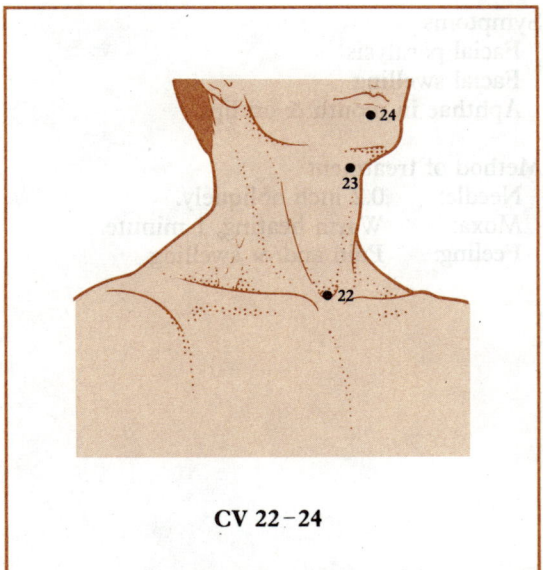

CV 22-24

Experience and skill in needle technique are essential.

Symptoms
  Dyspnoea
  Difficulty in swallowing
  Swelling of subglossal region
  Coughing
  Aphasia with stiff tongue

Method of treatment
  Needle: 0.3 inch perpendicularly.
  Moxa: **Forbidden.**
  Feeling: Pain and/or swelling.

CV 23; *Lian-Quan*; 'Clear Fountain'

Location
  On midline of neck, halfway between laryngeal prominence and border of mandible, on superior border of hyoid bone.

Regional anatomy
  Geniohyoid muscle;
  Anterior jugular vein;
  Branch of cutaneous cervical nerve;
  Hypoglossal nerve;
  Branch of glossopharyngeal nerve.

Functions
  Dispels sputum;
  Expels heat;
  Regulates energy flow.

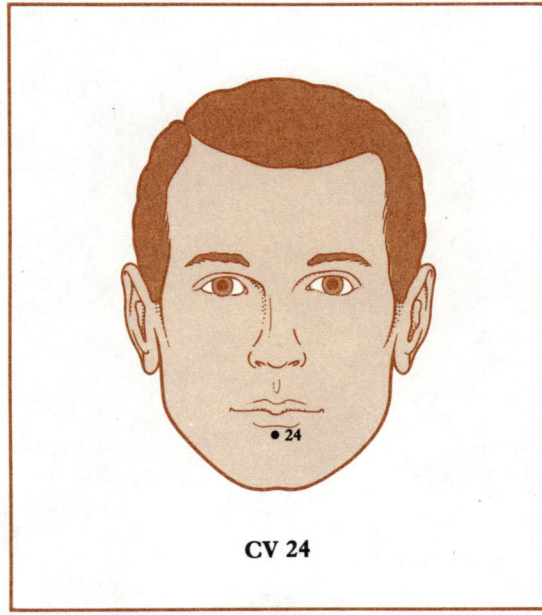

CV 24

CV 24; *Cheng-Jian*; 'Containing the Fluid'

Location
  On midline of face between chin and lower lip, in depression of mentolabial groove.

Regional anatomy
  Depressor muscle of lower lip;
  Chin muscle;
  Branches of inferior labial artery & vein;
  Branch of facial nerve.

FOURTEEN MERIDIANS AND ACUPUNCTURE POINTS

Connecting point
    Meeting point of Hand and Foot Yang-*Ming* Meridians and Conception Vessel Meridian.

Functions
    Balances energy flow of Yin and Yang Meridians;
    Frees energy obstruction in face and mouth;
    Dispels wind.

Symptoms
    Facial paralysis
    Facial swelling
    Aphthae in mouth & on lips

Method of treatment
    Needle: 0.2 inch obliquely.
    Moxa: Warm heating, 1 minute.
    Feeling: Pain and/or swelling.

5 ACUPUNCTURE AND MOXIBUSTION TECHNIQUES

MOXIBUSTION

In Chinese medicine, because acupuncture and moxibustion are usually used together to balance each other, the treatment is always referred to as 'acupuncture and moxibustion'.

Moxibustion is the application of heat to the points of acupuncture and to certain regions of the body by means of an ignited moxa stick or moxa cone. Depending upon the amount of heat/herbs which is able to penetrate the body and follow the Meridian energy circulation, moxibustion can warm the blood and energy flows, alleviate certain disorders and strengthen the body's defense against disease. Moxibustion can be applied separately or in combination with the acupuncture needle.

Moxa wool (or moxa stick) is made of dry moxa or mugwort leaves (*Artemisia vulgaris*) and has been used in China for several thousands of years. Indeed, the history of moxibustion is older than that of the acupuncture needle.

Classification of moxibustion

Moxa cone
  Direct
    Scarring
    Non-scarring
  Indirect
    Ginger insulation
    Garlic insulation
    Salt insulation

Moxa stick
  Pure moxa stick
  Tai-I moxa stick
  Nien-Ying moxa stick

Other methods of warm heating
  Sunshine
  Infrared lamp
  Some herbs (pepper, etc.)

Moxibustion with moxa sticks

There are two different types of moxa sticks: one is made of pure moxa; the other is a mixture of moxa and herbs. The difference between them is that the latter has a stronger effect in treatment, especially for rheumatism/arthritis.

Methods of application
Generally speaking, a lit moxa stick applied about 2 *cun* above the selected point gives a mild warm feeling. If the point is kept heated for about one to two minutes, the skin becomes hot and pink. However, application varies depending on the region of the body and type of disorder being treated. For example, for a cold ache in the hip region, it will take longer to heat point GB 30 (three to five minutes or more) before achieving a warm/hot feeling than it will at point LI 4, which takes about one minute to heat.

In practice, a moxa stick is held for a few seconds on top of the point, then moved in a circling motion or up and down 'like a sparrow picking'. This helps the heat penetrate the point

ACUPUNCTURE AND MOXIBUSTION TECHNIQUES

and increase blood and energy flows. It also removes cold and damp from the body.

As well as increasing blood and energy flows in the Meridians, moxibustion is used for strengthening the Yang energy flow, such as at points Bl 43, St 36 and CV 6. A fatigued person, an elderly patient, someone with great body weakness or after a chronic disease, all are good candidates for moxa treatment. As the head, face, and front and back of the neck (more Yang regions) should not be given too much heat, they are areas not often subjected to moxibustion, except for special reasons. Some of the acupuncture points, for example, St 9 and St 30 where the blood and energy flows are strong, are also unsuitable, and particular attention should be given to the 'Moxibustion: **Forbidden**' warning given for certain points. Above all, it must be remembered that moxa treatment is forbidden at many of the acupuncture points during pregnancy.

Heat by moxibustion can be concentrated on specific regions of the body to remove cold, damp and wind attacks which have created a stasis in the blood circulation and obstructed the energy flow. In these cases, moxa treatment is far more effective than the needle, as the heat of the moxa wool warms the blood and makes it flow again. Only when the blood moves freely does the energy flow follow.

In some circumstances, the needle is used in combination with moxibustion. Using the moxa stick at an acupuncture point produces only a mild heat but, if the needle is retained, the moxa heat can follow the deeper needle penetration and concentrate on that spot. Once the blood has been warmed by moxa, it is the needle which helps the energy flow to move freely. Thus, when used together, the needle and moxa are complementary.

When the body has too much heat (Fire), it is an indication that moxibustion must not be used as this will increase the disorder and harm the body. These are cases for needle treatment only.

When a young patient has a cold condition in the hip region, moxa is necessary for removing the cold even though the patient may react strongly to it. Use of the needle then balances the treatment by reducing the reaction.

After moxibustion treatment, quietude and rest are essential; the patient should also avoid cold drinks, alcohol, over-heating and extreme conditions (of heat and cold). It is also advisable to wait one or two hours before eating a meal.

NEEDLE TECHNIQUE

Acupuncture treatment embraces several different needle manipulation methods to regulate the blood and energy flows in the Meridians, to balance the body's internal organs and external tissue functions, to treat disorders of the body and to prevent diseases from occurring. Treatment is substantially effective and good results are accomplished with skilled needle technique.

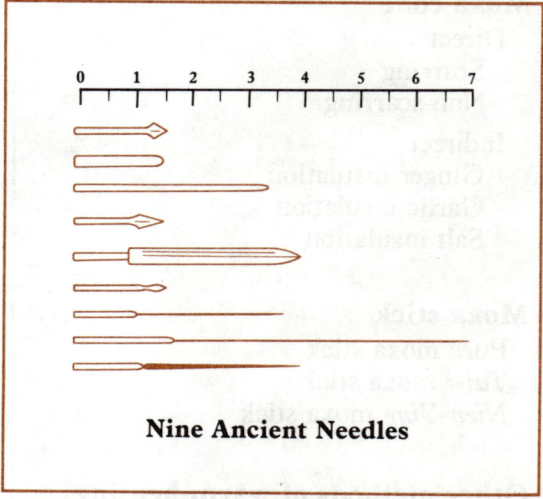

Nine Ancient Needles

The *NEI-JING* refers to the use of nine different types of needles: arrowheaded; blunt; puncturing; spear-pointed; ensiform; round; capillary; long; and big. Originally made of flint, they were later made of gold, silver or steel. Chinese philosophy attributed a 'stimulating power' to the yellow Yang metals such as gold and copper, and a 'calming, dispersing power' to the white Yin metals such as silver and chrome.

The most commonly used needles today are the Filiform needle, the Three-edged needle, the Plum-blossom needle and the Intradermal needle.

Filiform needle

This needle is made of high-quality stainless steel mixed with other metals.

Filiform Needle Dimensions

Length								
Inches	0.5	1.0	1.5	2.0	2.5	3.0	4.0	5.0
mm	12.7	25.4	38.1	50.8	63.5	76.2	101.6	127.0

Diameter				
Gauge	26	28	30	32
mm	0.46	0.38	0.32	0.26

Structurally, the needle is divided into five parts: tail; handle; root; body; and tip.

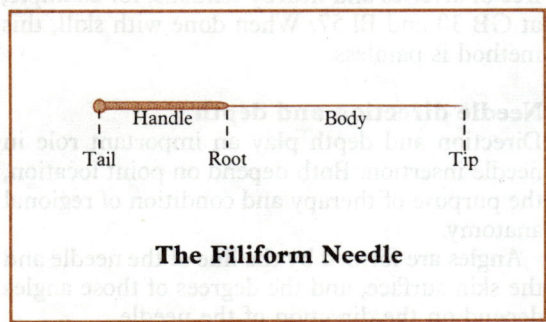

The Filiform Needle

A good needle is strong, fine and flexible with a round smooth body and a sharp tip. (The tip itself is shaped rather like the tip of a pine needle).

To avoid accidents, a thorough inspection of the needle should be made before use to check for rust, bent sections or 'hooks'.

To minimize the feeling of pain to the patient, appropriate finger force must be mastered through practice. It is advisable to begin practising with a short (1.0 inch) and thick (gauge 28 or 30) needle and progress to the longer (2.0 inches) and finer (gauge 32) needles. Practise can be on sheets of paper or small cotton cushions and then progress to one's own body to gain personal experience of the acupuncture sensation.

Sterilization

Strict sterilization of needles is imperative. Although disposable needles can be used, there are many methods available in clinical practice for needle sterilization (see Appendix, page 283). The area on the body surface selected for needle insertion must be sterilized with seventy to eighty percent alcohol solution, and the practitioner's fingers must also be routinely sterilized.

Patient posture

Correct posture is essential to ensure that the patient is comfortable and that the practitioner is able to locate easily the appropriate acupuncture points. If the patient is kept in an awkward position, undue fatigue or fainting may ensue; accidents, such as needles bending or breaking, may also occur should the patient change position abruptly.

- The **supine** position is preferable for needling points of the facial and frontal regions (chest, abdomen) and the anterior aspect of the extremities.

- The **prone** position is preferable for occipital, neck, back, lumbodorsal regions and the posterior aspect of the lower extremities.

The **recumbent** position facilitates needling of points on the lateral aspect of the body, such as those for shoulder pain or sciatica.

Needle insertion techniques

Generally, the needle is held in one hand (left or right), called the 'puncturing hand', with the thumb and index finger holding the handle of the needle, and the middle finger backing the index finger near the root of the needle. The other hand, called the 'pressing hand', presses upon the area close to the point. Coordination of the two hands is essential.

Usually, pain will be felt when the needle breaks the skin surface but, once the needle penetrates beyond the skin, the pain is marginal and will give what is known as an 'acupuncture sensation'. In order to minimize the initial pain, the movement of puncturing the skin should be swift.

The choice of technique for needle insertion depends on the length of the needle and the location of the point.

1. Aided by finger pressing

The point is pressed with the nail of the thumb or index finger of the pressing hand before insertion. The needle is quickly plunged, alongside the nail, into the point.

This method is suitable for short needles (1.0 inch) when puncturing points such as LI 4 or TH 3.

2. Coordination of fingers of both hands

The pressing hand holds the tip of the needle on the selected point while the puncturing hand holds the handle of the needle. The needle is pressed quickly through the skin at the same time that the puncturing hand twirls the needle downwards to the required depth.

This method can be used for short or long needles at points such as GB 29 or Bl 54.

3. With fingers stretching the skin

The skin over the point is stretched with the thumb and index finger of the pressing hand to cause tension, which facilitates insertion of the needle.

This method is used for points where the skin is loose, such as at LI 20 or CV 4.

4. Pinching up the skin

The thumb and index finger of the pressing hand pinch the skin up around the point and the puncturing hand inserts the needle rapidly into the point.

This method is adopted for points where the tissue is thin, such as on the head, face, and neck (GB 14 or Bl 2).

5. Injection method

The point is marked with the pressing hand. The body of the needle is held with the thumb and index finger of the puncturing hand and 0.5 cm of its tip is swiftly punctured into the point. Once the needle is through the skin, it must remain still. Holding the lower section of the needle with the pressing hand, the puncturing hand manipulates the needle to the desired depth.

This method can be used for both short and long needles, but only at points in muscular regions free of arteries and nearby tendons, for example, at GB 30 and Bl 57. When done with skill, this method is painless.

Needle direction and depth

Direction and depth play an important role in needle insertion. Both depend on point location, the purpose of therapy and condition of regional anatomy.

Angles are formed by the line of the needle and the skin surface, and the degrees of those angles depend on the direction of the needle.

When the needle is inserted **perpendicularly**,

ACUPUNCTURE AND MOXIBUSTION TECHNIQUES

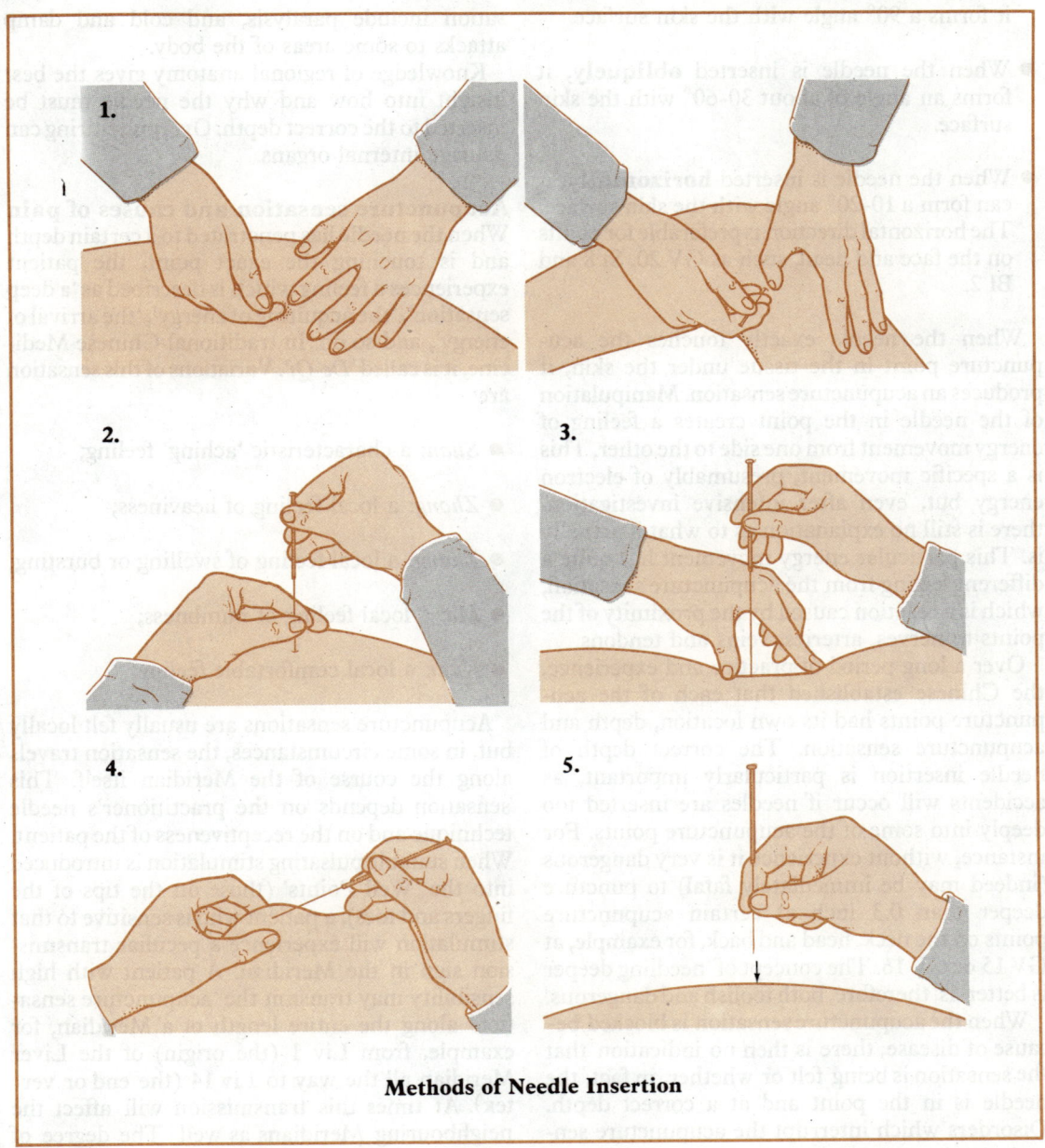

Methods of Needle Insertion

ACUPUNCTURE AND MOXIBUSTION TECHNIQUES

it forms a 90° angle with the skin surface.

- When the needle is inserted **obliquely**, it forms an angle of about 30-60° with the skin surface.

- When the needle is inserted **horizontally**, it can form a 10-20° angle with the skin surface. The horizontal direction is preferable for points on the face and head, such as GV 20, St 8 and Bl 2.

When the needle exactly touches the acupuncture point in the tissue under the skin, it produces an acupuncture sensation. Manipulation of the needle in the point creates a feeling of energy movement from one side to the other. This is a specific movement, presumably of electron energy but, even after intensive investigation, there is still no explanation as to what it actually is. This particular energy movement has quite a different feeling from the acupuncture sensation, which is a reaction caused by the proximity of the points to nerves, arteries, veins and tendons.

Over a long period of practice and experience, the Chinese established that each of the acupuncture points had its own location, depth and acupuncture sensation. The correct depth of needle insertion is particularly important, as accidents will occur if needles are inserted too deeply into some of the acupuncture points. For instance, without experience it is very dangerous (indeed may be immediately fatal) to puncture deeper than 0.3 inch at certain acupuncture points on the neck, head and back, for example, at GV 15 or GV 16. The concept of 'needling deeper is better' is, therefore, both foolish and dangerous.

When the acupuncture sensation is blocked because of disease, there is then no indication that the sensation is being felt or whether, in fact, the needle is in the point and at a correct depth. Disorders which interrupt the acupuncture sensation include paralysis, and cold and damp attacks to some areas of the body.

Knowledge of regional anatomy gives the best insight into how and why the needle must be inserted to the correct depth. Overpuncturing can damage internal organs.

Acupuncture sensation and causes of pain

When the needle has penetrated to a certain depth and is touching the exact point, the patient experiences a feeling which is described as 'a deep sensation', 'the acquiring of energy', 'the arrival of energy', and so on. In traditional Chinese Medicine, it is called '*De-Qi*'. Variations of this sensation are:

- *Suan*: a characteristic 'aching' feeling;

- *Zhong*: a local feeling of heaviness;

- *Zhang*: a local feeling of swelling or bursting;

- *Ma*: a local feeling of numbness;

- *Kuai*: a local comfortable feeling.

Acupuncture sensations are usually felt locally but, in some circumstances, the sensation travels along the course of the Meridian itself. This sensation depends on the practitioner's needle technique and on the receptiveness of the patient. When suitable pulsating stimulation is introduced into the 'Well Points' (those on the tips of the fingers and toes), a patient who is sensitive to that stimulation will experience a peculiar transmission sign in the Meridian. A patient with high sensibility may transmit the 'acupuncture sensation' along the entire length of a Meridian, for example, from Liv 1 (the origin) of the Liver Meridian all the way to Liv 14 (the end or vertex). At times this transmission will affect the neighbouring Meridians as well. The degree of sensibility varies according to the individual. Generally, the sensitive patient will have better results from acupuncture treatment than the less sensitive.

The acupuncture sensation also varies in different regions of the body; for example, ear points always feel sore and hot while points on the foot feel sore and swollen.

When inserting a needle into a point, the practitioner should be able to gauge the correct amount of stimulation by the resistance travelling up the needle; it will feel caught or sucked in by something in the tissues.

Ostensibly to abolish pain, acupuncture may also create pain if the needle technique is unskilled. The skin surface has many sensory neurons or receptors (microscopic sense organs) scattered generously over almost every part of the body. This is demonstrated when the skin is pricked with a fine needle; mild pain is followed by a hot or cold sensation or simply by pressure. If, however, the point is pressed with the fingernail before needling, the sensitivity of the sensory neurons is diminished and subsequent needling will be free of pain, providing the skin is penetrated quickly.

Alternatively, the practitioner may talk to the patient to allay his fears and distract him from nervous apprehension. With experience the practitioner will discover what action is best suited to himself and his patients. The primary requirement, however, is to insert the needle quickly enough to diminish pain coming from the skin surface.

After penetration, needle manipulation is necessary in order to find the exact point. When this has been located, there will be a feeling of *De-Qi* ('acquiring of energy'). If there is pain, it is a warning of danger, as the needle may have entered an artery wall, the periosteum, the peritoneum or a tendon. The needle should be lifted until it lies just beneath the skin surface and its direction changed before reinsertion.

Pain may also be felt in the muscle fibres if the tip of the needle is bent or the body of the needle is rough. This creates the sensation of the needle 'cutting' into the muscle; when the needle is rotated, it will catch in the fibres. To relieve the pain, the needle must be gently rotated back and forth until the fibres are released.

Pain will often arise if the needle is rotated too strongly and too quickly in one direction, causing it to twist the fibre tissues. The correctly rotated needle is a smooth movement 180° clockwise and the same number of degrees anticlockwise.

Pain will occur when inserting needles into the very sensitive areas of the body, such as the face, head, palm, foot, abdomen and the tips of the fingers and toes. These regions require skilled needle technique. Before needling in these areas, it is advisable either to ask the patient to breathe deeply or to distract him with a question before inserting the needle swiftly.

When the patient is emotionally distressed, nervous, lacking confidence or troubled with premenstrual tension, the internal tension causes oversensitivity to pain. In these circumstances, before proceeding with needle treatment, the practitioner should relax the patients by taking the time to converse with them, especially with those who are having acupuncture treatment for the first time.

Manipulation techniques

As a result of long experience of acupuncture, the practitioners of ancient China developed many techniques of needle manipulation.

1. Point massage

Before inserting the needle, the pressing hand locates and feels the point. The point and Meridian are gently massaged and, pressing with the fingernail, a mark is made for needling.

ACUPUNCTURE AND MOXIBUSTION TECHNIQUES

2. Needle rotation

Holding the body of the needle with the pressing hand and the handle with the puncturing hand, the needle is rotated clockwise from 90°, 180° and 360°, then the same anticlockwise. At the same time, the needle is moved gently deep into the tissue and the exact depth of the point located, causing the needle sensation. The movement of the needle should be smooth and should not entwine with the fibrous tissue.

Needle rotation is of primary importance in manipulation and is the most frequently applied of all the needle techniques. It can be used for point location, increasing or decreasing energy flow in the Meridians, relieving muscle spasm, relieving pain in local areas and controlling needle sensation.

3. Needle lift and thrust

The needle is inserted until it touches exactly, or is close to, the acupuncture point. Using the pressing hand to hold the body of the needle, the puncturing hand holds the handle of the needle and lifts it from the deep position to the surface ('lifting the needle').

When the needle is in the deep position and is pressed downwards further, it is called 'thrusting the needle'. This movement is limited to a depth of 0.2-0.5cm only, with the needle direction either perpendicular (moving up and down in the same spot) or at an angle (moving up and down in an oblique direction).

The total maximum depth of lift and thrust of the needle must never exceed 0.5cm, and puncturing too strongly or at too great an angle must be avoided.

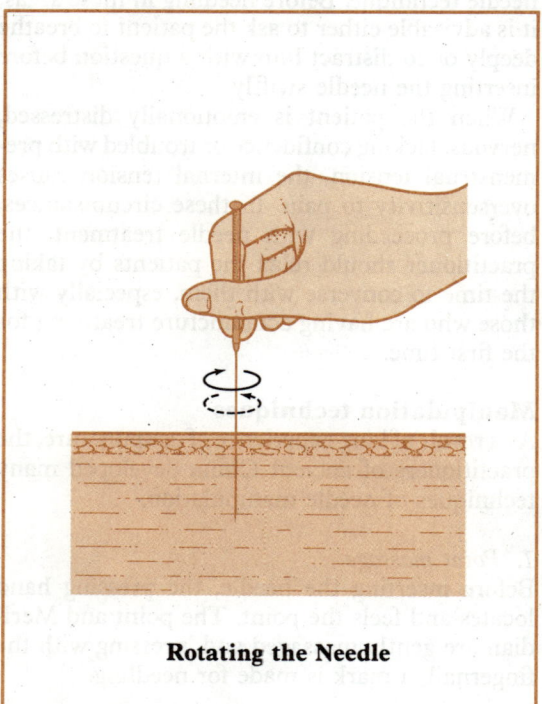

Rotating the Needle

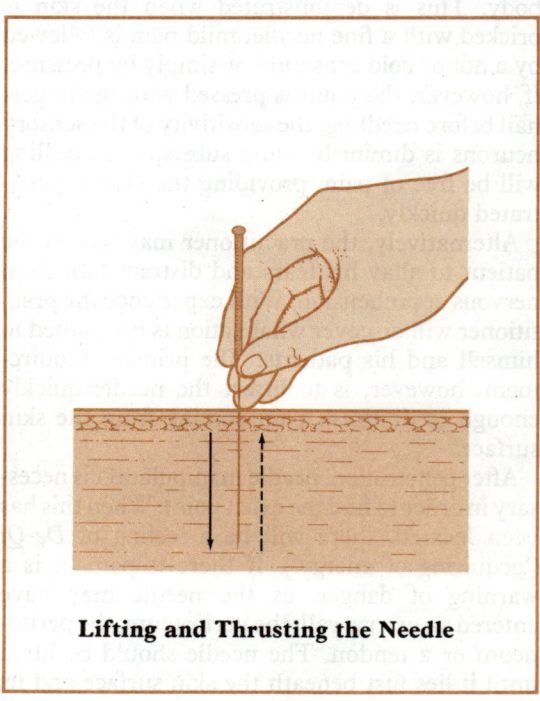

Lifting and Thrusting the Needle

ACUPUNCTURE AND MOXIBUSTION TECHNIQUES

The philosophy behind this needle technique is that, when the needle is lifted, it opens the 'gate' which allows energy to flow forward along the Meridian, while thrusting the needle closes the 'gate'. Hence, 'lifting the needle' increases energy flow and 'thrusting the needle' reduces it. This technique is used primarily for removing blood stases and energy obstructions in local regions. When puncturing deeper, closer to the bone periosteum, it can relieve swelling in the fibrous tissue. The lift and thrust technique is also very effective for needling cysts.

Note
It is just as safe to insert several needles at angles to lift and thrust as it is to use only one in different directions.

4. Needle scraping
After inserting the needle exactly into the point, it is kept in position. The tail of the needle is pressed with the thumb and, at the same time, the handle of the needle is scraped from bottom to top, several times, with the nail of the index finger. This action helps to increase both the needle sensation and the energy flow in the Meridian.

5. Needle trembling
On achieving the 'acquiring of energy' sensation, the needle is kept in that position. While holding the needle handle with the thumb, index and middle fingers, the needle is gently shaken. This technique, often used for those with body weakness, helps to give strength to the patient's energy flow (and a feeling of more control to the practitioner).

6. Needle vibration
This technique is useful when a disturbance to the

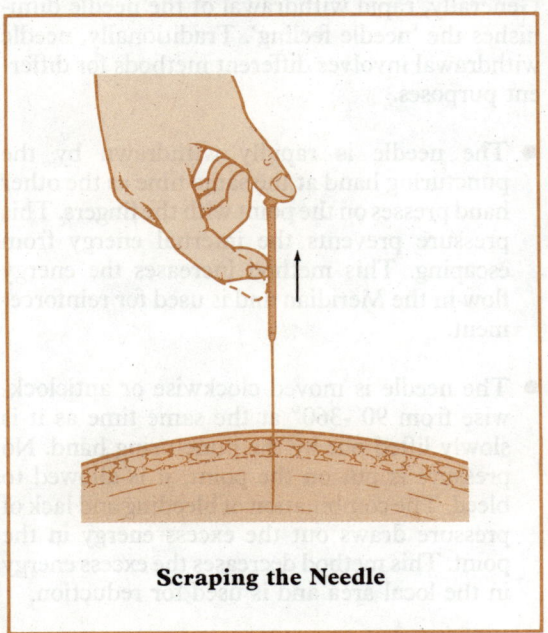

Scraping the Needle

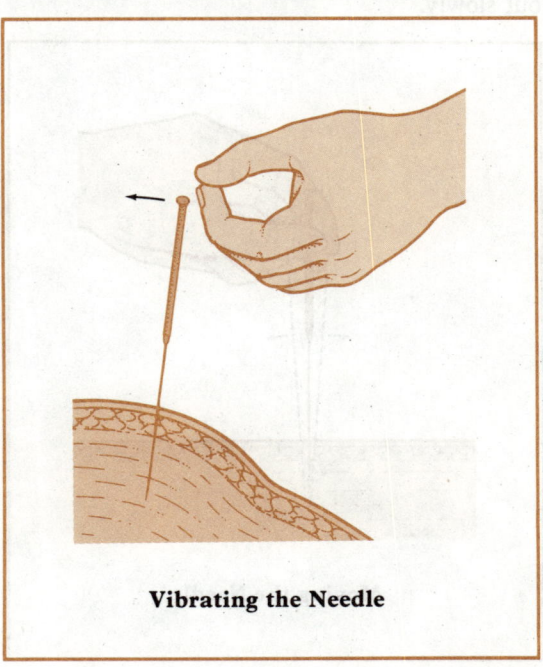

Vibrating the Needle

ACUPUNCTURE AND MOXIBUSTION TECHNIQUES

Meridian energy flow is not relieved by the needle touching the acupuncture point. Holding the needle in the point position, the index finger taps the handle of the needle, causing a gentle vibration from a different direction. This helps the Meridian energy to flow again and relieves pain in the local area.

7. Needle movement

Before withdrawal, the handle of the needle is held, keeping the tip in position deep in the point. The needle is moved clockwise or anticlockwise to enlarge the hole and increase stimulation at the point, thus removing excess energy in the local region or Meridian.

An additional manipulation technique, used especially for drawing out excess energy in local areas, involves moving the handle of the needle clockwise (or anticlockwise), then lifting the needle out slowly.

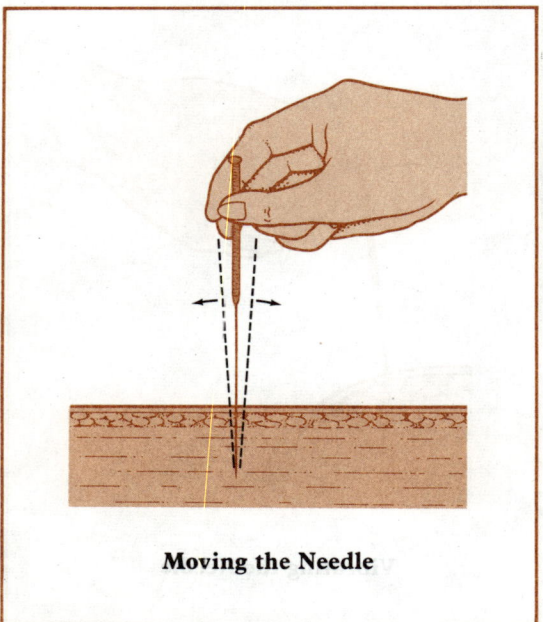

Moving the Needle

8. Needle retention

When the needle is stimulated by the acupuncture sensation, the practitioner knows it is working. Retention of the needle in the point for a specified time is dependent upon several factors: the nature of the disorder; method of needle manipulation; and the patient's condition. For a chronic disorder in a nervous patient, gentle manipulation is required and the needles are kept in the points for more than fifteen minutes. On the other hand, a relaxed patient with an acute disorder requires strong manipulation and needle retention is for a short time only, certainly less than fifteen minutes.

Normally, needle retention improves treatment, relaxes the patient and completely relieves pain. However, it is essential that the patient is in a comfortable position in a relaxing environment and is given the best care and attention.

9. Needle withdrawal

Generally, rapid withdrawal of the needle diminishes the 'needle feeling'. Traditionally, needle withdrawal involves different methods for different purposes.

- The needle is rapidly withdrawn by the puncturing hand at the same time as the other hand presses on the point with the fingers. This pressure prevents the internal energy from escaping. This method increases the energy flow in the Meridian and is used for reinforcement.

- The needle is moved clockwise or anticlockwise from 90°-360° at the same time as it is slowly lifted out by the puncturing hand. No pressure is put on the point; it is allowed to bleed. The combination of bleeding and lack of pressure draws out the excess energy in the point. This method decreases the excess energy in the local area and is used for reduction.

Withdrawing the needle too quickly and leaving the point unsealed leads to bleeding. Internal bleeding is dangerous, especially at points on the face. A usual method of needle withdrawal (either rapidly or slowly) from deep within the tissue is to bring it up to just under the skin surface and keep it there for a few seconds or, sometimes, minutes. It is then quickly withdrawn through the skin and the point is pressed with the fingers.

After needle withdrawal
During needle retention treatment, the patient must remain absolutely still in position; the needle and the patient together experience the acupuncture sensation. Needle withdrawal may create a little discomfort; thus, gentle massage helps the energy to flow more smoothly, relieves tension and creates greater relaxation.

NEEDLING THE LUO MERIDIAN (BLEEDING TECHNIQUE)

A very special needle technique is used to bleed surface blood vessels or acupuncture points in the *Luo* Meridian, for reviving from unconsciousness, for relief of fever and local blood congestion, and for skin disorders.

- Sore throat: bleed LI 1 or Lu 11.
- Conjunctivitis: bleed point *Tai*-Yang.
- Acute lumbar pain caused by trauma: bleed Bl 40.

This needle technique is one of the most important methods described in the *NEI-JING* and is used for 'expelling heat with bleeding' and for 'freeing energy obstruction with bleeding'. It follows the basic philosophy that 'only when the blood moves freely does the energy flow follow'.

The Meridian Complex or *Jing-Luo* System consists of the Twelve Main Meridians, Eight Extra Meridians, Twelve Divergent Meridians, Twelve Muscle Meridians and Twelve Derma Meridians. The *Jing* System on its own is a network of Meridians running perpendicularly (up or down) while the *Luo* System crosses between the Yin and Yang channels of the *Jing* System. To complete the *Jing-Luo* System, there are also fifteen *Luo*-Connecting Points, and countless blood *Luo* and Sun-*Luo* Points throughout body.

Needle techniques
Bleeding is accomplished using:

- A **Three-edged Needle** made of stainless steel; the head is triangular in shape with a sharp tip. There are two methods of insertion.

1. Prompt pricking method
As its name suggests, this is done swiftly, inserting the needle to a depth of 0.05-0.1 inch into the selected point. This method is used at the tips of the fingernails and toes, in the temporal region and at the apex of the ear.

2. Slow pricking method
This is used to bleed the superficial veins at selected points, such as Bl 40 or Lu 5. Before pricking, the local point is massaged to make the vein more prominent. The tip of the three-edged needle is placed close to the point just above the vein and pricked slowly through the wall of the vein to a depth of about 0.1 inch, followed by a slow withdrawal of the needle. The point is unsealed to allow a few drops of blood to escape; the point is then pressed gently to stop the bleeding.

This technique is used only when circumstances permit. It is not advisable for the elderly, for pregnant women, haemorrhagic diseases or when there is body weakness. Great care must be taken to avoid over-bleeding and injury to other tissues.

ACUPUNCTURE AND MOXIBUSTION TECHNIQUES

• A **Dermal Hammer** ('**Seven Star Needle**') is composed of seven short stainless steel needles inlaid onto a small round plate which is attached vertically to a handle about six inches long.

Holding the needle by the handle, the skin surface is tapped with a flexible movement of the wrist. With light tapping, there is no bleeding but the skin turns red or pink around the tapped area. Heavy tapping, however, draws a little blood and the skin becomes deep red. Locations for tapping can be on the acupuncture points, along the course of the Meridians or on the local pathological condition itself.

Although there are other bleeding techniques, only the dermal hammer method is discussed here for bleeding the *Luo* Meridian, in particular, for blood stases in the small veins and capillaries. The most frequently used acupuncture points for this bleeding method are:

1. *Shi-Xuan*; '**Ten Drains**'
   Extraordinary Point

   Location
   On tips of fingers about 0.1 *cun* distal to nails.

   Symptoms
   Fever   Numb fingertips
   Coma   Stiff fingers
   Sunstroke

   Method of treatment
   Prick with three-edged needle to cause bleeding.

2. *Si-Feng*; '**Four Fissures**'
   Extraordinary Point

   Location
   On palmar surface in transverse creases of proximal interphalangeal joints of index, middle, ring and little fingers.

   Symptoms
   Malnutrition & indigestion syndrome in children

   Method of treatment
   Prick with three-edged needle and extrude a small amount of yellowish viscous fluid.

3. *Tai-Yang*; '**The Sun**'
   Extraordinary Point

   Location
   In depression about 1 *cun* posterior to midpoint between lateral end of eyebrow and outer canthus.

   Symptoms
   Headache
   Conjunctivitis

   Method of treatment
   Insert filiform needle 0.3 inch obliquely and posteriorly, or prick with three-edged needle to cause bleeding.

4. *Yin-Tang*; '**Seal Room**'
   Extraordinary Point

   Location
   Midway between medial ends of eyebrows.

   Symptoms
   Infantile convulsions
   Frontal headache
   Conjunctivitis

   Method of treatment
   Insert filiform needle 0.3 inch horizontally along the skin, or prick with three-edged needle to cause bleeding.

ACUPUNCTURE AND MOXIBUSTION TECHNIQUES

5. Lu 11; *'Shao-Shang'*
   LI 1; *'Shang-Yang'*

Symptoms
   Fever   Numb fingers
   Coma   Sore throat
   Sunstroke

Method of treatment
   Prick with three-edged needle to cause bleeding.

6. Lu 5; *'Chi-Ze'*
   Pc 3; *'Qu-Ze'*

Symptoms
   Sunstroke   Restlessness
   Fullness in chest Palpitations

Method of treatment
   Prick with three-edged needle to cause bleeding.

7. Bl 40; *'Wei-Zhong'*

Symptoms
   Acute lumbar pain
   Spasm in gastrocnemius muscle

Method of treatment
   Prick with three-edged needle to cause bleeding.

8. Sp 6; *'San-Yin-Jiao'*
   Sp 10; *'Yin-Ling-Quan'*

Symptoms
   Abdominal distention
   Leg swelling
   Erysipelas

Method of treatment
   Prick with three-edged needle to cause bleeding.

9. GB 40; *'Qiu-Xu'*

Symptoms
   Acute ankle trauma

Method of treatment
   Prick with three-edged needle to cause bleeding.

10. GV 20; *'Bai-Hui'*

Symptoms
   Headache   Coma
   Dizziness   Hypertension

Method of treatment
   Prick with three-edged needle to cause bleeding.

11. TH 18; *'Qi-Mai'*

Symptoms
   Headache
   Epilepsy

Method of treatment
   Prick with three-edged needle to cause bleeding.

12. 'Tip of the Ear' Ear Point

Symptoms
   Fever
   Conjunctivitis
   Tonsillitis

Method of treatment
   Prick with three-edged needle to cause bleeding.

265

ACUPUNCTURE AND MOXIBUSTION TECHNIQUES

Warnings (for Three-edged Needle and Dermal Hammer)

- **Needle techniques to cause bleeding must never be used for body weakness, anaemia, blood disorders, before and after menstruation or before and after childbirth.**

- **Do not puncture too deeply or too hard.**

- **Avoid bleeding the artery.**

- **Sterilization and stopping of the blood flow must both be done with care.**

PRINCIPAL METHODS OF REINFORCEMENT AND REDUCTION

In clinical practice, acupuncture embraces two main ideas for treating disorders: 'to balance the body energy flow' and 'to reinforce deficiency and to reduce excess'. In using the needle to control and balance the body energy circulation, the practitioner should apply different techniques to 'acquire energy', 'remove energy obstruction', 'move the energy flow in a planned direction' and 'stimulate the energy flow to the organs and to other regions of the body'.

The chapter entitled *'Tiao Jing Lun'* from the *NEI-JING* expresses the theory that 'no matter what the disease, it will either be one of a deficient energy nature or of an excess energy nature'. The chapter *'Jing Mai Pian'* instructs that 'in the case of deficient energy, apply the reinforcement method and, in the case of excess energy, apply the reduction method'. The early practitioners created various techniques to achieve these two effects.

Simple needle techniques

1. Slow and rapid insertions

Reinforcement
The needle is slowly inserted through the skin surface until it reaches the point. This brings the Yang energy to the acupuncture point.

Reduction
The needle is rapidly inserted through the skin surface to the point, then drawn back to the superficial level. This removes the excess energy from the body.

2. Needle withdrawal

Reinforcement
The needle is withdrawn rapidly; the point is sealed and massaged gently. This allows the energy to remain in the point and within the Meridian.

Reduction
The needle is slowly withdrawn and the point left unsealed. This allows the excess energy to be drawn out.

3. Needle lift and thrust

Reinforcement
The needle is gently lifted, then thrust back firmly into the point. This gathers the energy.

Reduction
The needle is firmly lifted, then thrust back gently into the point. This reduces the energy.

4. Needle rotation

Reinforcement
The needle is inserted in the direction of Meridian

ACUPUNCTURE AND MOXIBUSTION TECHNIQUES

energy flow and gently rotated clockwise in an arc of 180°.

Reduction
The needle is inserted in the opposite direction to Meridian energy flow and rapidly rotated anti-clockwise in an arc of 360°.

5. *Needle direction*

Reinforcement
The needle is inserted in the direction of Meridian energy flow. Needling is from one point on the Meridian in the direction of the next point on that Meridian.

Reduction
The needle is inserted in the direction opposite to Meridian energy flow. Needling is from one point on the Meridian in the direction of the preceding point on that Meridian.

6. *Respiration*

Reinforcement
The needle is inserted during exhalation and withdrawn during inhalation. On occasions, the patient may be asked to cough for the initial insertion.

Reduction
The needle is inserted during inhalation and withdrawn during exhalation. The patient must always breathe deeply for the initial insertion.

7. *Timing of needle insertion*

Reinforcement
When energy flow is deficient, needling takes place at the time of day when the energy of the deficient organ has reached its minimum output. Following the Five Element theory, the practitioner should reinforce the 'Mother' element of the deficient organ.

Reduction
When energy flow is in excess, needling takes place at the time of day when the energy of the organ involved has reached its maximum output. The practitioner should reduce the 'Son' element of the organ in excess.

Complex needle techniques
These complex needle techniques were developed by the ancient philosophers and most of these are still used in clinical practice today.

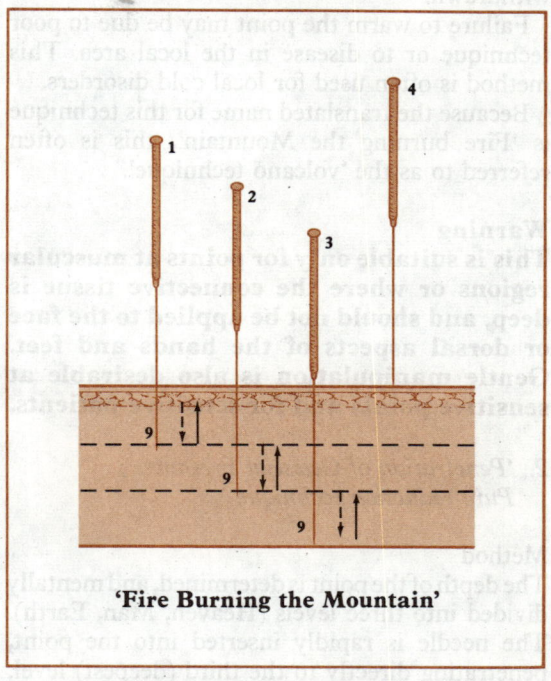

'Fire Burning the Mountain'

1. *'Fire Burning the Mountain'; Pure reinforcement technique*

267

ACUPUNCTURE AND MOXIBUSTION TECHNIQUES

Method
The depth of the point is determined and mentally divided into three levels: Heaven, Man and Earth. The needle is slowly inserted through the skin, thrust firmly into the first level and lifted gently back to just beneath the skin. At each of the three levels, the needle is firmly thrust and gently lifted nine times. On completion, the needle is quickly withdrawn from the third (deepest) level and the point sealed with the fingers.

If correctly applied, the patient feels a warm sensation at the local area. If this is not so, the entire procedure may be repeated, but not more than three times, before the needle is completely withdrawn.

Failure to warm the point may be due to poor technique or to disease in the local area. This method is often used for local cold disorders.

Because the translated name for this technique is 'Fire burning the Mountain', this is often referred to as the 'volcano technique'.

Warning
This is suitable only for points at muscular regions or where the connective tissue is deep, and should not be applied to the face or dorsal aspects of the hands and feet. Gentle manipulation is also desirable at sensitive points and for sensitive patients.

2. 'Penetration of Celestial Freshness'; Pure reduction technique

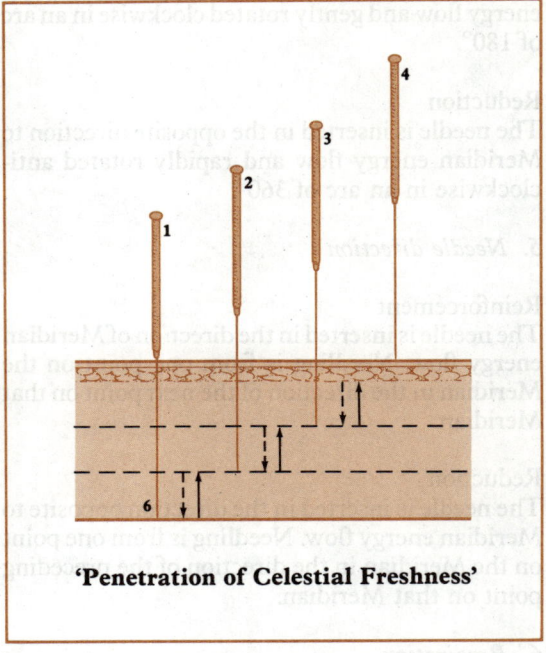

'Penetration of Celestial Freshness'

Method
The depth of the point is determined, and mentally divided into three levels (Heaven, Man, Earth). The needle is rapidly inserted into the point, penetrating directly to the third (deepest) level. The needle is then thrust gently and lifted firmly, a further six times at each level. On completion, the needle is withdrawn slowly through the skin surface from the first (most superficial) level and the point left unsealed.

After treatment, the tissue surrounding the point feels cold ('as cool as mountain air' according to the ancients). If not, the entire procedure may be repeated, but not more than twice, before the needle is withdrawn completely. This method is used for excessive heat in the body.

Warning
This method is suitable only for points at muscular regions or where the connective tissue is deep, and should not be applied to the face or dorsal aspects of the hands and feet. Gentle manipulation is also desirable at sensitive points and for sensitive patients.

3. 'Shadow of Yin between the Yang'; Combination of reinforcement and reduction techniques

ACUPUNCTURE AND MOXIBUSTION TECHNIQUES

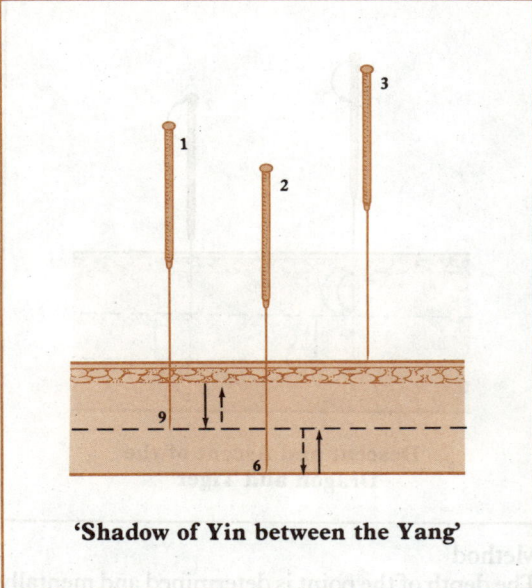

'Shadow of Yin between the Yang'

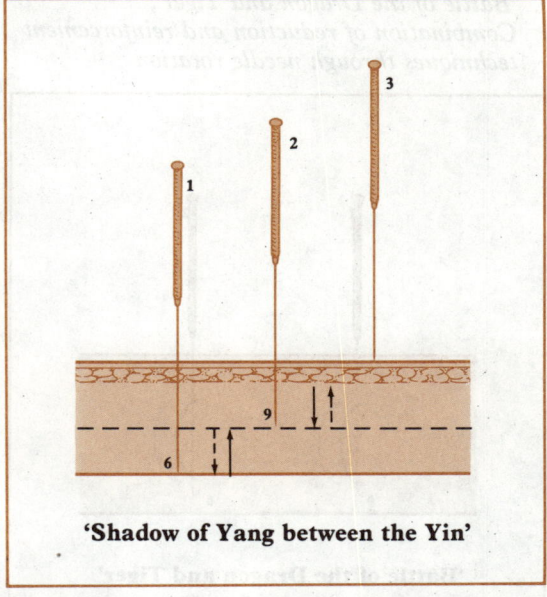

'Shadow of Yang between the Yin'

Method
The depth of the point is determined and mentally divided into two equal parts. The reinforcement aspect is applied at the upper level. The needle is thrust firmly and lifted gently and slowly nine times.

The reduction aspect is used at the lower level. The needle is thrust gently and lifted firmly six times, slowly retracted into the upper level, then slowly withdrawn. The point is left unsealed.

This method is used for treating a cold disorder which has been followed by heat symptoms or for a disease causing body weakness and giving rise to heat symptoms. The reinforcement aspect first strengthens the body and the reduction aspect then removes the excess heat.

4. *'Shadow of Yang between the Yin';*
Combination of reduction and reinforcement techniques

Method
The depth of the point is determined and mentally divided into two equal parts. Reduction is used in the lower half. The needle is inserted directly into the deeper level, then lifted firmly and thrust gently six times.

The needle is retracted into the upper level for reinforcement, which involves gently lifting and firmly thrusting the needle nine times. The needle is quickly withdrawn and the point sealed with the fingers.

This method is used for treating the patient who has suffered from a heat disorder which has weakened the body condition and created a cold disorder. The reduction aspect removes the excess heat, producing a cool sensation, after which the reinforcement aspect strengthens the body by providing warmth.

ACUPUNCTURE AND MOXIBUSTION TECHNIQUES

5. **'Battle of the Dragon and Tiger';** Combination of reduction and reinforcement techniques through needle rotation

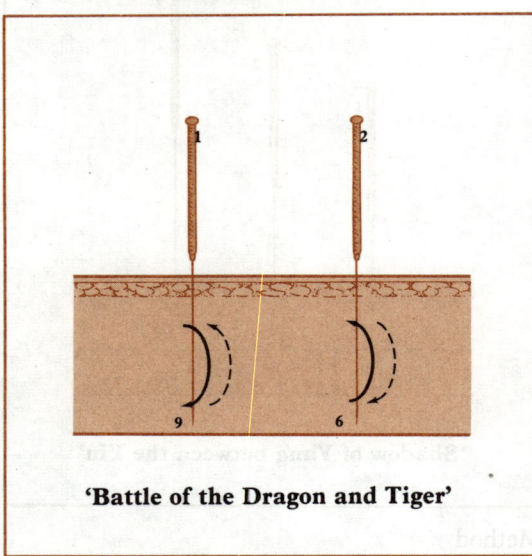

'Battle of the Dragon and Tiger'

6. **'Descent and Ascent of the Dragon and Tiger';** Combination of reinforcement and reduction techniques through needle rotation and lift and thrust

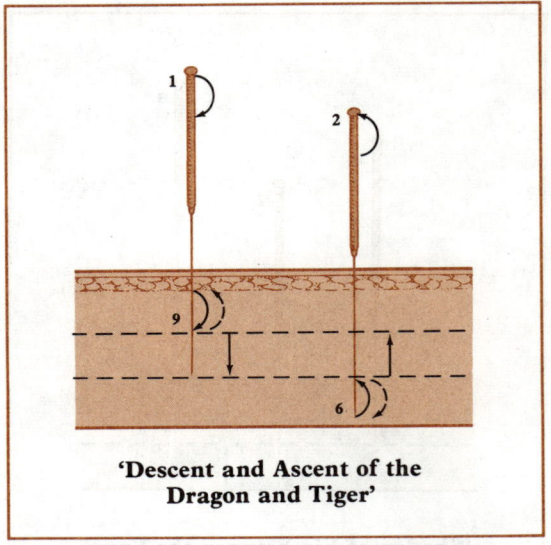

'Descent and Ascent of the Dragon and Tiger'

Method

The needle is inserted into the point. When it 'receives energy' and gives the 'acupuncture sensation', the needle is rotated clockwise nine times in the direction of Meridian energy flow; this is followed by rotation anticlockwise six times.

On completion, the needle is left in the point for twenty to thirty minutes. When pain has been relieved, the needle is quickly withdrawn and the point sealed.

Combining these two techniques through needle rotation balances the *Jing* and *Wei* energy flows and removes local energy obstructions. Clinically it is used for pain relief.

Method

The depth of the point is determined and mentally divided into three levels (Heaven, Man, Earth). The needle is inserted into the uppermost level and, following the direction of Meridian energy flow, rotated 180° clockwise.

The needle is then firmly thrust into the middle level, gently retracted back to the uppermost level, and rotated 180° clockwise. This procedure is repeated nine times and results in the Yang energy of the uppermost level being sent down to the middle level. The Chinese called this 'the dragon descending'.

The next step is for the needle to be gently thrust from the middle to the deepest level, rotated 360° anticlockwise, then firmly lifted back to the middle level. Holding the body of the needle, this procedure is repeated six times and results in the excess energy being brought to the surface. This the Chinese called 'the tiger ascending'. (While the dragon descends, the tiger ascends; in other words, Yang energy is sent downwards and the excess energy is brought upwards.) The needle is retracted to the surface, slowly withdrawn and the point left unsealed.

This strong needle stimulation is mostly used for balancing Yin and Yang energy flows, removing energy obstructions in the Meridians and, especially, removing any local blood stases and local energy obstructions. Clinically it is used for relieving severe pain and ache.

This needle technique is only applied in muscular regions and on patients with an ability to cope with strong needle manipulation. For a patient in severe pain, this type of stimulation balances the pain and quickly relieves it. Pain is not felt from the needle.

7. 'Pounding the Meridian in Mortar';
Combination of reinforcement and reduction techniques through needle rotation and simultaneous lift and thrust

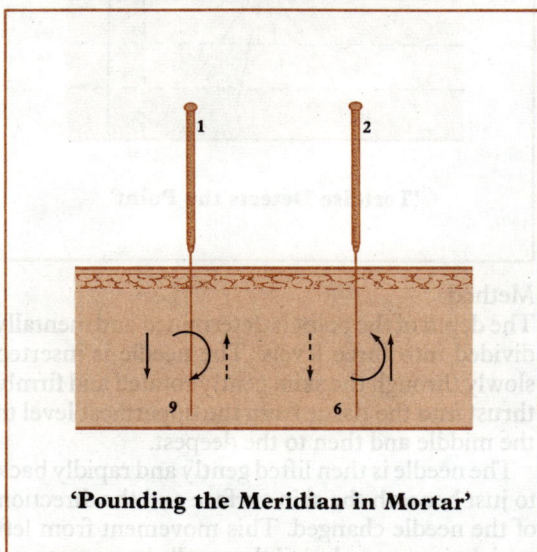

'Pounding the Meridian in Mortar'

Method
The needle is inserted into the point and manipulated until it receives the 'needle sensation'. The needle is then firmly thrust and gently lifted at the same time as it is rotated 180° clockwise in the direction of Meridian energy flow. This is repeated nine times.

The needle is then gently thrust and firmly lifted at the same time as it is rotated 360° anti-clockwise in the direction opposite to that of Meridian energy flow. After six repetitions, the needle is slowly withdrawn and the point left unsealed.

This method is used to balance Yin and Yang energy flows, remove energy obstruction in the Meridians and to treat water retention.

8. 'Wagging the Tail of the Dragon';
Reinforcement through manipulation of the tail of the needle

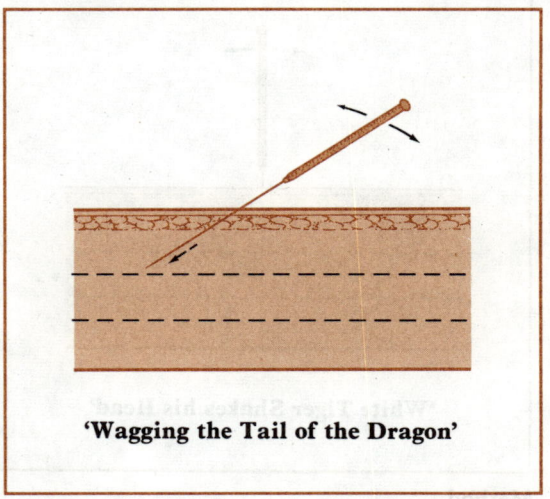

'Wagging the Tail of the Dragon'

Method
The needle is inserted into the point and, when it has 'acquired energy', its tip is turned obliquely in the direction of the disorder. The needle is left in the tissue, taking care not to move the body of the needle.

Holding the handle and tail only of the needle, a

ACUPUNCTURE AND MOXIBUSTION TECHNIQUES

slow and gentle movement is made from back to front (as in rowing a boat), twenty-seven (3 × 9) times. The needle is quickly withdrawn and the point sealed.

This method increases energy flow throughout the region of the disorder (which is caused by body weakness and energy obstruction in the local area).

9. 'White Tiger Shakes His Head'; Reduction through manipulation of the tail of the needle

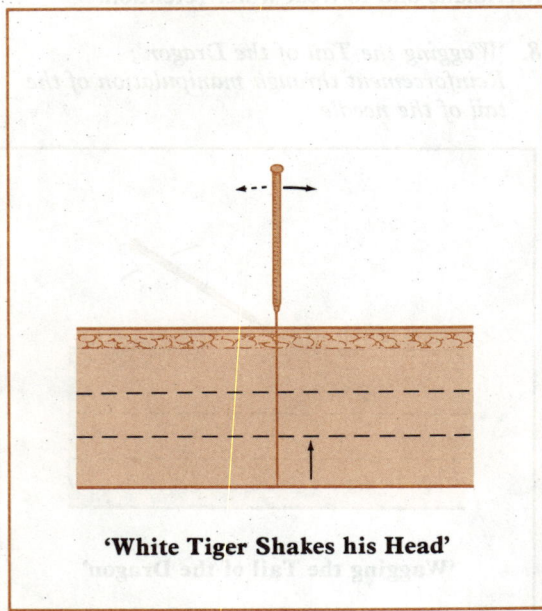

'White Tiger Shakes his Head'

Method
The needle is inserted straight into the point and gently thrust at the same time as it is rotated anticlockwise in the direction opposite to that of Meridian energy flow. The needle is then firmly lifted, at the same time as it is rotated anticlockwise, eighteen (3 × 6) times.

The needle is left in the point and, while holding

only its handle and tail, manipulated from left to right (as if ringing a bell) eighteen (3 × 6) times. The needle is slowly withdrawn and the point left unsealed. This technique is used for removing blood stasis in the *Luo* Meridian.

10. 'Tortoise Detects the Point'; Multidirectional placement of needle for reinforcement

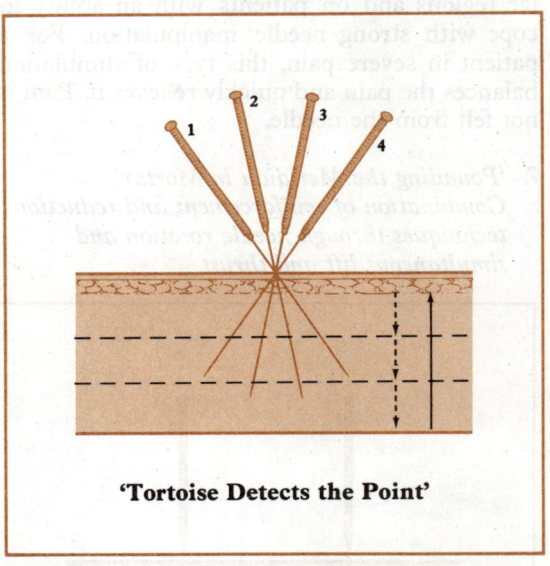

'Tortoise Detects the Point'

Method
The depth of the point is determined and mentally divided into three levels. The needle is inserted slowly through the skin, gently rotated and firmly thrust into the tissue from the uppermost level to the middle and then to the deepest.

The needle is then lifted gently and rapidly back to just beneath the skin surface and the direction of the needle changed. This movement from left to right is repeated until the needle has punctured a large area around the point. The needle is then quickly withdrawn and the point sealed.

This strong reinforcement technique is used for

ACUPUNCTURE AND MOXIBUSTION TECHNIQUES

increasing energy flow in the Meridian.

11. 'Peacock's Fantail'; Reinforcement technique

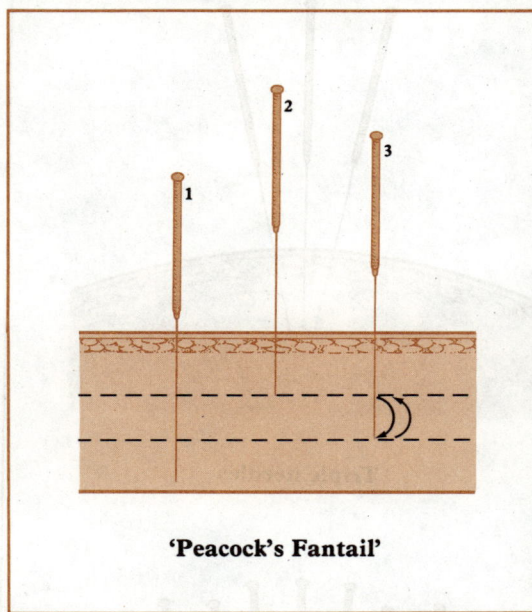

'Peacock's Fantail'

Method
The depth of the point is determined and mentally divided into three levels. The needle is inserted slowly through the skin and gently rotated and firmly thrust into the deepest level. When the needle acquires the 'needle sensation', it is retracted gently and rapidly to the uppermost level.

When the needle again responds, it is gently rotated and firmly thrust into the middle level, rotated 180° clockwise, then gently lifted and firmly thrust several times. Finally, the needle is withdrawn quickly and the point sealed.

When *Luo* Meridian energy is obstructed, this technique increases energy and starts it flowing again.

NEEDLE NUMBERS

Generally, one needle is used for each acupuncture point. Nevertheless, one needle may be used for more than one point, and more than one needle may be inserted into a single point.

The number of needles to be inserted at each point depends upon factors such as the condition of the disorder, body structure, the patient's response to needles and the experience of the practitioner. Usually, stimulation is stronger with more needles than with less. However, strong manipulation of one needle in a point can produce a stronger reaction than several unmanipulated needles in a single point.

Using fewer needles is not necessarily better, as some of the special needle combinations described below indicate.

Single needle

One needle in one point
A single needle manipulated in a very sensitive point (for example, GV 26, all the Well Points) creates a stronger reaction than several needles inserted in a less sensitive point. Stimulating Liv 1, for example, sometimes produces a sensation throughout the whole Meridian.

One needle can also be used for two or more points:

- Needling Pc 6 to TH 5 uses one needle for two points;

- Needling LI 4 to SI 3 uses one needle for five points.

Double needles

Two needles in one point
One needle perpendicularly and one needle obliquely in the same point are used for treating a chronic disorder in a local region.

ACUPUNCTURE AND MOXIBUSTION TECHNIQUES

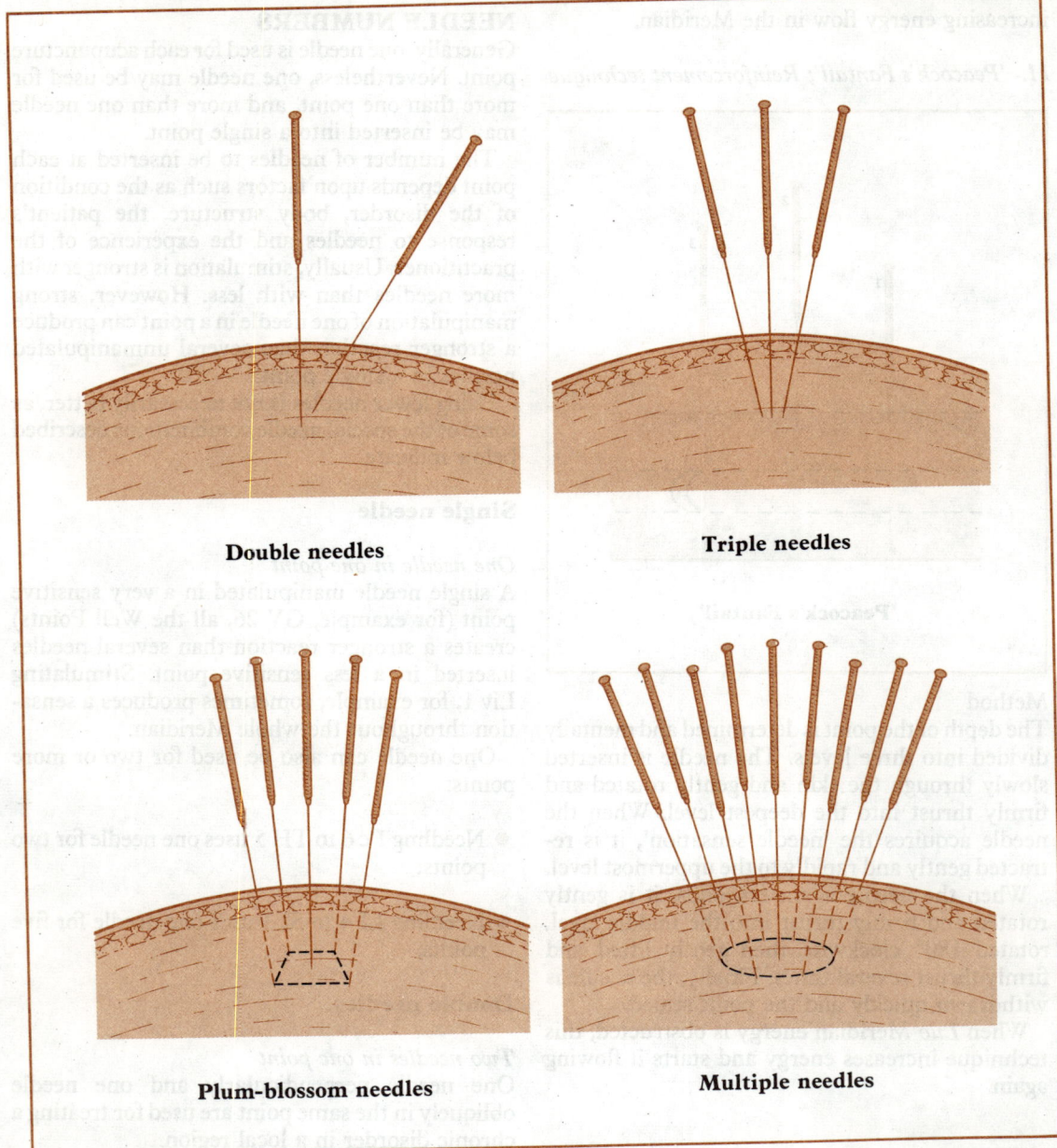

Double needles

Triple needles

Plum-blossom needles

Multiple needles

ACUPUNCTURE AND MOXIBUSTION TECHNIQUES

Triple needles

Three needles in one point
One needle perpendicularly and two needles obliquely in the same point are used for treating pain deep in a local area.

Plum-blossom needles

Five needles in one area
One needle perpendicularly in the centre surrounded by four others obliquely are used to treat local pain which has spread further than the one spot.

Multiple needles

More than seven needles in one area
This method is used mostly for skin problems or where local pain is not concentrated in one spot but is dispersed among several separate foci.

ACCIDENT MANAGEMENT

Accidents are rare during acupuncture treatment, but precautions should always be taken against their occurrence. Unskilled needle technique, lack of clinical experience or inconsideration for the patient can all lead to accidents. The possibilities include:

Needle sticks in tissue

The patient feels pain after puncturing and the needle cannot be moved.

Causes
- Muscle spasm is usually the main reason, often created by the patient's nervous tension.
- Rough manipulation of the needle.
- Body of the needle is not smooth.

Rectification
- The needle is retained in the point while the practitioner talks to the patient.
- The muscle around the needle is gently massaged.
- The needle is slowly turned back to its correct position until it is loose, then withdrawn.

Prevention
- Before insertion, the needle is carefully checked.
- Improvement of needle technique: do not rotate the needle too strongly in one direction.
- The point is massaged before needling.

Needle bends in tissue

The patient feels pain after puncturing because the needle has changed direction, is bent and cannot be moved.

Causes
- The patient changes position after needle insertion.
- A sudden muscle spasm is caused by too strong a manipulation of the needle.
- An external force presses on the needle.
- Poor needle technique, such as needling with uneven finger force.

Rectification
- Do not pull strongly at or twist the needle while it is bent.
- The patient is moved to the original position.
- The muscle is relaxed.
- After careful examination, the needle is gently removed, following the direction in which it is bent.

Prevention
- Careful attention should be paid to puncturing and to gentle needle manipulation.
- The patient must be in a comfortable position and be warned not to move against the needle after insertion.

275

ACUPUNCTURE AND MOXIBUSTION TECHNIQUES

Needle breaks in tissue
The needle breaks during or after insertion and one end is left in the tissue.

Causes
- The needle is of poor quality and/or may have cracks or erosions on its body, especially at the root.
- The patient changes position either too frequently or too abruptly.
- A strong muscular spasm due to faulty manipulation.
- A bent needle has been incorrectly withdrawn.

Rectification
- This accident is serious; surgery is the only course of action.

Prevention
- Always inspect carefully the quality of the needle before use.
- Do not insert the needle to the hilt; the needle body should be exposed at least 0.3 inch above the skin.

Fainting
During acupuncture treatment, the patient has symptoms such as dizziness, an oppressive feeling in the chest, nausea, a pale complexion, cold sweating, cold extremities, loss of consciousness and a weak pulse. Sometimes, the feeling of faintness occurs after acupuncture treatment.

Causes
- Body weakness (due to, for example, diarrhoea, menstruation or hunger).
- Nervousness (fear of the needle).
- Unskilled needle technique (for example, unnecessarily strong manipulation of the needle).

Rectification
- The needles are removed immediately.
- The patient lies flat with the head slightly lower and is kept warm.
- Moxibustion may be applied to acupuncture point St 36.
- If the symptoms are unrelieved, further emergency measures must be taken.

Prevention
- Do not manipulate the needle too strongly if the patient is nervous, emotionally disturbed, distressed, hungry, fatigued or has a chronic illness.
- After needle insertion, the patient must be carefully observed for changes in complexion colour or any other reactions.

Needle punctures vital organ
If a vital organ is accidentally injured during acupuncture treatment, the practitioner must assume complete responsibility and immediately send the patient to a hospital.

Brain and Spinal Cord
If the needle is inserted too deeply, or inappropriately manipulated at acupuncture points in the head and spine (such as GV 15, GV 16, GV 17, GB 20), injuries to the brain or spine may occur. Clinical symptoms include convulsions, paralysis and coma.

Lungs
Many acupuncture points in the chest, back and supraclavicular fossa are very close to the lungs. Needling those points too deeply or with incorrect needle direction may injure the lungs, especially of patients with cough and asthma. Clinical symptoms include pain in the chest, cough, dyspnoea, a pale complexion, cyanosis and coma.

Heart
Acupuncture is of possible help to patients with cardiac disorders, but such treatment requires

special expertise; otherwise, the treatment may cause heart failure.

Liver and Spleen
A needle inserted into an enlarged liver or spleen can easily cause rupture by bleeding, followed by symptoms of abdominal pain, rigidity of abdominal muscle, rebound pain upon pressure and, in severe cases, coma. Before needling abdominal acupuncture points, therefore, it is very important to make a physical examination of the liver and spleen.

Blood vessels
Some acupuncture points lie very close to the larger arteries and veins (for example, CV 22, St 9, St 25, St 30, Sp 12), and careful attention must be paid when needling these points. Great care must also be taken when puncturing in regions close to the eyes, ears, bladder, gall bladder, stomach and intestines, as any mishandling can lead to accidents.

It must be impressed that pregnant women, elderly patients or young children should not be given acupuncture treatment except by experienced and skilled practitioners.

CLINICAL NEEDLE TECHNIQUES

The ancient Chinese philosophers always reminded practitioners that, before they could treat patients, they must fully understand not only needle techniques but the humanitarian aspect of treatment as well. They believed that treating a patient was not to be considered merely a job or a technique, but that it also required other attributes, such as a general knowledge of the Universe and, especially, love of Mankind.

Acupuncture is only one method of medical treatment. To attempt to cure all things by a single method is impossible; instead, all fields of medicine should work together towards the treatment of disease.

Criteria
In the *NEI-JING* and other ancient Chinese books on acupuncture, descriptions are given of standards to uphold, the necessary precautions to be taken, and the circumstances in which acupuncture and moxibustion are forbidden. These important aspects have been maintained for many centuries and must continue to be carefully adhered to in clinical practice today.

When Acupuncture and Moxibustion are Forbidden
Many points are classified as 'forbidden' for acupuncture and moxibustion treatment and, even though this may seem obvious from the anatomy and physiology of the points, nevertheless, a completely satisfactory explanation is yet to be found. Likewise, there is still no explanation for the Meridians or, indeed, how acupuncture itself works.

Various theories have been put forward in an attempt to break with the traditional idea of forbidden acupuncture points, but meaningful discussion of this subject is difficult. It is important to realize, however, that a single or short-term experience is insufficient for full assessment of medical results. There is no doubt that these forbidden acupuncture points must be recognized as such in clinical practice.

There are five severe disorders for which acupuncture treatment cannot be used:

- major blood loss;
- severe and frequent diarrhoea;
- after childbirth (especially after major blood loss);
- severe sweating;
- extreme body weakness.

In these conditions, the blood and energy flows are out of control; needling patients who have these disorders is very dangerous.

In addition, there are many other disorders

which are unsuitable for acupuncture treatment, including acute infectious diseases and severe heart diseases.

To avoid accidents in clinical practice, some conditions require either very careful needling or no needle treatment at all:
- Fatigue
- Diarrhoea
- After a big meal
- Hunger
- After alcohol consumption
- Needle phobia

Treatment can be given to all patients, but care must be taken to select the right treatment at the right time.

Depth of needle insertion
NEEDLING MAIN MERIDIAN POINTS
Although all acupuncture points have an average depth depending on the point sensation and the body's physioanatomical structure, it is largely experience which marks the depth of each point. When the needle correctly reaches the exact point, it reacts with the acupuncture sensation. This sensation, however, can sometimes be blocked, such as in cases of paralysis or when the local area has been attacked by cold, damp or wind disorders. Because of this, the practitioner cannot depend solely on receiving the acupuncture sensation to help determine the exact depth/location of the point.

Needle depth varies with each patient; for example, patients who are obese, very muscular or slow to react to the needle sensation all require deeper than average needle insertion. For children and patients who are thin, weak or sensitive, insertion should be shallow.

The Seasons also influence the depth of needle insertion. In Spring and Summer, when Yang energy floats near the body surface, needling more easily increases energy flow. In these Seasons, therefore, needle insertion is shallow. Conversely, in Autumn and Winter, when Yang energy is deep in the body and energy flow is slower, needle insertion must be deeper.

Because heat increases energy flow, needling is shallow for treating a 'heat' syndrome. With a 'cold' syndrome, because energy flow is slow, needling is deeper and needle retention time longer.

For disorders in the Main Meridians, needling is applied to the acupuncture points of the Main Meridians; for disorders in the *Luo* Meridians, treatment involves needling only those Meridians or bleeding the surface of the skin with a Dermal Hammer or a Three-edged needle.

NEEDLING REGIONS OF LOCAL DISORDER
A region of local disorder may or may not be in a Meridian acupuncture point. The particular technique of needling into such an area (and the concept for treatment) is different from needling into the Main Meridian acupuncture point. There are five needle techniques in this category:

1. Needle insertion into skin surface only
The technique is shallow and fast. One needle can be inserted in different directions or several needles can be concentrated in one spot.

This technique is used to free energy obstruction in the Derma (skin) Meridians, to expel local blood congestion and to treat skin disorders and numbness in the skin.

Bleeding the surface of the skin is done with a Dermal Hammer or a Three-edged needle.

2. Subcutaneous needle insertion
After pinching the skin up around the point, the needle is inserted rapidly through the skin at an angle of about 10°–20°. The tip and body of the needle is then lying beneath the superficial layer of skin. Care must be taken to avoid puncturing muscle or an artery.

This technique is widely used for treating cold which has penetrated beneath the skin, disorders in the fascia, and especially for treating scar tissue, adhesions between skin and muscle, trauma in the soft tissues and fluid retention in the local subcutaneous tissues.

3. Needle insertion into muscle
Insertion is directly into the muscle in any of three needle directions.

- Obliquely: two needles are inserted from opposite directions towards the region of disorder. This relieves local muscle spasm.

- Perpendicularly: the needle is inserted deep into the region of the muscular disorder. This is used after trauma, and when wind and cold have penetrated deep into the local muscle area, manifesting symptoms such as ache and pain in that region.

- Between the junction of two muscles: three needles are inserted in a line with the middle needle inserted perpendicularly and the side pair obliquely. This relieves pain in muscle after chronic trauma caused by local tissue adhesions and muscle spasm.

4. Needle insertion into tendon or ligament
There are two methods of needling into tendon:

- Perpendicularly, especially for tendons in the extremities;

- Obliquely, into the side of the tendon, usually using two needles.

This technique relieves spasm or inflammation in the tendon. Care must be taken to avoid needling into the joint and causing bleeding.

5. Needle insertion into periosteum
The needle is inserted perpendicularly, deeply and close to the bone into the periosteum, with gentle lift and thrust of the needle several times in the area. Inserting too deeply and rotating the needle are both to be avoided. This technique is used to treat disorders in the periosteum, such as osteoarthritis and osteoperiostitis.

Point selection
There are various ways to select acupuncture points for treatment and, in many instances, the same points may be used for different reasons. This is because the Chinese method of diagnosis is different from Western methods and because, often, the basis of point selection is largely dependent on the practitioner's experience.

FOLLOWING SPECIFIC POINTS
1. Five *Shu* (Five Element) Acupuncture Points
These sixty acupuncture points are frequently used to treat disorders in the Zang and Fu; the *He*-Sea Point in particular is used for disorders in the Fu. Treatment follows the theory of the Five Elements:

- 'For a deficiency of energy in the Meridian or Zang, reinforce the Mother.'
- 'For an excess syndrome in the Meridian or Zang, reduce the Son.'

For example, in an excess syndrome of the Liver, accompanied by headache and red eyes, the Fire point (Liv 2 or H 8) is reduced because Wood creates Fire and Fire is the 'Son' of Wood.

In a deficiency of Liver energy accompanied by dizziness, blurred vision and fatigue, the Water point (Liv 8 or K 10) is reinforced because Water creates Wood and Water is the 'Mother' of Wood.

2. Combination of *Yuan* and *Luo* Points
The *Yuan* and the *Luo* Points can be used singly or in combination. When combined, the result is better as both the internal and superficial energy flows are balanced. For example, for a

ACUPUNCTURE AND MOXIBUSTION TECHNIQUES

COMBINATION OF YUAN AND LUO POINTS

HOST	GUEST	YUAN	LUO	SYMPTOMS	
Lung	Large Intestine	Lu 8	LI 6	Fullness in chest Dyspnoea Coughing Throat swelling	Dry mouth Pain in chest & shoulder Perspiration
Large Intestine	Lung	LI 4	Lu 7	Facial swelling Toothache Dry mouth	Rhinitis Sore throat Shoulder pain
Spleen	Stomach	Sp 3	St 40	Stiff tongue Vomiting Gastric pain Body heaviness	Weight loss Constipation Swelling & pain in thigh & knee
Stomach	Spleen	St 42	Sp 4	Gastric pain Heartburn Fear	Epistaxis Pain in leg & foot Restlessness
Heart	Small Intestine	H 7	SI 7	Cardiac pain Pain in arm	Dry mouth Palpitations
Small Intestine	Heart	SI 4	H 5	Cheek swelling Pain in shoulder & arm	Stiff neck Deafness
Kidney	Bladder	K 3	Bl 58	Darkened complexion Lower back pain Pain in foot Fear	Fullness in chest Drowsiness Loss of appetite Blurred vision Fever
Bladder	Kidney	Bl 64	K 4	Stiff neck Ophthalmalgia Pain in lower back, leg & foot	Restlessness Stiff spine Epistaxis Haemorrhoids

ACUPUNCTURE AND MOXIBUSTION TECHNIQUES

HOST	GUEST	*YUAN*	*LUO*	SYMPTOMS	
Three Heater	Pericardium	TH 4	Pc 6	Deafness Sore throat Dry mouth Red eyes Constipation	Pain in back of ear, back, shoulder & arm Enuresis
Pericardium	Three Heater	Pc 7	TH 5	Pain in forearm, arm & chest Red complexion	Restlessness Cardiac pain
Liver	Gall Bladder	Liv 3	GB 37	Pain in groin & lower back Abdominal distention	Fullness in chest Diarrhoea
Gall Bladder	Liver	GB 40	Liv 5	Pain in chest & rib Headache Ophthalmalgia	Swelling & pain in axilla region Fever

disorder in the Lung Meridian which has affected the Large Intestine, the *Yuan* Point of the Lung Meridian, Lu 8, is combined with the *Luo* Point, LI 6, to complete the treatment. The Chinese call this the 'Host-Guest Combination'.

3. Combination of Back-*Shu* and Front-*Mu* Points

Good results are obtained when Front-*Mu* or Back-*Shu* Points are selected (singly and not in combination) for treating disorders in the Zang and Fu. Only when the disorder is severe does the combination of Back-*Shu* and Front-*Mu* Points improve treatment, such as needling points CV 12 and Bl 21 for gastric pain. This method of combination is called 'Needling Yin and Yang'.

4. Other specific points

The *Xi* (Cleft) Points, Eight Confluent Points, Eight Influential Points and Meeting Points all are of clinical value (see **Specific Points**, p 67).

SELECTING POINTS CLOSE TO REGION OF DISORDER

Selecting points close to the region of disorder is one of the most simple and effective treatments. It is mainly used to treat disorders in local areas and for diseases which have not yet penetrated the internal organs. Often, the Meridian points near the area of disorder are used, sometimes the *Ah-Shi* Points and, in many instances, the points on the opposite side, for example, a right elbow point is needled for a left elbow disorder. Generally, however, the points are selected by following the direction of the Meridian:

ACUPUNCTURE AND MOXIBUSTION TECHNIQUES

LAW OF 'MOTHER' AND 'SON'

Meridian	Syndrome	Meridian Points Own	Meridian Points Other
Lung	Deficiency Excess	Lu 9 Lu 5	Sp 3 K 10
Pericardium	Deficiency Excess	Pc 9 Pc 7	Liv 1 Sp 3
Heart	Deficiency Excess	H 9 H 7	Liv 1 Sp 3
Spleen	Deficiency Excess	Sp 2 Sp 5	H 8 Lu 8
Liver	Deficiency Excess	Liv 8 Liv 2	K 10 H 8
Kidney	Deficiency Excess	K 7 K 1	Lu 5 Liv 1
Large Intestine	Deficiency Excess	LI 11 LI 2	St 36 Bl 66
Three Heater	Deficiency Excess	TH 3 TH 10	GB 41 St 36
Small Intestine	Deficiency Excess	SI 3 SI 8	GB 41 St 36
Stomach	Deficiency Excess	St 41 St 44	SI 5 LI 1
Gall Bladder	Deficiency Excess	GB 43 GB 38	Bl 66 SI 5
Bladder	Deficiency Excess	Bl 65 Bl 67	LI 2 GB 41

- For nasal obstruction, use LI 20 for the local point, and LI 4 and St 36 for the distal points of the Meridian.

Using the five different needle techniques for needling into the region of the local disorder not only provides effective treatment but also assists in point selection.

SELECTING POINTS THROUGH EXPERIENCE
Certain acupuncture points have been successfully used clinically for particular diseases. Some of these have been developed, through experience, by the practitioner himself; others have come into use through longstanding practice [for example, LI 4 and Sp 6 (for miscarriage) date back to the *Sung* Dynasty (circa 1026)].

Formula
Although a good prescription for success depends upon the correct diagnosis, correct point selection and personal experience of the practitioner, there are other factors which should be taken into account.

NATURE OF DISEASE
For acute and simple disorders, little treatment may be necessary. A single session may be sufficient, using few needles but strong manipulation technique, for example, the reduction needle technique at LI 4 for toothache.

For chronic and more complicated disorders, extra treatment may be required. In each session, it is then more appropriate to use more needles and a gentle reinforcement technique, for instance, LI 11 + St 25 + GV 25 + CV 12 + CV 4 + St 36 + St 37 + Sp 6 for chronic colitis.

PATIENT'S PHYSICAL CONDITION
The patient with good blood and energy flows who is sensitive to acupuncture will need less treatment. With each successive session, fewer

needles should be used and more gentle needle technique required.

The patient with body weakness who is sensitive to the needle will need more treatment to increase body energy. With each successive session, fewer needles and gentle reinforcement needle technique should be used.

The patient who is obese or slow to react to the needle also needs more treatment. With each session, more needles should be used, possibly in a combination of reinforcement and reduction techniques.

In acupuncture treatment, the use of many needles or few needles is not an issue; one method is not better than the other. Each patient must be treated individually. The responsibility of the practitioner is to diagnose the patient's disorder(s), select the appropriate points, concentrate on needling technique, watch for reactions and, above all, treat the patient as a whole.

ACUPUNCTURE AS PREVENTION

Preventive treatment by acupuncture is far more important than the treatment of symptoms. Furthermore, acupuncture should treat the body as a whole. Acupuncture is able to balance the mind and the body as well as strengthen the physical body against attack by disease.

- 'Keep the physical body healthy;
- Strengthen the mind and Spirit;
- Let the body, mind and Spirit live in harmony.'

These are the main principles of traditional Chinese Medicine and explain why acupuncture was used in ancient China primarily as preventive treatment.

'Hence, the sages did not treat those who were already ill; instead, they **instructed** those who were not yet ill.

They did not wish to rule those who were already rebellious; instead, they **guided** those who were not yet rebellious.

To administer medicines for diseases which have already developed is comparable to the behaviour of those who start to dig a well after they have become thirsty, or those who begin to cast weapons after they have already engaged in battle. Would not these actions then be too late?'

HUANG-DI NEI-JING
(The Yellow Emperor's
Classic of Internal Medicine,
300–500 BC)

Appendix

Ultrasonic decontamination unit:
1. Use Sonidet detergent for ten minutes. Rinse well.
2. Use Soaic in Wavercide-aide (glutaraldehyde) for ten minutes. Soak and rinse well.
3. Insert needles in a cotton-wool sponge cushion.
4. Sterilize needles in dry heat sterilizer for two hours at 160°C or twenty minutes at 180°C.

INDEX

Balance, importance in Yin and Yang, 2–4
Bladder
    disorders of Kidney and, 31
    philosophy of, 30–31
Bladder Meridian, 140 (fig.)
    organs associated, 139
    pathway, 30, 139
    points
        Connecting, 139
        description
            1–10, 140–144
            11–20, 145–150
            21–30, 150–154
            31–40, 154–158
            41–50, 158–162
            51–60, 162–164
            61–67, 164–168
    symptomatology, 139–140
Bleeding, internal, avoidance of, 263
Bleeding needle technique see Needling, Luo Meridian
Blood, circulation of, 7
Brain, philosophy of, 34

Chong Meridian, 34
Climate, effect on pulse, 44–45
    see also Season
Conception Vessel Meridian, 241 (fig.)
    pathway, 240
    points
        Connecting, 240
        description
            1–10, 240–246
            11–20, 246–250
            21–24, 250–252
    symptomatology, 240

Dermal hammer, 264
Disease
    role in prevention of, 283

Yin and Yang in, 2, 4
Disorder
    Bladder, 31
    Gall Bladder, 16
    Heart, 9–10, 11–12
    Kidneys, 26, 31
    Large Intestine, 24–25
    Liver, 13, 16
    Lung, 24–25
    pulse and depth of, 39
    Small Intestine, 19–20
    Spleen, 19–20
    Stomach, 19–20

Emotion
    disease and, 45–46
    Heart, 7
    Kidneys, 30
    Liver, 13
    Lung, 23
    Spleen, 17–18
    Zang, 6
Extra Meridians, 34
Energy
    blood, 20
    Extra Fu, 33–34
    Heart, 8–9
    Kidneys, 25–26, 28–30
    Liver, 12
    Lung, 20, 23
    moxibustion's effect, 254
    reduction, 266–273
    reinforcement, 266–273
    source of, 2
    Spleen, 19
    Stomach, 19
    Three Heater, 32–33, 39
    Zang, 6

Finger-length measurement, 66
Fourteen Meridians, and acupuncture points, 59–252
Fu, Extra
    Brain, 33–34
    philosophy of, 33–34

Uterus, 34

Gall Bladder
    disorders of Liver and, 16
    philosophy of, 15–16
Gall Bladder Meridian, 200 (fig.)
    organs associated, 199
    pathway, 199
    points
        Connecting, 199
        description
            1–10, 201–204
            11–20, 205–208
            21–30, 208–213
            31–40, 214–218
            41–44, 218–219
    symptomatology, 199–201
Governor Vessel Meridian, 229 (fig.)
    pathway, 228
    points
        Connecting, 228
        description
            1–10, 228–233
            11–20, 233–237
            21–28, 237–240
    symptomatology, 228

Heart
    circulatory system, 7
    disorder, 9–10, 11
    effect on
        complexion, 8
        emotion, 7
        perspiration, 9
        tongue, 8
    Pericardium and, 8
    Small Intestine and, 11
    Spirit (*Shen*), 7
    Yin and Yang, 9
Heart Meridian, 124 (fig.)
    organs associated, 123
    pathway, 123
    points 1–9, 125–129
    symptomatology, 123

Intestine, Large *see* Large Intestine
Intestine, Small *see* Small Intestine

Jing-Luo system *see* Meridian, Complex

Kidney
    Ching, 34
    disorders of Bladder and, 30
    effect on
        body fluid metabolism, 29
        bone and marrow, 29
        breathing, 29
        ear, 29
        emotion, 30
        growth cycle, 27
        hair, 29
        sex drive, 30
        teeth, 29
    energy location controversy, 28–29
    Yin and Yang powerhouse, 25–27
Kidney Meridian, 169 (fig.)
    organs associated, 168
    pathway, 168
    points
        Connecting, 168
        description
            1–10, 168–175
            11–20, 175–178
            21–30, 178–181
    symptomatology, 168

Large Intestine
    disorders of Lung and, 24–25
    philosophy of, 23–24
Large Intestine Meridian, 81 (fig.)
    organs associated, 82
    pathway, 80–82
    points description
        1–10, 82–87
        11–20, 87–91
    symptomatology, 82
Liver
    blood storage, 14

condition revealed by eyes, 15
disorders of, 13, 16
effect on
  bile, 14
  emotion, 13
  energy, 12
  tendon, 15
Gall Bladder and, 15–16
Yin and Yang, 14
Liver Meridian, 220 (fig.)
organs associated, 219
pathway, 219
points
  Connecting, 221
  description
    1–10, 221–226
    11–14, 226–228
symptomatology, 221
Lower Heater, 32–33, 39
Lung
disorders of Large Intestine and, 24–25
effect on
  body fluid metabolism, 22
  emotion, 23
  energy, 20–21, 23
  hair, 22
  nose, 22
  skin, 21–22
  sweat gland, 22
  voice, 22–23
Lung Meridian, 74 (fig.)
organs associated, 73–74
pathway, 73
points description, 1–11, 75–80
symptomatology, 74
Luo Meridian, needling, 263–266

Meridian
Chong, 34
Complex (*Jing-Luo* system), 59–61
  Extra, 34
  see also Bladder, Conception Vessel, Gall Bladder, Governor Vessel, Heart, Kidney, Large Intestine, Liver, Lung, Pericardium, Small Intestine, Spleen, Stomach, Three Heater

Middle Heater, 32–33, 39
Ming Men Huo (Kidney Yang), 25–26
Moxa
cone, 253
stick, 253
wool, 253
Moxibustion
application, 253–254
classification, 253
contraindication, 254
effect, 253–254
other methods of warm heating, 253
pregnancy and, 254
Mugwort, for moxa wool, 253

Needle
broken, 276
filiform, 255
number used
  double, 273
  multiple, 275
  plum-blossom, 275
  single, 273
  triple, 275
sterilization, 255, 283
three-edged, 263
Needling
acupuncture sensation, 255, 256, 258
adverse symptoms during, 276
broken needle, 276
depth, 258, 278–279
direction, 256–258
disorders unsuitable, 277–278
internal bleeding, 263
Luo Meridian
  dermal hammer, 264
  points, 264–265
  three-edged needle methods, 263
  warning, 266
manipulation
  lift and thrust, 260–261
  movement, 262
  point massage, 259
  retention, 262
  rotation, 260

scraping, 261
trembling, 261
vibration, 261–262
withdrawal, 262–263
muscle, 279
organ damage, 276–277
pain during, 259
patient posture, 255–256
periosteum, 279
point selection, 279–282
reduction energy methods, 266–273
reinforcement energy methods, 266–273
skin surface, 278
subcutaneous, 278–279
tendon, 279
warning, 268
Yin and Yang, 280

Obesity, effect on treatment, 283
Organ, damage during needling, 276–277
Overpuncturing, dangers of, 258

Pain, during needling, 259
Patient, effect on treatment, 282–283
Pericardium
    disorders compared with those of Three Heater, 32
    philosophy of, 31–32
Pericardium Meridian, 182 (fig.)
    organs associated, 181
    pathway, 181
    points description, 1–9, 182–187
    symptomatology, 181
Pin, Dr Hoo Lee, pulse reading method, 36–37
Points
    Ah-Shi, 62
    definition of, 62
    Extraordinary, 62
    location methods, 63–66
    massage, 259
    Meridian
        Bladder, 139–168
        Conception Vessel, 240–252
        Gall Bladder, 199, 201–219
        Governor Vessel, 228–240
        Heart, 125–129
        Kidney, 168–181
        Large Intestine, 82–91
        Liver, 221–228
        Lung, 75–80
        Luo, 264–265
        Pericardium, 182–187
        Small Intestine, 129–139
        Spleen, 114–123
        Stomach, 93–110
        Three Heater, 187, 189–199
    naming of, 63
    New, 62
    selection, 279–282
    specific, 67–73
Pregnancy
    moxibustion in, 254
    pulse, 43, 48, 55
Proportional measurement, 64–66
Pulse
    character in
        abdomen, 41
        child, 42, 48
        female, 42–43
        foot, 42
        head, 40–41
        internal organ, 97
        neck, 41
        pregnancy, 43, 48, 55
    diagnosis, 35–58
    effect of
        climate, 44
        season, 41, 43–44, 55
    location of, 35
    radial artery
        death foreshadowed, 40
        Floating, 39–40
        health, 36
        influencing factors, 37–38
        level comparison, 38–39
        patient preparation, 38
        reading, 36–37
        rhythm, 38
        Sunken, 40
        Three Heater energy and, 39
reading method

Dr Pin Hoo Lee, 36
Twelve Main Meridians, 36–37
type of
    Bowstring, 52–53
    Choppy, 49
    death foreshadowed, 42, 47, 48, 54, 56–58
    Empty, 49–50
    Fine, 55
    Firm, 53–54
    Floating, 46
    Full, 50
    Hasty, 56
    Hidden, 55–56
    Hollow, 52
    Hurried, 57–58
    Intermittent, 57
    Knotted, 56–57
    Leather, 52
    Long, 50
    Minute, 51
    Moving, 56
    Overflowing, 51
    Rapid, 48
    Scattered, 55
    Short, 50
    Slippery, 48
    Slow, 47
    Sunken (Deep), 47
    Tight, 51–52
    Unhurried, 52
    Weak, 54–55
    Weak Floating, 54

Sea of all Yang Meridians *see*
    Governor Vessel Meridian
Sea of Yin Meridians *see*
    Conception Vessel Meridian
Season, effect on pulse, 41, 43–44, 45
    see also Climate
Shen Ching (Kidney Yin), 24
Shen, and Heart *see* Spirit
Small Intestine
    disorders of Heart and, 11–12
    philosophy of, 9
Small Intestine Meridian, 130 (fig.)

organs associated, 129
pathway, 129
points
    Connecting, 129
    description
        1–10, 129–135
        11–18, 136–139
    symptomatology, 129
Spirit (*Shen*), and Heart, 7
Spleen
    disorders of Stomach and, 19–20
    effect on
        blood formation, 17
        digestion, 17
        emotion, 17–18
        energy, 19
        lip colour, 18
        mouth, 18
        muscle, 18
        water metabolism, 17
Spleen Meridian, 113 (fig.)
    organs associated, 114
    pathway, 112–114
    points
        Connecting, 114
        description
            1–10, 114–119
            11–21, 119–123
    symptomatology, 114
Stomach
    disorders of Spleen and, 19–20
    energy, 19
    Spleen relationship, 19
Stomach Meridian, 92 (fig.)
    organs associated, 92
    pathway, 92
    points
        Connecting, 93
        description
            1–10, 93–98
            11–20, 98–102
            21–30, 102–105
            31–40, 105–110
    symptomatology, 93
Sex, of fetus by pulse, 43

T'ai Chi t'u', symbol of life force, 1 (fig)
Three Heater
    philosophy of, 32–33
    pulse, 39
    regions of, 32–33
Three Heater Meridian, 188 (fig.)
    organs associated, 187
    pathway, 187
    points
        Connecting, 187
        description
            1–10, 189–193
            11–23, 194–199
    symptomatology, 189

Upper Heater, 32–33
Uterus, philosophy of, 33–34

Warm heating, methods of, 253
    see also Moxibustion
Well point, and acupuncture sensation, 258

Yang, and Yin, description, 1–2
Yin, and Yang, 1–4
    disease, 2, 4
    heart, 9
    importance of balance, 2–4
    Kidney as powerhouse of, 25–27
    liver, 14
    needling, 280–281
    principle of, 1
    relationship to
        blood, 7
        energy, 7
Yin, centre of, 34

Zang, and Fu, 5–34
    organ pairs, 5
    relationship with elements, 6
Zang
    emotion, 6
    energy, 6